**1990
YEAR BOOK OF
DIGESTIVE DISEASES®**

From the library of

Dr. _____

_____

_____

*Compliments of REED & CARNRICK,
Ethamolin® (ethanolamine oleate)
and Colyte® (PEG-3350 and Electrolytes
for Oral Solution)*

The 1990 Year Book® Series

Year Book of Anesthesia®: Drs. Miller, Kirby, Ostheimer, Roizen, and Stoelting

Year Book of Cardiology®: Drs. Schlant, Collins, Engle, Frye, Kaplan, and O'Rourke

Year Book of Critical Care Medicine®: Drs. Rogers and Parrillo

Year Book of Dentistry®: Drs. Meskin, Ackerman, Kennedy, Leinfelder, Matukas, and Rovin

Year Book of Dermatology®: Drs. Sober and Fitzpatrick

Year Book of Diagnostic Radiology®: Drs. Bragg, Hendee, Keats, Kirkpatrick, Miller, Osborn, and Thompson

Year Book of Digestive Diseases®: Drs. Greenberger and Moody

Year Book of Drug Therapy®: Drs. Hollister and Lasagna

Year Book of Emergency Medicine®: Dr. Wagner

Year Book of Endocrinology®: Drs. Bagdade, Braverman, Halter, Horton, Kannan, Korenman, Molitch, Morley, Odell, Rogol, Ryan, and Sherwin

Year Book of Family Practice®: Drs. Rakel, Avant, Driscoll, Prichard, and Smith

Year Book of Geriatrics and Gerontology®: Drs. Beck, Abrass, Burton, Cummings, Makinodan, and Small

Year Book of Hand Surgery®: Drs. Dobyns, Chase, and Amadio

Year Book of Hematology®: Drs. Spivak, Bell, Ness, Quesenberry, and Wiernik

Year Book of Infectious Diseases®: Drs. Wolff, Barza, Keusch, Klempner, and Snydman

Year Book of Infertility: Drs. Mishell, Paulsen, and Lobo

Year Book of Medicine®: Drs. Rogers, Des Prez, Cline, Braunwald, Greenberger, Wilson, Epstein, and Malawista

Year Book of Neonatal and Perinatal Medicine: Drs. Klaus and Fanaroff

Year Book of Neurology and Neurosurgery®: Drs. Currier and Crowell

Year Book of Nuclear Medicine®: Drs. Hoffer, Gore, Gottschalk, Sostman, Zaret, and Zubal

Year Book of Obstetrics and Gynecology®: Drs. Mishell, Kirschbaum, and Morrow

Year Book of Occupational and Environmental Medicine: Drs. Emmett, Brooks, Harris, and Schenker

Year Book of Oncology: Drs. Young, Longo, Ozols, Simone, Steele, and Weichselbaum

Year Book of Ophthalmology®: Drs. Laibson, Adams, Augsburger, Benson, Cohen, Eagle, Flanagan, Nelson, Reinecke, Sergott, and Wilson

Year Book of Orthopedics®: Drs. Sledge, Poss, Cofield, Frymoyer, Griffin, Hansen, Johnson, Springfield, and Weiland

Year Book of Otolaryngology — Head and Neck Surgery®: Drs. Bailey and Paparella

Year Book of Pathology and Clinical Pathology®: Drs. Brinkhous, Dalldorf, Grisham, Langdell, and McLendon

Year Book of Pediatrics®: Drs. Oski and Stockman

Year Book of Plastic, Reconstructive, and Aesthetic Surgery: Drs. Miller, Bennett, Haynes, Hoehn, McKinney, and Whitaker

Year Book of Podiatric Medicine and Surgery®: Dr. Jay

Year Book of Psychiatry and Applied Mental Health®: Drs. Talbott, Frances, Frances, Freedman, Meltzer, Schowalter, and Yudofsky

Year Book of Pulmonary Disease®: Drs. Green, Loughlin, Michael, Mulshine, Peters, Terry, Tockman, and Wise

Year Book of Speech, Language, and Hearing: Drs. Bernthal, Hall, and Tomblin

Year Book of Sports Medicine®: Drs. Shephard, Eichner, Sutton, and Torg, Col. Anderson, and Mr. George

Year Book of Surgery®: Drs. Schwartz, Jonasson, Peacock, Shires, Spencer, and Thompson

Year Book of Urology®: Drs. Gillenwater and Howards

Year Book of Vascular Surgery®: Drs. Bergan and Yao

1990
The Year Book of DIGESTIVE DISEASES®

Editor
Norton J. Greenberger, M.D.
Peter T. Bohan Professor and Chairman, Department of Internal Medicine, University of Kansas Medical Center, Kansas City

Frank G. Moody, M.D.
Denton A. Cooley Professor and Chairman, Department of Surgery, The University of Texas Medical School at Houston; Chief of Surgery, Hermann Hospital, Houston

Contributing Editor
Philip B. Miner, Jr., M.D.
Associate Professor of Medicine, Director, Division of Gastroenterology, University of Kansas Medical Center, Kansas City

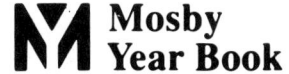

St. Louis   Baltimore   Boston   Chicago   London   Philadelphia   Sydney   Toronto

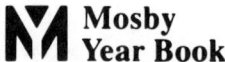
**Mosby
Year Book**
Dedicated to Publishing Excellence

Editor-in-Chief, Year Book Publishing: Nancy Gorham
Sponsoring Editor: Gretchen C. Templeton
Manager, Medical Information Services: Edith M. Podrazik
Senior Medical Information Specialist: Terri Strorigl
Assistant Director, Manuscript Services: Frances M. Perveiler
Assistant Managing Editor, Year Book Editing Services: Wayne Larsen
Production Coordinator: Max F. Perez
Proofroom Supervisor: Barbara M. Kelly

Copyright © October 1990 by Mosby-Year Book, Inc.
A Year Book Medical Publishers imprint of Mosby-Year Book, Inc.

Mosby-Year Book, Inc.
11830 Westline Industrial Drive
St. Louis, MO 63146

All rights reserved. No part of this publication may be reproduced, stored in a retrieval system, or transmitted, in any form or by any means, electronic, mechanical, photocopying, recording, or otherwise, without prior written permission from the publisher.
Printed in the United States of America.

Permission to photocopy or reproduce solely for internal or personal use is permitted for libraries or other users registered with the Copyright Clearance Center, provided that the base fee of $4.00 per chapter plus $.10 per page is paid directly to the Copyright Clearance Center, 21 Congress Street, Salem, MA 01970. This consent does not extend to other kinds of copying, such as copying for general distribution, for advertising or promotional purposes, for creating new collected works, or for resale.

Editorial Office:
Mosby-Year Book, Inc.
200 North LaSalle St.
Chicago, IL 60601

International Standard Serial Number: 0739-5930
International Standard Book Number: 0-8151-3887-3

Table of Contents

The material in this volume represents literature reviewed through December 1989.

Journals Represented xiii

Introduction xv

THE ESOPHAGUS

1. MOTOR DISORDERS 3
   A. Achalasia 3
   B. Diffuse Esophageal Spasm 8
   C. Cricopharyngeal Dysphagia 13
2. REFLUX ESOPHAGITIS 15
   A. Pathophysiology 15
   B. Medical Therapy 16
   C. Surgical Therapy 17
3. BARRETT'S ESOPHAGUS 25
   A. Dysplasia and Flow Cytometry 25
   B. Complications 28
4. CARCINOMA OF THE ESOPHAGUS 31
5. MISCELLANEOUS TOPICS 33
   A. Spontaneous Rupture 33
   B. Paraesophageal Hernia 34

THE STOMACH AND DUODENUM

6. PHYSIOLOGY AND PATHOPHYSIOLOGY 39
   A. Alcohol Metabolism 39
   B. Gastric pH After Cholecystectomy 42
7. PEPTIC ULCER DISEASE 45
   A. Medical Therapy for Duodenal Ulcer 45
   B. Medical Therapy for Gastric Ulcer 47
   C. Recurrent Ulcer and Maintenance Therapy 50
   D. Nonoperative Therapy for Perforated Ulcer 52
8. SURGICAL THERAPY FOR PEPTIC ULCER DISEASE 55
9. ZOLLINGER-ELLISON SYNDROME 59
10. POSTGASTRIC SURGERY SYNDROMES 65
11. GASTRIC SURGERY FOR MORBID OBESITY 69
12. UPPER GASTROINTESTINAL BLEEDING 73

13. GASTRIC AND DUODENAL NEOPLASMS 75
    A. Gastric Cancer 75
    B. Leiomyosarcoma 76
    C. Carcinoids 77
14. HELICOBACTER (CAMPYLOBACTER) PYLORI 79
15. GASTRIC EMPTYING PROBLEMS 85
16. MISCELLANEOUS 87

THE SMALL INTESTINE

17. PATHOPHYSIOLOGIC AND RADIOGRAPHIC CONSIDERATIONS 93
    A. Food Hypersensitivity and Histamine 93
    B. Segmental Dilatation of the Small Bowel 94
    C. Intestinal Defect in Hemochromatosis 96
    D. The "Ileal Brake" 98
18. MICROVILLUS INCLUSIONS DISEASE 101
19. AIDS AND RELATED PROBLEMS IN HOMOSEXUAL MEN 105
20. SHORT BOWEL SYNDROME 109
    A. In Neonates 109
    B. Somatostatin Analogues 110
21. ALIMENTARY TRACT DUPLICATIONS AND ATRESIA 115
22. ILEAL BYPASS FOR HYPERCHOLESTEROLEMIA 119
23. NEOPLASMS 121
    A. Inpatients With Familial Polyposis 121
    B. Recognition at Emergent Laparotomy 122
24. SMALL BOWEL OBSTRUCTION 125
    A. Diagnosis by Enteroclysis 125
    B. Postoperative 126
25. MESENTERIC INFARCTION 129
26. CROHN'S DISEASE AND RELATED TOPICS 133
    A. Radiologic Considerations 133
    B. Immunosuppressive Therapy 134
    C. Strictureplasty 140
    D. Recurrence and Reoperation 140
    E. Cancer 141
27. NUTRITION 145
    A. Enteral and Parenteral Nutrition; Tube Feedings 145
    B. Percutaneous Endoscopic Gastrostomy and Jejunostomy 154
    C. Miscellaneous Considerations 155

THE COLON

28. Physiology and Pathophysiology 159
    A. Studies on Mechanisms of Diarrhea 159
29. Infectious Colitis and Related Disorders 165
    A. Hemorrhagic Colitis and *Escherichia coli* 0157:H7 165
    B. Shigella 166
    C. Associated With Drinking Water 169
    D. *C. difficile* and Antibiotic-Associated Diarrhea 171
    E. Typhoid Enteritis and Perforation 173
30. Lymphocytic ("Microscopic") Colitis 175
31. Diversion Colitis 179
32. Ileal-Anal Anastomoses 181
33. Rectal Injuries and Colonic Trauma 185
34. Rectal Prolapse and Sigmoid Volvulus 189
    A. Rectal Prolapse 189
    B. Sigmoid Volvulus 190
35. Colorectal Carcinoma and Other Neoplasms 191
    A. Radiologic and Imaging Studies 191
    B. Polyps: Cancer Sequence 194
    C. Clinical Studies 194
    D. Radioimmunolocation and Ablation Studies 200
36. Irritable Bowel Syndrome 203
    A. Clinical Studies 203
37. Appendicitis 207
    A. Clinical Studies 207
38. Colonic Ischemia 213
39. Miscellaneous Topics 217
    A. Total Colectomy for Aganglionosis 217
    B. Colon Surgery Without Nasogastric Decompression 218

THE LIVER

40. Jaundice and Disorder of Bilirubin Metabolism 221
41. Fulminant Hepatitis and Liver Failure 227
42. Viral Hepatitis Type B 233
    A. Clinical Studies 233
    B. Chronic Hepatitis B 236
43. Non-A, Non-B Hepatitis (Hepatitis C) 241

　　　　A. Development of Specific Tests for Hepatitis C 241
　　　　B. Clinical Studies 242
　　　　C. Treatment With Interferon 247
　　　　D. Hepatitis C and Hepatocellular Carcinoma 250
44. ALCOHOLIC HEPATITIS 253
45. CIRRHOSIS AND RELATED PROBLEMS 255
　　　　A. Ascites 255
　　　　B. Portal Hypertension, Bleeding Varices, Sclerotherapy, and Shunts 258
　　　　C. Portal Systemic Encephalopathy 266
46. DRUG-ASSOCIATED HEPATIC INJURY 271
47. LIVER NEOPLASMS 273
　　　　A. Primary Liver Cancer 273
　　　　B. Metastatic Liver Disease 274
　　　　C. Imaging Studies 275
48. LIVER TRANSPLANTATION 277
49. PRIMARY BILIARY CIRRHOSIS 283
50. MISCELLANEOUS TOPICS 289
　　　　A. Major Hepatic Resection 289
　　　　B. Wilson's Disease 290
　　　　C. Hepatic Hemangiomas 292
　　　　D. Hydatid Cysts 293
　　　　E. Blunt Trauma 295

THE GALLBLADDER AND BILIARY TRACT

51. PHYSIOLOGY AND PATHOPHYSIOLOGY 299
　　　　A. Bile Acid Kinetics After Cholecystectomy 299
　　　　B. Cholecystokinin and Analogues 302
52. RADIOGRAPHIC AND IMAGING CONSIDERATIONS 305
53. GALLSTONES AND RELATED PROBLEMS 309
　　　　A. Pathophysiology 309
　　　　B. Gallstone Dissolution and Fragmentation 315
　　　　C. Gallstone Recurrence After Dissolution 322
　　　　D. Percutaneous Cholecystostomy 323
54. SPHINCTER OF ODDI DYSFUNCTION AND SPHINCTEROTOMY 327
55. BILE DUCT PROBLEMS 335
　　　　A. Common Duct Stones 335
　　　　B. Sclerosing Cholangitis 341
　　　　C. AIDS-Related Cholangiopathies 343
　　　　D. Bile Duct Strictures and Atresia 346

56. CARCINOMA OF THE GALLBLADDER 349

THE PANCREAS

57. PHYSIOLOGY AND PATHOPHYSIOLOGY 353
58. RADIOGRAPHIC CONSIDERATIONS 359
59. CYSTIC FIBROSIS 367
60. ACUTE PANCREATITIS 369
    A. Gallstone Pancreatitis..369
    B. Severe Acute Pancreatitis and Complications..370
61. CHRONIC PANCREATITIS 377
    A. Pancreatitis Stone Protein..377
    B. Clinical Studies...379
    C. Surgical Therapy..381
62. PANCREATIC NEOPLASMS 385
    A. Evaluation of Ca19-9..385
    B. Clinical Studies...387
63. PANCREATIC TRAUMA 395
64. PANCREAS TRANSPLANTATION 397

CAPSULES AND COMMENTS 399

VISUAL VIGNETTES 415

SUBJECT INDEX 431

AUTHOR INDEX 447

Journals Represented

Year Book Medical Publishers subscribes to and surveys nearly 850 U.S. and foreign medical and allied health journals. From these journals, the Editors select the articles to be abstracted. Journals represented in this YEAR BOOK are listed below.

American Journal of Clinical Nutrition
American Journal of Gastroenterology
American Journal of Medicine
American Journal of Physiology
American Journal of Roentgenology
American Journal of Surgery
American Journal of Surgical Pathology
American Surgeon
Annals of Internal Medicine
Annals of Surgery
Annals of Thoracic Surgery
Annals of the Royal College of Surgeons of England
Archives of Internal Medicine
Archives of Surgery
Blood
British Journal of Surgery
Cancer
Clinical Radiology
Critical Care Medicine
Digestive Diseases and Sciences
Diseases of the Colon and Rectum
Gastroenterology
Gastrointestinal Radiology
Gut
Hepatology
Human Pathology
Journal of Clinical Investigation
Journal of Computer Assisted Tomography
Journal of Laboratory and Clinical Medicine
Journal of Parenteral and Enteral Nutrition
Journal of Pediatric Gastroenterology and Nutrition
Journal of Pediatric Surgery
Journal of Perinatology
Journal of Thoracic and Cardiovascular Surgery
Journal of Trauma
Journal of the American Geriatrics Society
Journal of the American Medical Association
Journal of the Canadian Association of Radiologists
Journal of the Royal College of Surgeons of Edinburgh
Lancet
New England Journal of Medicine
Quarterly Journal of Medicine
Radiology
Science
Surgery
Surgery, Gynecology and Obstetrics
World Journal of Surgery

STANDARD ABBREVIATIONS

The following terms are abbreviated in this edition: acquired immunodeficiency syndrome (AIDS), the central nervous system (CNS), cerebrospinal fluid (CSF), computed tomography (CT), electrocardiography (ECG), and human immunodeficiency virus (HIV).

Introduction

The format for the 1990 YEAR BOOK OF DIGESTIVE DISEASES is similar to that of the previous six editions. We have reviewed more than 4,000 articles and selected 243 for inclusion with abstracts and comments, 29 for capsules and comments, and 8 for the visual vignettes section. The selections again include a mix of basic advances, new insights into mechanisms of disease, clinical studies dealing with diagnosis and therapy, and unusual manifestations of common disorders. Emphasis has been placed on soliciting papers with clinical manifestations.

We thank Shirley Sears, Ruth Stricklen, Charlotte Johnson, and Flora Roeder for their continued fine efforts in preparation of the manuscript and Gretchen Templeton of Mosby-Year Book, Inc. for her editorial and administrative support.

Norton J. Greenberger, M.D.
Frank G. Moody, M.D.

The Esophagus

Chapter 1.	**Motor Disorders**
	Achalasia
	Diffuse Esophageal Spasm
	Cricopharyngeal Dysphagia
Chapter 2.	**Reflux Esophagitis**
	Pathophysiology
	Medical Therapy
	Surgical Therapy
Chapter 3.	**Barrett's Esophagus**
	Dysplasia and Flow Cytometry
	Complications
Chapter 4.	**Carcinoma of the Esophagus**
Chapter 5.	**Miscellaneous Topics**
	Spontaneous Rupture
	Paraesophageal Hernia

1 Motor Disorders

Achalasia

Radiographic and Manometric Correlation in Achalasia With Apparent Relaxation of the Lower Esophageal Sphincter
Ott DJ, Richter JE, Chen YM, Wu WC, Gelfand DW, Castell DO (Wake Forest Univ)
Gastrointest Radiol 14:1–5, 1989   1–1

Typically, manometric studies show esophageal aperistalsis and incomplete relaxation of the lower esophageal sphincter (LES) in achalasia. The characteristic radiographic findings are absent peristalsis, dilatation of the esophagus, and smooth tapering at its lower end, indicating LES dysfunction. Over a 2-year period 5 men and 5 women were seen with clinical and radiologic findings of achalasia but with apparent complete LES relaxation at manometric study. Thirty-nine other patients with the usual manometric findings were seen in the same period.

Patients with atypical achalasia (Fig 1–1) were younger, had lost less weight, and had dysphagia of shorter duration than those with classic findings (table). The mean caliber of the esophagus was significantly smaller in the atypical patients (Fig 1–2). All patients in both groups had delayed emptying of a labeled test meal.

The findings were normal for 4 patients with atypical achalasia after pneumatic dilatation. All but 1 of the atypical patients responded to pneumatic dilatation. Twenty-six (81%) of 32 patients with classic achalasia had symptomatic relief afer dilatation or Heller myotomy.

A functional abnormality of the LES is likely in patients with atypical achalasia; these cases may represent an early stage of the disorder. Complete relaxation of the LES does not exclude achalasia in a patient with typical radiologic findings.

▶ Typical achalasia is diagnosed by manometric findings of aperistalsis of the esophagus with incomplete relaxation of the LES. In this study, patients with atypical achalasia had incomplete relaxation of the LES although it was of shorter duration than in healthy persons. As a group, patients with atypical achalasia that were younger had a shorter period of dysphagia and less weight loss. These findings suggest it is possible to identify early achalasia by supplementing esophageal manometry, radionuclide, and radiographic esophageal studies. The authors speculate that this represents a spectrum in achalasia, and the demographic details presented support this opinion. Because patients are symptomatic, the option for early treatment of achalasia by dilatation should be considered. Adams, Roberts, and Smith (1) reported nine patients (15%) with esophageal tears during the

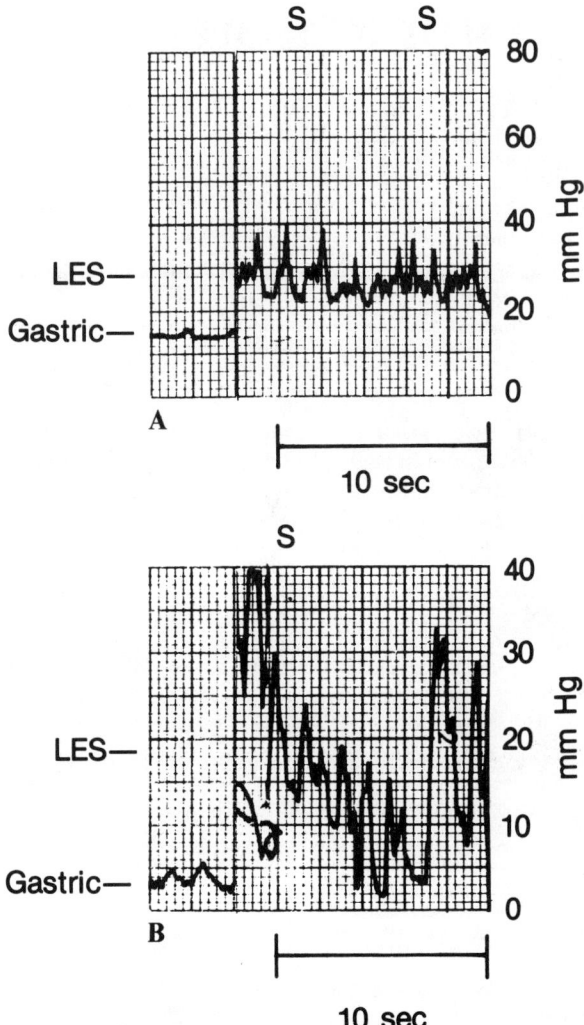

Fig 1–1.—A, failure of relaxation of LES with several swallows (S) in classic achalasia. *Gastric,* gastric baseline. **B,** complete LES relaxation within 4 seconds of swallowing (S) in atypical achalasia. Tracing irregularity represents respiratory and cardiac activity in both figures. (Courtesy of Ott DJ, Richter JE, Chen YM, et al: *Gastrointest Radiol* 14:1–5, 1989.)

Comparison of Clinical, Manometric, and Radiologic Findings in the 2 Groups of Achalasia Patients

Finding	Atypical achalasia	Classic achalasia	Statistics (p values)
Age (years)	46.1 ± 7.3*	60.6 ± 3.3	0.057
Dysphagia (months)	18.7 ± 5.0	45.7 ± 9.3	0.014
Weight loss (lbs)	8.2 ± 2.3	21.5 ± 3.1	0.021
LESP† (mmHg)	34.5 ± 4.2	37.7 ± 3.7	0.642
Esophageal caliber (cm)	2.8 ± 0.3	3.9 ± 0.2	0.020
EGJ† caliber (mm)	4.5 ± 0.7	4.8 ± 0.3	0.689

*Values are mean ± standard error of the mean.
†LESP, lower esophageal sphincter pressure; EGJ, esophagogastric junction.
(Courtesy of Ott DJ, Richter JE, Chen YM, et al: *Gastrointest Radiol* 14:1–5, 1989.)

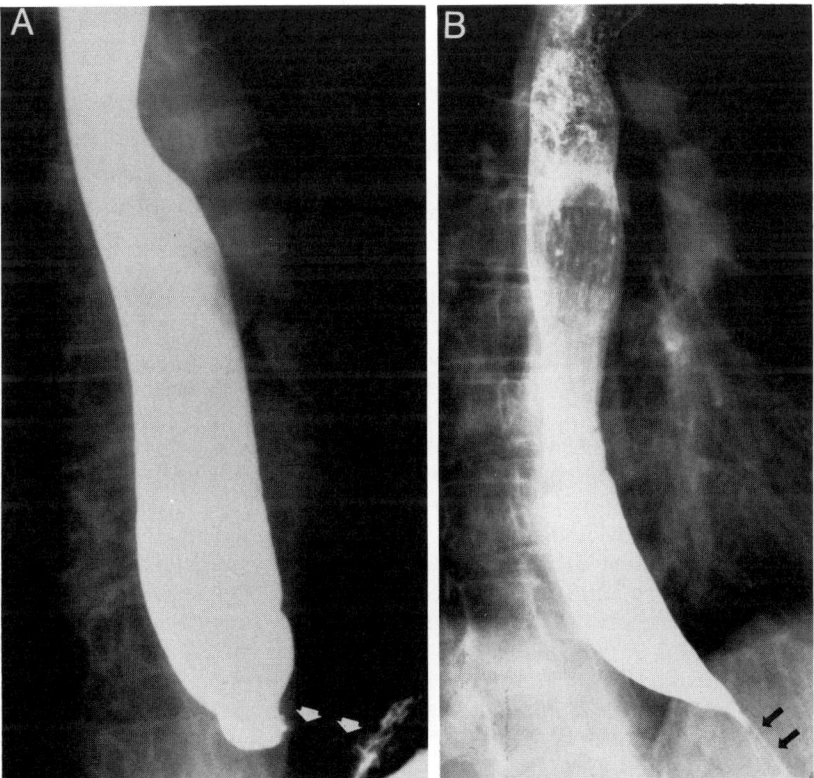

Fig 1–2.—**A,** classic achalasia with esophageal caliber measuring 3.5 cm. Typical beaking at lower end of esophagus *(arrows)*. **B,** atypical achalasia with 2.5-cm esophageal caliber. There is distal beaking similar in appearance to classic achalasia *(arrows)*. (Courtesy of Ott DJ, Richter JE, Chen YM, et al: *Gastrointest Radiol* 14:1–5, 1989.)

treatment of 58 patients being dilated for achalasia. Tears were indicated by diverticulum, linear tear, or complete rupture of the esophagus. All patients, including those with esophageal rupture were given conservative treatment without any complications. Conservative therapy included management with antibiotics, intravenous feeding, and abstinence from food and drink.—P.B. Miner, Jr., M.D.

Reference

1. Adams, Roberts, Smith: *Clin Radiol* 40:53, 1989.

The Treatment of Achalasia: A Current Perspective
Sauer L, Pellegrini CA, Way LW (VA Med Ctr; Univ of California, San Francisco)
Arch Surg 124:929–932, August 1989   1–2

Until about 10 years ago, the modified Heller's myotomy used to be the primary treatment for achalasia. However, pneumatic dilatation has since replaced operation as the primary treatment for esophageal achalasia. The effectiveness and complications of pneumatic dilatation in 40 women and 39 men aged 20–87 years, in whom achalasia was diagnosed in 1977–1988, were reviewed.

Pneumatic dilatation was the primary therapy in 66 patients (84%). Presenting symptoms included dysphagia in 91%, weight loss in 44%, and regurgitation in 52%. Duration of symptoms ranged from 8 months to 25 years (mean duration, 8.7 years). All 79 patients underwent contrast radiography, 71 had endoscopy, and 64 had manometry. Late follow-up data were available for 67 patients who were contacted by telephone to assess their present functional status.

Dilatation was uncomplicated in 53 patients (80%), all of whom had immediate improvement in swallowing. After an average follow-up of 4 years, 50% of the patients had no problems with swallowing, but 30% had symptoms of gastroesophageal reflux and 20% reported recurrent or persistent dysphagia. Four patients with dysphagia underwent repeat pneumatic dilatation, and 2 patients underwent a Heller myotomy procedure. Of the 66 patients who underwent dilatation, 10 had early complications, including pulmonary aspiration, which was fatal in 1 patient, and esophageal perforation in 8 patients; 3 patients who had immediate failure underwent repeat dilatation on the next day. A modified Heller cardiomyotomy was performed in 8 patients; in 3 as initial treatment, in 3 after acute perforation during dilatation, and in 2 after uncomplicated dilatation. Of the 8 patients, 7 had immediate improvement in swallowing. After an average follow-up of 4.3 years, 6 of the 8 patients had remained asymptomatic, 1 patient reported episodic mild heartburn, and 1 mentally retarded patient had died of massive pulmonary aspiration after operation.

Although pneumatic dilatation has been described as safe and effective, a 12% perforation rate and a 30% gastroesophageal reflux rate, coupled with overall good results in only 50% of the patients who had the procedure, do not support that opinion. If reviews from other institutions support the findings of this study, a return to Heller's myotomy for the treatment of achalasia may be advisable.

▶ The digestive surgeons at the University of California, San Francisco, have carefully documented the effectiveness and safety of pneumatic dilatation for the treatment of achalasia. I agree with the authors that a perforation rate of 12% is too high, and a less than 50% symptom-free rate is too low to be considered acceptable. Their patients would be better served by a standard Heller myotomy where the perforation rate will be nil and symptom-free rate greater than 80% in appropriately selected patients.—F.G. Moody, M.D.

Esophageal Resection for Achalasia: Indications and Results
Orringer, MB, Stirling MC (Univ of Michigan, Ann Arbor)
Ann Thorac Surg 47:340–345, March 1989
1–3

The effectiveness of forceful dilation or esophagomyotomy relieving esophageal obstruction in achalasia is well established. However, neither procedure is consistently reliable in the treatment of patients with either recurrent symptoms after a previous esophagomyotomy or a megaesophagus. Total thoracic esophagectomy was performed in 26 patients aged 15–84 years (average age 49 years) with achalasia; 18 patients had had previous esophagomyotomies and 14 had had megaesophagus.

A transhiatal esophagectomy without thoracotomy was performed in 24 patients and a transthoracic esophagectomy was necessary in 2 because of periesophageal adhesions from previous operations. In all patients, the stomach was positioned in the posterior mediastinum and a cervical anastomosis was performed. The average intraoperative blood loss was 765 mL (range, 150–3,000 mL). Postoperative complications included mediastinal bleeding requiring thoracotomy in 2 patients, chylothorax in 2, anastomotic leak in 1, transient laryngeal nerve paresis in 2, and a subdiaphragmatic abscess in 1. There were no postoperative deaths. The average postoperative hospital stay was 10 days. Follow-up was complete for the 254 suviving patients and averaged 30 months (range, 3–91 months). Except for 1 patient with severe psychiatric disease, all other patients ate regular, unrestricted diets without postprandial regurgitation. Ten patients required early postoperative anastomotic dilation. The dumping syndrome occurred in 5 patients. None of the patients had pulmonary complications secondary to aspiration.

Total thoracic esophagectomy and a cervical esophagogastric anastomosis can be performed in patients with megaesophagus or a failed previous esophagomyotomy with far more reliable and favorable long-term functional results than esophagomyotomy, cardioplasty procedures, or limited esophageal resection.

▶ At first glance, esophagectomy would appear to be a medical approach to a disease that primarily involves the lower esophageal sphincter. Orringer and his colleagues, relying on their extensive experience with blunt esophagectomy, provide convincing evidence that the procedure is not only safe, but also effective in this population of patients who have failed more conservative therapeutic attempts. That there were no deaths attests to the skill of the surgical team and those who cared for the patients in the postoperative period. Their success, however, is not a justification for the simpler and well-established approach of hydrostatic bougienage, which can be carried out with minimal morbidity on an ambulatory basis early in the disease process. A Heller myotomy is also effective when bougienage fails. Extirpation of the esophagus should be reserved for patients for whom these well-established measures have failed.—F.G. Moody, M.D.

Diffuse Esophageal Spasm

Diffuse Esophageal Spasm: Radiographic and Manometric Correlation
Chen YM, Ott DJ, Hewson EG, Richter JE, Wu WC, Gelfand DW, Castell DO (Wake Forest Univ)
Radiology 170:807–810, March 1989   1–4

Only 5% to 15% of patients with disordered esophageal motility have diffuse esophageal spasm (DES). The manometric and radiographic findings were reviewed in 9 men and 8 women with a mean age of 62 years and a diagnosis of DES who were seen in a 6-year period. All had chest pain or dysphagia and 10 had both of these symptoms. Intermittently normal primary peristalsis, with simultaneous contractions on more than 10% of swallowing function studies with water (Fig 1–3), was the major manometric criterion for DES.

The mean manometric frequency of primary peristalsis was 46% in these patients. The mean frequency of nonperistaltic events was 30%. Four patients had normal primary motility, and the other 13 had disordered primary peristalsis (Fig 1–4). In 2 patients DES was seen on radiographic study and achalasia was seen in 1 (Fig 1–5). The mean estimated width of the esophageal wall in patients with diffuse spasm (Fig 1–6) was 2.6 mm. Twelve patients had a hiatal hernia, and 2 had reflux esophagitis. The presence and degree of tertiary activity did not correlate with the percentage of primary peristalsis.

Primary peristalsis was disrupted in three fourths of the patients with a diagnosis of DES in this study. Simultaneous manometry and radiography are concordant in most cases in predicting normal or abnormal primary peristalsis. Tertiary activity is not synonymous with a diagnosis of DES. Fluoroscopic study of single barium swallows is a useful approach to patients with DES.

▶ The abnormalities seen in esophageal motility studies and barium studies have been difficult to reconcile. Recent efforts have been made to identify radiographic abnormalities that correlate with the manometric studies that have been done.

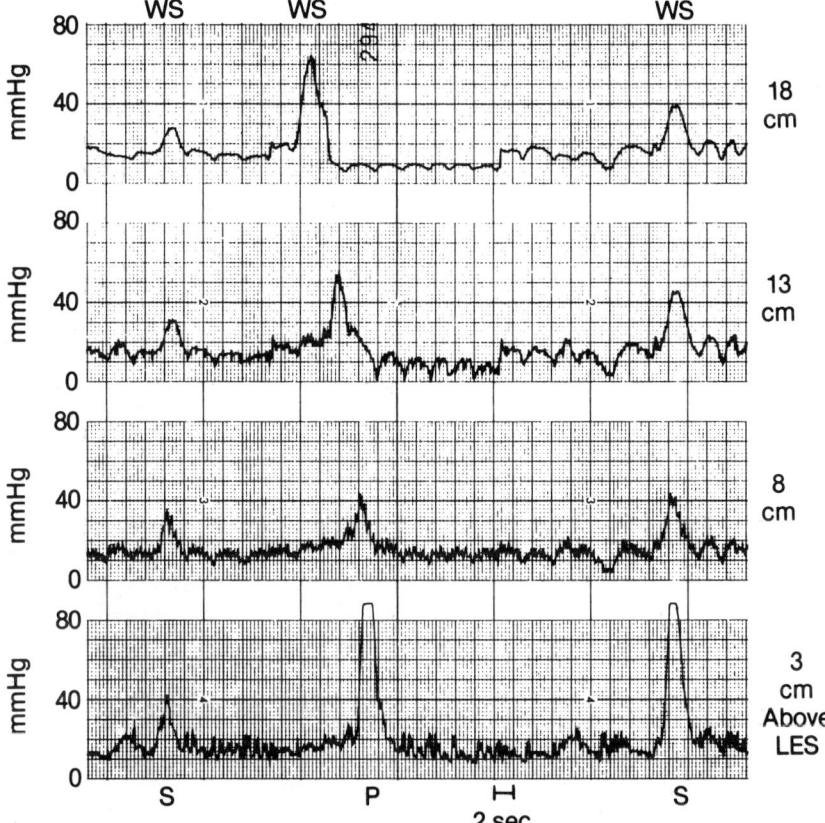

Fig 1–3.—Typical manometric appearance of DES shows normal peristalsis (P) interspersed with simultaneous (S) waves. Pressures in mm Hg are shown at left, and distance above lower esophageal sphincter (LES) is shown at right. WS, water swallow. (Courtesy of Chen YM, Ott DJ, Hewson EG, et al: *Radiology* 170:807–810, March 1989.)

Recently, studies have addressed a correlation between radiographic videotape recordings and esophageal motility tracings. In this study, tertiary contractions (nonprimary contractions of the esophagus ranging from mild distortion of esophageal contour to lumina-obliterating contractions) were seen most often with DES (70% of patients), though they are not specific for DES. Intermittent absence of primary peristalsis was the most common abnormality, occurring in 76% of the patients. The third traditional criteria for esophageal spasm is esophageal wall thickening, which was not evident in this study, raising questions as to its impor-

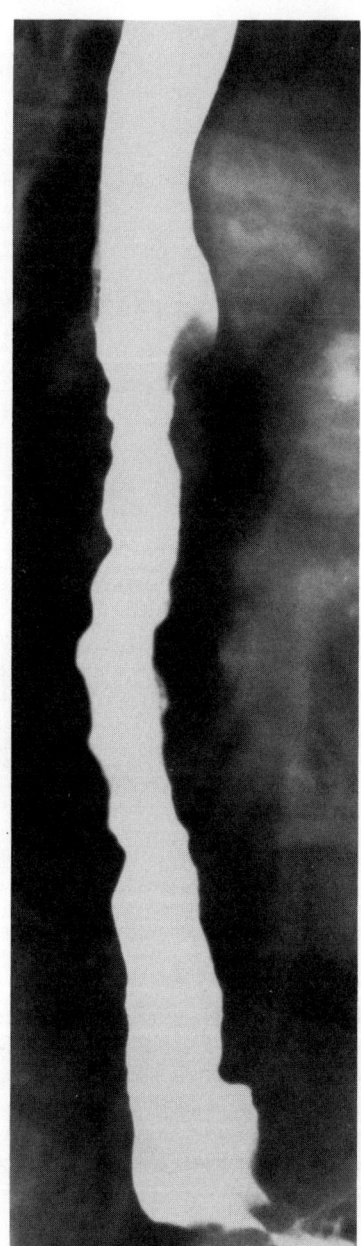

Fig 1–4.—Fluoroscopic study of man aged 56 years with chest pain and odynophagia shows intermittent absence of primary peristalsis with moderate tertiary activity. Specific diagnosis of DES was made on basis of radiographic and clinical findings. (Courtesy of Chen YM, OTT DJ, Hewson EG, et al: *Radiology* 170:807–810, March 1989.)

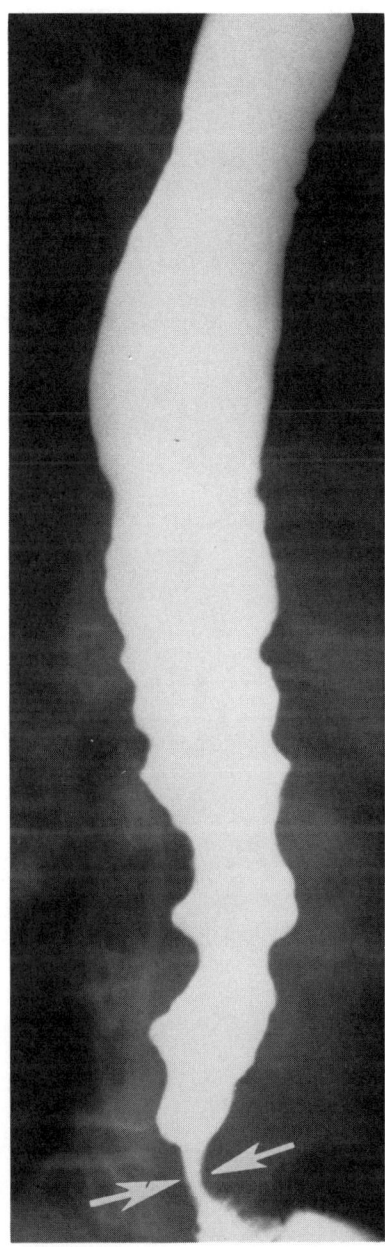

Fig 1–5.—Fluoroscopic study of man aged 64 years with chest pain and dysphagia shows absence of primary peristalsis with moderate tertiary activity and lower esophageal tapering *(arrows)*. These findings prompted a diagnosis of achalasia. Repeat manometry 30 months later showed achalasia, suggesting that the patient had an evolving esophageal motility disorder. (Courtesy of Chen YM, Ott DJ, Hewson EG, et al: *Radiology* 170:807–810, March 1989.)

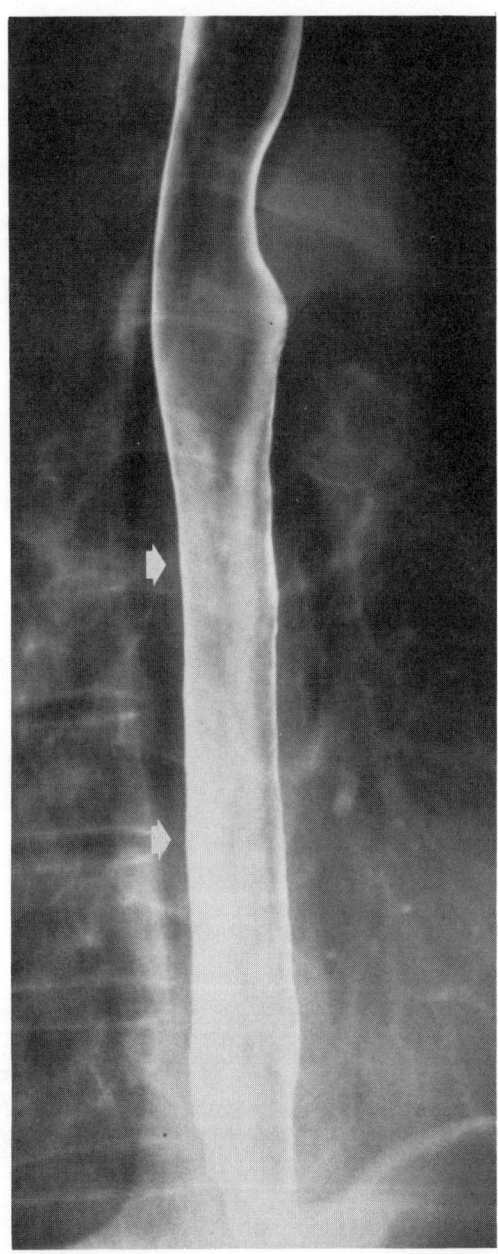

Fig 1-6.—Fluoroscopic study of woman aged 65 years with chest pain and diagnosis of DES on basis of manometry shows normal esophageal wall thickness *(arrows)*. (Courtesy of Chen YM, Ott OJ, Hewson EG, et al: *Radiology* 170:807–810, March 1989.)

tance in DES. The final important point the authors make concerns the difficulty in making the diagnosis with radiographic studies alone. In only 2 of 17 patients could the diagnosis of diffuse esophageal spasm be made with radiographic studies alone, pointing to the necessity of using clinical manometric and radiographic studies to make this diagnosis.—P.B. Miner, Jr., M.D.

Cricopharyngeal Dysphagia

Myotomy for Reflux-Induced Cricopharyngeal Dysphagia: Five-Year Review
Henderson RD, Hanna WM, Henderson RF, Marryatt G (Univ of Toronto)
J Thorac Cardiovasc Surg 98:428–433, September 1989   1–5

Reflux may induce cricopharyngeal dysphagia with symptoms severe enough to require surgical management. During a 5-year period, 4 men and 21 women aged 24–86 years (average age, 61.1 years) were first seen with severe cricopharyngeal symptoms. Overall symptoms included food sticking caused by eating solids in 84% of the patients and by consuming liquids in 60%. Regurgitation or choking was present in 80%. Ten patients had lost significant amounts of weight before surgery. No patient had mechanical dysphagia. All patients underwent preoperative manometry, which demonstrated cricopharyngeal incoordination in 90% of them.

Twelve patients with reflux-induced cricopharyngeal dysphagia as the main symptom underwent cricopharyngeal myotomy, which was extended proximally to the pharynx and distally to the intrathoracic esophagus (Fig 1–7).

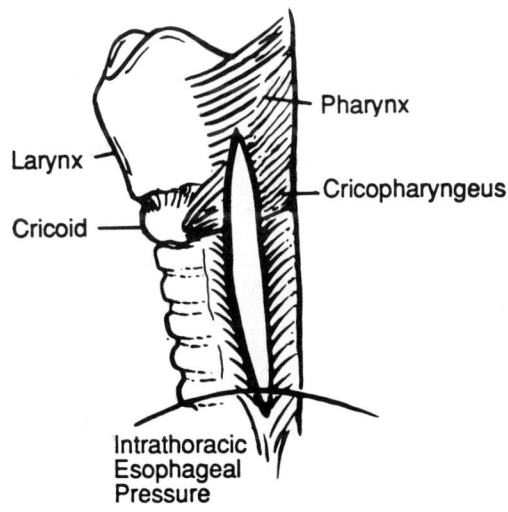

Fig 1–7.—Cricopharyngeal myotomy crossing the cricopharyngeal muscle. The myotomy extends 0.5 cm into the pharynx, approximately 5 cm into the cervical esophagus, and 1–2 cm into the intrathoracic esophagus to be within the negative intrathoracic pressure zone. (Courtesy of Henderson RD, Hanna WM, Henderson RF, et al: J Thorac Cardiovasc Surg 98:428–433, September 1989.)

Their symptoms were not severe, and they were not physically suitable for more extensive reflux-control operations. Six patients with severe cricopharyngeal dysphagia who had not responded to previous medical treatment also underwent cricopharyngeal myotomy only, because reflux symptoms were not severe enough to warrant antireflux operations. The remaining 7 patients had previously undergone total fundoplication gastroplasty. All had severe cricopharyngeal dysphagia that had not responded to gastroplasty, although they had responded well to reflux control. Also, the eophagus had been dilated after gastroplasty, revealing no evidence of distal obstructive disease. These patients also had treatment by cricopharyngeal myotomy.

Outcomes were excellent to satisfactory for 24 of the 25 patients. Only 1 operation was a definite failure (4%), as the patient had persistent significant dysphagia and has not responded to repeated dilation. Pathologic examination of the cricopharyngeal muscle specimens showed fibrosis ranging from mild to severe.

Cricopharyngeal myotomy is a useful and safe procedure for the treatment of cricopharyngeal dysphagia and aspiration, particularly in elderly patients with reflux.

▶ This is an interesting report of a unique approach to cricopharyngeal dysphagia from reflux esophagitis. Fibrosis of the cricopharyngeus was an unusual and, I suspect, an unexpected finding. The excellent results obtained with division of the cricopharyngeus, a procedure of low morbidity, is encouraging. That esophagopharyngeal reflux did not occur further substantiates the value of the procedure.—F.G. Moody, M.D.

2 Reflux Esophagitis

Pathophysiology

Sensitivity of the Esophageal Mucosa to pH in Gastroesophageal Reflux Disease
Smith JL, Opekun AR, Larkai E, Graham DY (VA Med Ctr; Baylor College of Medicine, Houston)
Gastroenterology 96:683–689, March 1989

The relationship between the sensation of pain and pH of the refluxed gastric contents was studied in 25 patients with symptomatic gastroesophageal reflux disease and a positive result of the Bernstein test. The timed Bernstein test was used to quantify the sensitivity of the esophageal mucosa to pain during intraesophageal infusions of different HCl solutions with pH 1, 1.5, 2, 2.5, 3, 4, 5, and 6 in a double-blind, randomized fashion. Twenty-four-hour intraesophageal pH monitoring was performed to correlate pH with duration and severity of pain.

Overall, the time to pain onset correlated positively with the pH of the solution infused (Fig 2–1). The time-to-pain onset was significantly longer

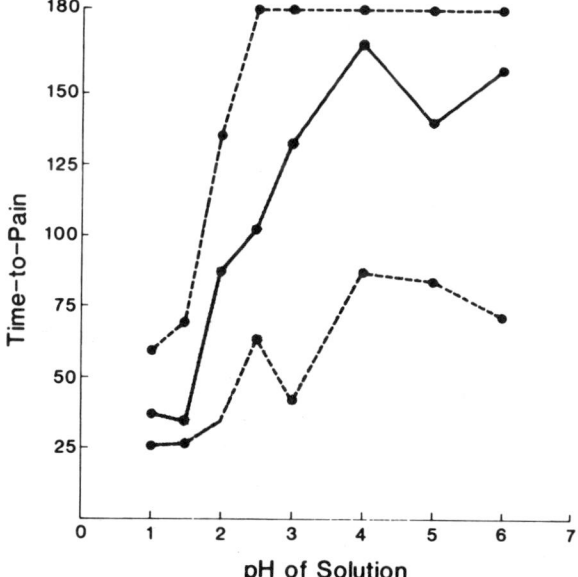

Fig 2–1.—Results of timed Bernstein test. *Solid line,* median; *dotted lines,* upper and lower quartiles. (Courtesy of Smith JL, Opekum AR, Larkai E, et al: *Gastroenterology* 96:683–689, March 1989.)

with increasing pH. However, the pain-pH response was curvilinear, so that pain appeared most rapidly with pHs of 1 and 1.5, increasing progressively and reaching a plateau of more than pH 4. An additional infusion of pH 1 solution was given to 14 patients after the randomized infusion test. The time-to-pain onset was significantly more rapid after the additional infusion than was recorded with the initial pH 1 solution, suggesting that sensitization for pain perception was produced by exposure to pain. Of the group, 15 underwent 24-hour intraesophageal pH monitoring. Only 64% of the pain episodes were associated with pH drop of less than 4. Compared with nonpainful episodes, reflux episodes associated with pain had a significantly longer duration of reflux and were more often associated with a recent painful episode. Painful episodes were not associated with lower pH or shorter time since reflux. Except for the number of recent painful episodes, none of the data from the 24-hour pH monitoring consistently predicted pain.

Pain in gastroesophageal reflux disease is more likely to be perceived with more severe reflux and with episodes that follow other painful episodes. Episodes of pain may sensitize the patients for subsequent pain.

▶ This interesting study indicates that gastroesophageal reflux disease (GERD) is a complex disease process. Some key findings in this study are restated below:

1. 24-hour pH monitoring was not that useful in predicting painful episodes, as 36% of the time that the intraesophageal pH decreased to ≤4, pain was not perceived.
2. Reflux episodes resulting in pain were significantly longer in duration than asymptomatic reflux episodes.
3. Episodes of pain sensitize patients with GERD to subsequent pain.

This latter observation underscores the need to bring painful GERD episodes under control using optimal dosages of medication as well as other support measures and "breaking the cycle," so to speak. In this regard, I have observed that patients with GERD periodically may require large doses of histamines H_2-receptor blockers, e.g., ranitidine, 150–300 mg 3 times daily, to effect control of their symptoms; after this is accomplished, the dosage of medication can be reduced carefully.—N.J. Greenberger, M.D.

Medical Therapy

Cimetidine Treatment of Reflux Esophagitis in Children: An Italian Multicentric Study
Cucchiara S, Gobio-Casali L, Balli F, Magazzú G, Staiano A, Astolfi R, Amarri S, Conti-Nibali S, Guandalini S (Univ of Naples; Modena; Messina; Mantova, Italy)
J Pediatr Gastroenterol Nutr 8:150–156, February 1989

Most previous treatment trials with gastroesophageal reflux of children have been open. In this study, the efficacy of cimetidine in dosages of 30–40 mg/kg daily was examined with 32 children having reflux disease complicated by esophagitis. The random double-blind trial lasted 12 weeks. Seventeen children received cimetidine, and 15 received a placebo. Intensive postural treatment was used with all children.

Both clinical and histologic scores improved significantly in cimetidine-treated patients but not in placebo recipients. All patients with mild or moderate esophagitis who received cimetidine had healing. Seven of 8 with severe esophagitis improved or were cured, compared with 2 of 8 placebo recipients. Most patients who had no response did have improvement when given ranitidine. Side effects from cimetidine were not significant.

Gastroesophageal reflux disease in infants is self-limited when conservative measures, including postural adjustment and thickened feedings, are used. If, however, esophagitis is present, drug treatment is appropriate. An H_2-receptor antagonist can be effective, but a motility-enhancing drug might also be helpful through improving gastroesophageal defenses.

▶ This controlled trial establishes the role of H_2-blockers in the treatment of regurgitation esophagitis of childhood. As pointed out, reflux esophagitis is a self-identified illness in the young, in contradistinction to adults, in whom it is progressive and relatively unresponsive to H_2 blockade. Total ablation of acid secretion with omeprazole, an inhibitor of proton translocation, however, continues to yield promising results in experimental trials.—F.G. Moody, M.D.

Surgical Therapy

Late Subjective and Objective Evaluations of Antireflux Surgery in Patients With Reflux Esophagitis: Analysis of 215 Patients
Csendes A, Braghetto I, Korn O, Cortés C (Univ of Chile, Santiago)
Surgery 105:374–382, March 1989
2–3

Posterior gastropexy is one of the definitive antireflux operations for the treatment of reflux esophagitis. Late subjective and objective outcome of a modified posterior gastropexy in 215 patients aged 18–72 years who were operated on for reflux esophagitis over an 11-year period were prospectively reviewed. A special protocol designed to assess outcome included analysis of reflux symptoms, radiology, endoscopy, esophageal manometry, and a standard acid reflux test. Operation consisted of highly selective vagotomy, closure of the hiatus, calibration of the cardia, posterior gastropexy, and fixation of the gastric fundus to the diaphragm (Fig 2–2).

Postoperative complications occurred in 11 patients, including intestinal obstruction, wound infection, pneumonia, and iatrogenic postoperative stricture that required reoperation. One patient died of an esophagogastric fistula caused by an esophageal tear after the stitches were placed too deep into the mucosa. The postoperative course in the other 203 patients was uneventful. Follow-up data were available for 202 patients, 150 of whom underwent reexamination 5 or more years after operation.

Reflux symptoms were greatly decreased after gastropexy. Radiologic examinations were normal in 93% of the patients, and endoscopy revealed long-standing healing of macroscopic esophagitis in 83% of the patients. Manometric studies confirmed that lower esophageal sphincter pressure was significantly

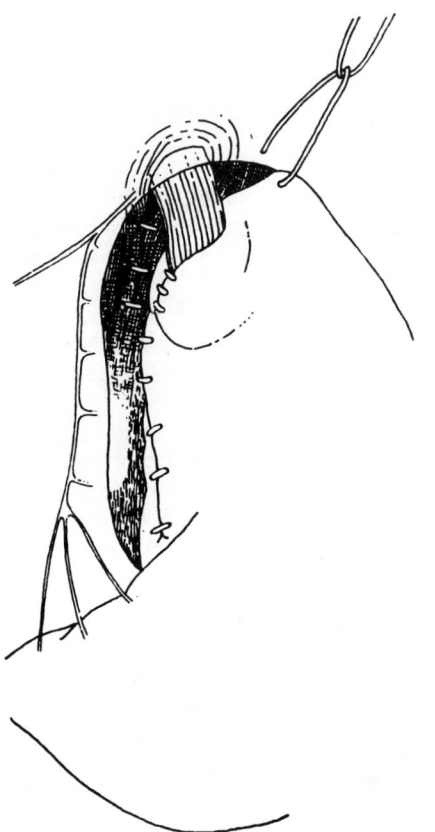

Fig 2–2.—Final aspect of surgical technique with highly selective vagotomy completed, the calibration of the cardia, posterior gastropexy to the median arcuate ligament, and 2 stitches of an anterior gastropexy of the greater curvature to the diaphragm, to avoid an anterior paraesophageal hernia. (Courtesy of Csendes A, Braghetto I, Korn O, et al: *Surgery* 105:374–382, March 1989.)

increased. Sphincter competence was maintained in 46 patients who underwent follow-up manometry 1 and 5 years after operation. The late results of antireflux gastropexy were excellent in 71% of patients, good in 14%, and average in 7%. The remaining 8% were considered surgical failures. Antireflux gastropexy adequately controls reflux esophagitis, particularly in patients with long-standing disease and in those in whom medical treatment has failed.

▶ Csendes and his associates have carefully documented their experience with a posterior gastropexy combined with parietal cell vagotomy for the treatment of reflux esophagitis. There was 1 death and minimal early or late morbidity. Only two thirds of the patients, however, were completely relieved of symptoms. This is somewhat lower than that reported for Nissen fundoplication, the preferred surgical approach in the United States. The proximal gastric vagotomy, which was most likely not an essential adjunct in most of the cases, possibly contributed to new symptomatology. I use proximal gastric vagotomy only in reoperations or when there is a history or documentation of peptic ulcer disease of the duodenum.—F.G. Moody, M.D.

Late Results of Fundoplication for Gastroesophageal Reflux in Infants and Children
Turnage RH, Oldham KT, Coran AG, Blane CE (Univ of Michigan)
Surgery 105:457–464, April 1989   2–4

The long-term results of the Nissen fundoplication operation for severe gastroesophageal reflux were studied in 46 infants and children available for follow-up more than 5 years after surgery. The mean follow-up was 6.7 years, and the mean age at operation was 4.1 years. Nearly half the patients in the series had cerebral palsy, and 11 patients had congenital anomalies, including esophageal atresia in 6 patients

One-fourth of the patients died during follow-up. All deaths but 1 were related to underlying medical problems. Twenty-six of 35 surviving patients are without symptoms, and 5 others have only mild symptoms requiring little or no treatment. Four patients have had repeat fundoplication for symptomatic recurrences of reflux, and 3 did well. Nearly half the patients had postoperative complications. There were 2 esophageal complications and 1 gastric perforation at surgery. Three patients each had the "gas bloat" syndrome, early dysphagia, and persistent stricture. Six had atelectasis/pneumonia. Small bowel obstruction was a problem in 4 patients and delayed gastric emptying caused a problem in 3.

The Nissen fundoplication procedure yielded good results in 88% of these patients. Both neurologically impaired children and others had a good outlook. Deaths are related primarily to associated disorders.

▶ This report establishes the perioperative complications and long-term outcome of Nissen fundoplication for the treatment of esophageal reflux in children. The majority of children had severe associated neurologic deficits or congenital defects that led to a high rate of attrition (25%) in the early follow-up. Survivors were relatively symptom free, thereby benefiting greatly from the procedure.—F.G. Moody, M.D.

Fifteen- to Twenty-Year Results After the Hill Antireflux Operation
Low DE, Anderson RP, Ilves R, Ricciardelli E, Hill LD (Virginia Mason Med Ctr, Seattle)
J Thorac Cardiovasc Surg 98:444–450, September 1989   2–5

Although antireflux operations are an important component in the treatment of reflux esophagitis, many physicians remain wary of surgical intervention because of published reports of operative failure. The longevity of surgical control of reflux also has been questioned. The long-term results of the Hill repair performed by 1 surgeon in 447 patients aged 18–79 years in 1968–1973 was assessed (Fig 2–3).

All patients had refractory gastroesophageal reflux, and 29 patients also had dysphagia. Of the 447 patients, 370 underwent primary operation and 77

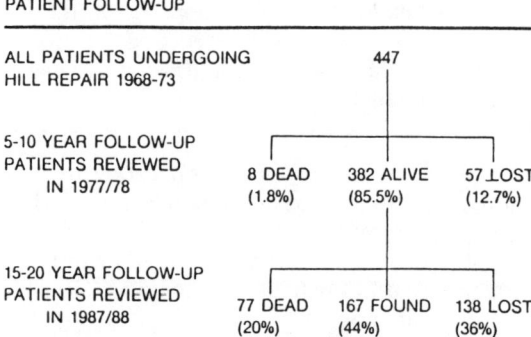

Fig 2–3.—Outcome of 447 consecutive patients undergoing the Hill repair for refractory esophageal reflux during the 5-year period between June 1968 and June 1973. (Courtesy of Low DE, Anderson RP, Ilves R, et al: J Thorac Cardiovasc Surg 98:444–450, September 1989.)

underwent secondary operations subsequent to a previous antireflux procedure. Follow-up data were collected through mailed questionnaires and personal interviews 5–10 years and 15–20 years after operation. Patients were asked to rate the results of operation on a scale of excellent, good, fair, or poor.

At the late follow-up attempt in 1987–1988, 167 of the 447 patients were located, 77 had died, and 138 were unavailable. The late group consisted of 88 men and 79 women with a mean age at operation of 53.7 years and a mean age at late follow-up of 71 years. Whereas 82% of the patients had rated their operative results as good or excellent at the short-term follow-up review, 88% of the patients rated their results as good or excellent at the late review. Only 4 patients from the original operative series had required reoperation for recurrent symptoms during the follow-up period. None of the patients reported late complications such as fistula, bleeding, or obstruction. The Hill antireflux operation, when properly performed in correctly selected patients, provides durable results in both the short and long term.

▶ The surgical group at the University of Michigan provides an update on its experience with the neoesophageal lengthening procedure and fundoplication (Collis-Nissen). Surgeons would be well advised to adapt their recommendations to use a large (54 French) dilator during construction of the gastroplasty and a complete wrap that encompasses only the gastroplasty. The large number of cases reported in the series suggests that not all patients needed such a complicated approach to their problem. Symptoms of reflux esophagitis are adequately treated most often by a standard floppy Nissen procedure with intraoperative dilatation of a stricture, if present.—F.G. Moody, M.D.

Continued Assessment of the Combined Collis-Nissen Operation
Stirling MC, Orringer MB (Univ of Michigan, Ann Arbor)
Ann Thorac Surg 47:224–230, February 1989

A complete fundoplication provides better reflux control than a partial gastric wrap in patients undergoing an antireflux operation especially after construction of a Collis gastroplasty. The effectiveness of the Collis-Nissen operation in the long-term control of gastroesophageal reflux was evaluated in 353 patients who underwent the Collis-Nissen operation between August 1976 and June 1988. Of the patients, 261 were followed up for an average of 43.8 months.

Success was achieved in 75% of the patients having the Collis-Nissen operation. Patients with spasm, scleroderma, previous antireflux operation, stricture or paraesophageal hernia were significantly less likely to have satisfactory results than patients without these features. Additionally, the recent classification in surgical technique has influenced results. A 54 French dilator in women and 56 French dilator in men have been used for construction of both the gastroplasty and the fundoplication; the fundoplication has been limited to 3 cm in length and encircles only the distal gastroplasty tube. With this modification, overall clinical status has improved, and subjective reflux control has improved significantly. Postoperative dysphagia is also less. Obesity, age greater than 70 years, or Barrett's epithelium had no significant effects on clinical outcome.

With both recurrent and persistent reflux and dysphagia, especially in patients with complicated esophageal disease, operation treatment of gastroesophageal reflux remains a challenge. Careful long-term follow-up and meticulous analysis of results of antireflux operations are necessary for future improvements.

▶ Hill and his associates at the Virginia Mason Clinic provide a long-term follow-up on the results of the operation devised and performed by the senior author over a 15-year period. A third of 447 were available for evaluation; 77 had died. A high percentage of those evaluated were satisfied with the results of the procedure, but what about those not traceable or who died during the interval of follow-up? Did they fare as well, or did the procedure contribute in some way to their demise or unavailability for evaluation? Unfortunately, long-term follow-up is difficult to achieve in our mobile society, precluding a precise statement as to the effectiveness of our surgical therapies.—F.G. Moody, M.D.

Relationship of a Satisfactory Outcome to Normalization of Delayed Gastric Emptying After Nissen Fundoplication
Hinder RA, Stein HJ, Bremner CG, DeMeester TR (Creighton Univ, Omaha)
Ann Surg 210:458–465, October 1989   2–7

Delayed emptying of the stomach in patients with gastroesophageal reflux may be caused by either an incompetent distal esophageal sphincter or a gastric abnormality. The effects of the Nissen fundoplication operation on gastric emptying were examined in 25 patients with proved gastroesophageal reflux disease. Of the patients, 9 had acid hypersecretion, 5 had gastritis, and 2 had significant duodenogastric reflux. In addition to fundoplication, the acid hypersecretors had a proximal gastric vagotomy, and the patients with duodenogastric reflux had a bile diversion procedure.

Gastric emptying, as estimated with a technetium-99m-sulfur coloid-labeled meal, was delayed in 17 patients before fundoplication, most often in those with gastric pathology (Fig 2–4). The mean emptying rate was significantly greater after operation (Fig 2–5).

Emptying became normal in 6 of 7 patients with markedly delayed emptying preoperatively. Significant symptoms were present in 5 patients with postoperative abnormal emptying and 2 with normal emptying. No patient believed that surgery had made things worse, and all those without gastric pathology were satisfied with the outcome.

Side effects from the Nissen fundoplication operation reflect a failure to normalize gastric emptying. Associated gastric pathology must not be ignored, as it may delay gastric emptying and cause persistent postoperative symptoms;

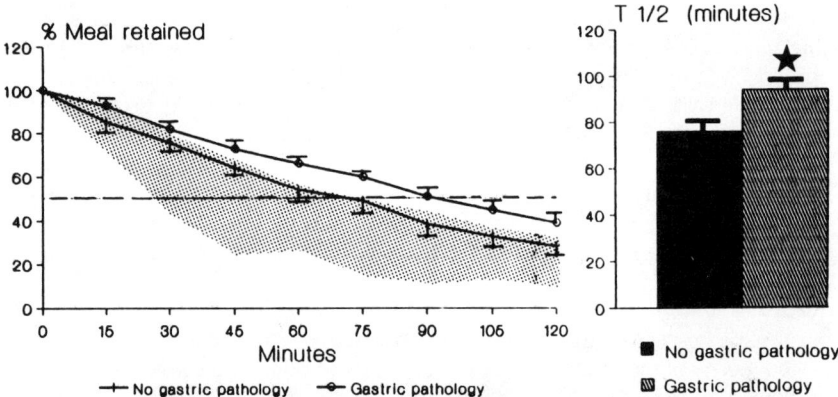

Fig 2–4.—Preoperative gastric emptying in 16 patients with gastric pathology *(open circles)* and in 9 patients without gastric pathology *(solid line)*. The *shaded area* represents the 10th to 90th percentiles of normal. The mean T½ is illustrated in the *bar graph* and shows delayed gastric emptying in patients with gastric pathology *(asterisk* indicates $P < .05$). (Courtesy of Hinder RA, Stein HJ, Bremner CG, et al: *Ann Surg* 210:458–465, October 1989.)

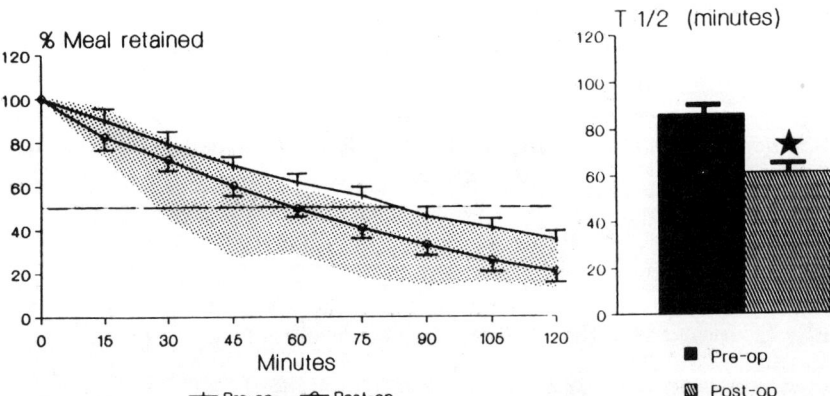

Fig 2–5.—Preoperative vs. postoperative gastric emptying in all 25 patients. The *shaded area* represents the 10th to 90th percentiles of normal. The mean T½ is illustrated in the *bar graph* and shows the speeding of postoperative emptying *(asterisk* indicates $P < .05$). (Courtesy of Hinder RA, Stein HJ, Bremner CG, et al: *Ann Surg* 210:458–465, October 1989.)

however, surgery for gastric pathology may itself alter gastric emptying.

▶ The authors make a good point. Some patients with reflux esophagitis may have an associated defect in gastric emptying. Gastric emptying possibly should be evaluated in selected patients who are candidates for antireflux procedure. Those who have acid peptic symptoms or gastritis or peptic ulcer identified at the time of gastroduodenal endoscopy are obvious candidates. I doubt whether routine emptying studies would be of much help, however, and believe they only would add to the expense of the preoperative assessment. Furthermore, it is unlikely that the occasional patient who has gastric emptying problems after fundoplication would be identified in this way.—F.G. Moody, M.D.

A Prospective Randomized Trial of Angelchik Prosthesis Versus Nissen Fundoplication
Stuart RC, Dawson K, Keeling P, Byrne PJ, Hennessy TPJ (St James's Hosp, Dublin)
Br J Surg 76:86–89, January 1989
2–8

Recent reviews of the Angelchik gastroesophageal antireflux prosthesis have reported low mortality and morbidity with this device. However, most clinical trials of the Angelchik device were uncontrolled studies, and the role of this prosthesis in antireflux procedures is not yet clear. Opinion on the Nissen fundoplication procedure also is divided. A prospective controlled trial was conducted to compare the Angelchik prosthesis with Nissen fundoplication in the treatment of esophageal reflux in 61 patients with gastroesophageal reflux unresponsive to medical treatment.

A total of 30 patients with a mean age of 51.4 years were randomly assigned to insertion of an Angelchik prosthesis and 31 patients with a mean age of 50.1 years underwent fundoplication. Both groups had similar preoperative pH profiles and manometric findings. Esophageal strictures were present in 8 patients in the Angelchik group and 7 patients in the fundoplication group. The mean postoperative follow-up was 38 months. All patients underwent endoscopy, 24-hour pH monitoring, and manometry 3–6 months after operation. Long-term endoscopic follow-up was performed as indicated by symptoms.

No operative deaths occurred in either group, and there were no complications specific to the Angelchik prosthesis such as migration and erosion into the gastrointestinal tract. In the Angelchik group, 23 (77%) and 29 (94%) patients in the fundoplication group were either symptom free (Visick I) or had occasional mild symptoms that did not require treatment (Visick II). Of the 7 patients in the Angelchik group with poor results, 7 reported severe, persistent dysphagia. Assessment 3–6 months after operation confirmed that both procedures were equally effective in reducing reflux and increasing lower esophageal sphincter pressure. However, long-term follow-up endoscopic examinations revealed that 7 patients in the Angelchik group but none in the fundoplication group had grade III esophagitis. The Nissen fundoplication yields better results than the Angelchik prosthesis as fundoplication appears to provide more permanent control of gastroesophageal reflux and is associated with less frequent and less persistent dysphagia.

▶ Randomized trials, when carried out in a well-controlled environment that does not have an interest bias, can yield useful and truthful information. The surgeons in Dublin sought the truth with a controlled clinical trial and learned that a Nissen fundoplication gets results superior to the Angelchik prosthesis. I have expressed over the last several years my bias against the Angelchik approach because of its tendency to migrate. The surgeons in Dublin found out how to keep it in place, but learned that it cannot provide protection as effective against gastroesophageal reflux as the upper stomach when appropriately wrapped around the lower esophagus.—F.G. Moody, M.D.

3 Barrett's Esophagus

Dysplasia and Flow Cytometry

Discordance Between Flow Cytometric Abnormalities and Dysplasia in Barrett's Esophagus
Fennerty MB, Sampliner RE, Way D, Riddell R, Steinbronn K, Garewal HS (VA Med Ctr; Univ of Arizona, Tucson; McMaster Univ, Hamilton, Ont)
Gastroenterology 97:815–820, October 1989   3-1

Barrett's esophagus, characterized by metaplastic columnar rather than stratified squamous epithelial lining of the esophagus, occurs in up to 12% of all patients with symptomatic gastroesophageal reflux disease. Adenoma is the most serious clinical consequence of Barrett's esophagus, but its true incidence as a complication of Barrett's esophagus is not known. Dysplasia and flow cytometric abnormalities have been implicated as markers of the premalignant state. This study was done to assess the relationship between histologic dysplasia and abnormal flow cytometry, including aneuploidy and increased G_2 as markers of the premalignant state, in 108 tissue specimens obtained from the upper gastrointestinal tract. Of the specimens, 86 were obtained from 25 men with endoscopically confirmed Barrett's esophagus, and 22 control specimens were obtained from 10 men without Barrett's esophagus.

Thirteen specimens obtained from 6 patients with Barrett's esophagus had a histologic diagnosis of dysplasia; 7 were low grade and 6, high grade. Two of the 6 high-grade but none of the 7 low-grade dysplasia specimens were aneuploid, and only 2 low-grade dysplastic specimens had increased G_2. Eight of the 73 nondysplastic specimens were aneuploid, and another 15 specimens had increased G_2.

The 86 specimens from patients with Barrett's esophagus were classified into 4 subgroups based on histology and flow cytometry findings. Sixty-five specimens (76%) were type 1, defined as Barrett's epithelium without dysplasia or aneuploidy; 8 (9%) were type 2, defined as Barrett's epithelium without dysplasia but with aneuploidy; 11 (13%) were type 3, defined as Barrett's epithelium with dysplasia but no aneuploidy (Fig 3–1), and 2 (2%) were type 4, defined as Barrett's epithelium with dysplasia and aneuploidy.

Thus dysplasia and aneuploidy are often discordant. Whether the presence of both in patients with Barrett's epithelium reflects an increased risk for adenocarcinoma remains to be determined. For now, the validity of aneuploidy as an independent marker of cancer risk remains unconfirmed.

▶ I would like to restate the major findings and the author's conclusion from this study in patients with Barrett's esophagus:

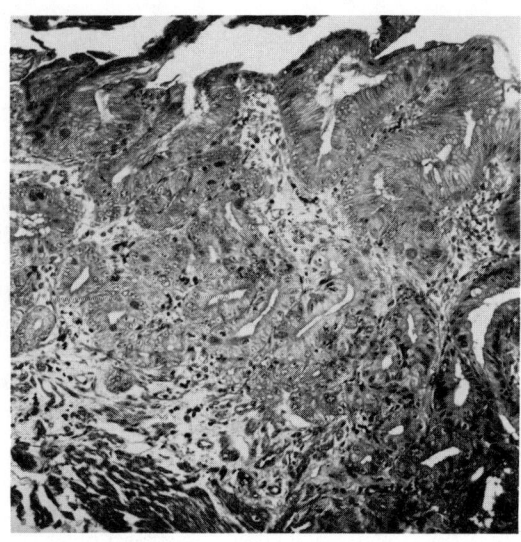

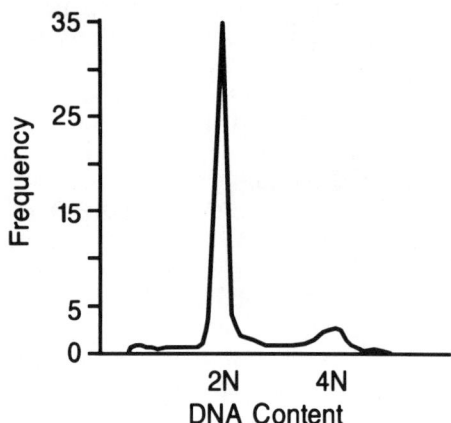

Fig 3–1.—Histology reveals dysplasia, but the DNA histogram is normal (type 3 classification). (Courtesy of Fennerty MB, Sampliner RE, Way D, et al: *Gastroenterology* 97:815–820, October 1989.)

1. Histologic evidence of dysplasia and aneuploidy as demonstrated by flow cytometry may be discordant findings.
2. The findings of dysplasia and aneuploidy may identify different subgroups at risk for the development of cancer.
3. The findings of *both* dysplasia and aneuploidy may reflect an *increased* cancer risk.
4. Further study is necessary to define the role of histology and flow cytometry in the screening and management of patients with Barrett's esophagus.

Although there is not a uniform opinion, most authorities now recommend that patients with either dysplasia or dysplasia plus aneuploidy undergo surgical resection of the involved esophagus.—N.J. Greenberger, M.D.

Barrett's Esophagus: Development of Dysplasia and Adenocarcinoma
Hameeteman W, Tytgat GNJ, Houthoff HJ, van den Tweel JG (Univ of Amsterdam)
Gastroenterology 96:1249–1256, May 1989   3–2

Barrett's esophagus is considered a premalignant condition. Long-term surveillance with careful histologic examination of multiple biopsy specimens is warranted to detect dysplasia or developing carcinoma. A prospective endoscopic and histologic follow-up study investigated the development of dysplasia and carcinoma in 50 patients with Barrett's esophagus without carcinoma. Barrett's epithelium was classified as fundic, junctional or cardia, or specialized columnar, and intermediate when the epithelium could not be classified in any of the first 3 types. The mean follow-up period was 5.2 years (range, 1.5–14 years).

At entrance into the study, 7 patients (14%) had dysplasia, low grade in 6 and high grade in 1. During follow-up, dysplasia increased in frequency and severity. At the end of the observation period, 13 patients had dysplasia — low grade in 10 and high grade in 3 — and in 5 patients adenocarcinoma had developed. Both dysplasia and adenocarcinoma were seen in the specialized columnar and intermediate types of epithelium. In the 5 patients with carcinoma, an increase in the severity of dysplasia was observed (Fig 3–2). The time between findings of low-grade dysplasia and carcinoma varied from 1.5 to 4 years.

Carcinoma was limited to the mucosa or submucosa in 3 patients who underwent surgery.

This study underscores that Barrett's esophagus is a premalignant condition. The incidence of carcinoma in this group of patients was 1 in 52 patient-years, corresponding to 1,920 Barrett's carcinoma per 100,000 patients. This relates to a 125-fold increased risk compared with the general Dutch population. The presence of high-grade dysplasia should be considered an ominous sign of potential malignancy, and patients with specialized columnar- or intermediate-type epithelium are especially at risk of dysplasia or carcinoma. A long-

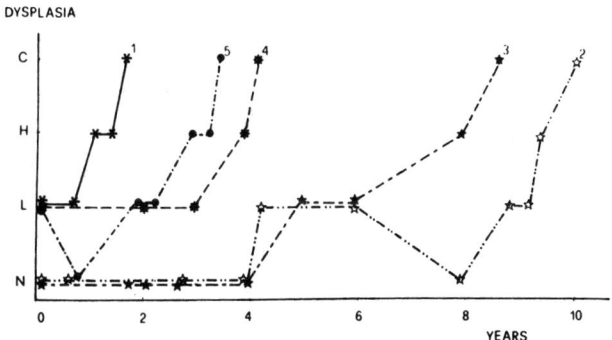

Fig 3–2.—Progression of dysplasia in 5 patients with BE in whom carcinoma developed. *N*, negative for dysplasia; *L*, low-grade dysplasia (including indefinite for dysplasia); *H*, high-grade dysplasia; *C*, carcinoma. (Courtesy of Hameeteman W, Tytgat GNJ, Houthoff JH, et al: *Gastroenterology* 96:1249–1256, May 1989.)

term clinical, endoscopic, and histologic follow-up program in patients with Barrett's esophagus is necessary.

▶ The management of Barrett's esophagus continues to be problematic, especially so because of the risk of carcinoma developing in dysplastic epithelium. The study by Hameeteman and colleagues indicates that the incidence and severity of dysplasia increase over time, and that dysplasia is most likely to develop in specialized columnar epithelium. It would appear that an objective of medical management is to effect regression of Barrett's epithelium. A recent letter to the editor (1) describes regression of Barrett's epithelium in 3 patients treated with omeprazole in high doses. These patients had previously been treated unsuccessfully with H_2 blockers and had resistant Barrett's ulcers. Omeprazole was given in a dosage of 60 mg/day in an attempt to induce complete inhibition of acid secretion. After 3 months of therapy there was no evidence of Barrett's esophagus in 2 patients and gastric metaplasia had regressed from 32 cm to 36 cm in the third. These observations confirm the role of acid reflux in the pathogenesis of Barrett's esophagus and emphasize the need for further prospective studies to confirm the effectiveness of omeprazole in the treatment of this lesion. Further, it will be important to determine whether patients can be given lower doses of omeprazole or switched from omeprazole to H_2 blockers after regression of Barrett's esophagus.—N.J. Greenberger, M.D.

Reference

1. DeViere J, et al: Regression of Barrett's epithelium with omeprazole. *N Engl J Med* 320:1497, 1989.

Complications

Alkaline Gastroesophageal Reflux: Implications in the Development of Complications in Barrett's Columnar-Lined Lower Esophagus
Attwood SEA, DeMeester TR, Bremner CG, Barlow AP, Hinder RA (Creighton Univ, Omaha)
Surgery 106:764–770, October 1989   3–3

Barrett's esophagus is a frequent finding in patients with gastroesophageal reflux and is associated with high rates of stricture formation, ulceration, and carcinoma. It is not clear why only some patients with reflux have this disorder. Endoscopy, manometry, and 24-hour pH monitoring were performed in 23 consecutively seen patients with histologic diagnoses of Barrett's esophagus. Complications in 12 patients included stricture, giant ulcer, and dysplasia. Fifty-three patients with reflux esophagitis and 50 healthy persons also were assessed.

Eleven patients with Barrett's esophagus and 13 of those with esophagitis had increased esophageal exposure to a pH above 7. Barrett's patients with complications had greater exposures to alkaline than those without complications. The finding of duodenogastric reflux at endoscopy was associated with complications of Barrett's esophagus. Positive results on hepatoiminodiacetic acid scanning also were associated with symptoms of duodenogastric reflux. The manometric findings were similar for patients with and those without complications.

Complications in patients with Barrett's esophagus result from the damaging effects of refluxed duodenal juice. Complications of the Roux-en-Y duodenal diversion may be avoided by preserving gastroduodenal continuity while diverting the flow of bile and pancreatic juice through the duodenal switch operation.

► The authors propose that duodenogastric reflux plays a role in the pathogenesis of the Barrett's variant of reflux esophagitis. Their study design of matching endoscopic, manometric, and pH monitoring data of Barrett's patients to those with non-Barrett's esophagitis offers circumstantial evidence for this novel hypothesis. I am not prepared, however, to adopt the duodenal diversion procedure they propose as a substitute for a Nissen fundoplication, which, when properly performed, relieves the inflammatory component of Barrett's esophagitis. Unfortunately, the potential for malignancy remains, as it probably will even when duodenogastric reflux is prevented.—F.G. Moody, M.D.

Adenocarcinoma Arising in Barrett's Esophagus
Ovaska J, Miettinen M, Kivilaakso E (Helsinki Univ Central Hosp, Helsinki)
Dig Dis Sci 34:1336–1339, September 1989   3–4

Retrospective studies have shown an association between Barrett's esophagus and esophageal adenocarcinoma. To determine the incidence of adenocarcinoma among patients who lack neoplastic disease when first seen, data on 134 patients with endoscopically marked esophagitis or Barrett's esophagus, or both, who were seen in a 10-year period, were studied. Thirty-two patients met gross and histologic criteria for Barrett's esophagus.

Three patients had adenocarcinoma during a follow-up of 166 patient-years, for an annual incidence of 1.8%. Two of the patients had dysplastic columnar epithelium 6 and 15 months, respectively, before carcinoma was diagnosed. Endoscopic follow-up showed unchanged Barrett's epithelium in all but 3 patients after a mean of 6.7 years of treatment. Initial treatment was operative in 12 of the patients with Barrett's esophagus.

Barrett's esophagus is a potentially precancerous condition, but the precise risk remains to be determined. Patients require close endoscopic follow-up for dysplastic columnar epithelium in the distal esophagus, even after antireflux surgery.

► The actuarial risk of cancer developing in a Barrett's epthelial-lined esophagus is not known. This prospective follow-up of 32 patients with Barrett's epithelium disclosed an annual increase of nearly 2%. Of note is that dysplasia preceded the histologic evidence of cancer in 2 of 3 patients and 1 case occurred in a patient who had previously undergone an antireflux procedure. In my experience, following up patients with Barrett's becomes difficult after a successful approach to their problem. Yearly or even more frequent endoscopies for biopsy and histologic monitoring become more difficult as the likelihood of dysplastic change becomes greater with time. Histologic evidence of dysplasia is an indication for resection of the involved segment of the esophagus, either before or after an antireflux procedure. Resection clearly would be the best way to prevent cancer in Barrett's epithelium, but the morbidity of such an approach exceeds the risk of neoplastic change. From a public health point of view, early effective control of gastroesophageal reflux offers the best prophylaxis.—F.G. Moody, M.D.

4 Carcinoma of the Esophagus

Endosonography and Computed Tomography of Esophageal Carcinoma: Preoperative Classification Compared to the New (1987) TNM System
Tio TL, Cohen P, Coene PP, Udding J, Den Hartog Jager FCA, Tytgat GNJ (Academic Med Ctr; The Netherlands Cancer Inst, Amsterdam)
Gastroenterology 96:1478–1486, June 1989   4–1

The accuracy and limitations of transesophageal endosonography (ES) and CT in preoperative staging of esophageal carcinoma were investigated in 74 patients. The results were correlated with the histology of resected specimens according to the new (1987) TNM classification.

Endosonography was significantly more accurate than CT in the evaluation of tumor depth, for an overall accuracy of 89% and 59%, respectively. Limited intramural carcinomas and nonresectable carcinoma were detected more accurately with ES than with CT. In addition, ES was superior to CT in the assessment of regional lymph node metastases, for overall accuracies of 80% and 51%, respectively. The incidence of lymph node metastasis increased with the progression of the depth of tumor infiltration. Inadequate ES examination occurred in 26% of patients because of the presence of severe stenosis. In these patients, CT was superior to ES in the diagnosis of lymph node metastasis, for overall accuracies of 82% with CT and 68% with ES.

Transesophageal ES is more accurate than CT in the preoperative TNM classification of esophageal carcinoma. However, inadequate ES examination can occur in the presence of severe stenosis, in which instance CT would prove beneficial.

Superficial Squamous Cell Carcinoma of the Esophagus: A Report of 76 Cases and Review of the Literature
Bogomoletz WV, Molas G, Gayet B, Potet F (Inst Jean Godinot, Reims, France; Hôpital Beaujon, Clichy, France)
Am J Surg Pathol 13:535–546, July 1989   4–2

Invasive squamous cell carcinoma of the esophagus still causes a significant number of cancer deaths, but an "early" form of superficial squamous cell cancer of the esophagus (SSCCE) recently was examined. These patients have much improved survival when treated in a timely manner. Studies were made in 76 patients with SSCCE seen in 1979–1987.

The patients had a mean age of 56 years. Dysphagia was the most frequent presenting feature, but several patients had no symptoms. Six tumors had spindle-cell features, and 5 were adenoid cystic carcinomas. Twelve percent of lesions were poorly differentiated. The mean tumor thickness was 0.3 cm. Multicentricity was noted in 17% of tumors. The resection margins were involved by tumor in 6 instances. Postoperative mortality was 17%. Half of the patients lived for a mean of 30 months after surgery, most of them without evidence of recurrent disease. Lymph node metastasis was most frequent in cases with submucosal involvement. Only 1 of 9 patients with encroachment onto the muscularis mucosae had node metastasis.

Among patients having SSCCE, those with intraepithelial or infiltrating disease limited to the mucosa have a good prognosis. Those with involvement of the submucosa are more likely to have nodal spread. Patients with SSCCE benefit markedly from early diagnosis and treatment.

▶ The surgeons in Clichy, France, were fortunate in being able to treat 76 cases of superficial and presumably early esophageal cancer. In spite of the low volume of tumor, multicentricity was common (17%), and the margins of the resected esophagus were involved in nearly 10% of cases. Furthermore, the operative mortality (17%) was surprisingly high, considering the superficial nature of the tumor. How to identify esophageal cancer before it can be seen through the endoscope or with radiographic imaging remains a problem, because once the tumors can be discovered by these means, they usually are incurable.—F.G. Moody, M.D.

5 Miscellaneous Topics

Spontaneous Rupture

Spontaneous Rupture of the Esophagus: A 30-Year Experience
Pate JW, Walker WA, Cole FH Jr, Owen EW, Johnson WH (Univ of Tennessee, Memphis)
Ann Thorac Surg 47:689–692, May 1989   5–1

Boerhaave's syndrome, rupture of the esophagus, is rare but associated with a high mortality. Diagnosis is difficult because patients do not necessarily have the classic symptoms: severe vomiting; epigastric or substernal pain, or both; collapse; and shock. Data on 35 patients with spontaneous rupture of the esophagus who were seen over a 30-year period were retrospectively reviewed.

The condition was more common among men (79%); the median age of the patients was 53 years. Rapid onset of pain (85%), vomiting (71%), or both were the most frequent presenting symptoms. Pain occurred in the abdomen in 16 patients, in the thoracic area in 9, and in the shoulder in 4. Physical examination yielded little specific information for diagnosis; the condition was correctly identified on admission for only 14 (41%) patients. Routine chest roentgenographic examinations revealed nondiagnostic abnormalities in 24 patients. Pleural effusions were noted in 18 patients, and mediastinal emphysema, in 9.

Twenty-six patients underwent primary surgical repair, and pleural flaps were used to cover suture lines in 20 patients. Multiple antibiotics were given intravenously to all patients. Thoracotomy was performed in all but 4 patients. Ruptures most commonly were located on the left wall of the distal esophagus.

The 14 patients (41%) who died included all 4 who did not have thoracotomy. Delay in treatment (24 hours or more) did not significantly affect mortality, but caused a significant increase in complications. Surgical repair, even when delayed, offers the best chance of recovery. When esophagograms were made, the suspected diagnoses were confirmed for all but 1 patient. Undigested food in pleural aspirates also strongly suggests esophageal rupture.

▶ Boerhaave's syndrome is a diagnosis that you must carry around in your memory and review the features of every once in a while. If you don't, you will miss its presence at a great cost to the patient who has it. Esophagogram is a simple, noninvasive test that should be done early for patients with unexplained pleural effusions or mediastinal widening. An operative repair of the torn esophagus at an early stage in the illness offers the only chance for survival. This is a serious complication of retching that carries with it a high mortality, even when treated in an optimal manner.—F.G. Moody, M.D.

Paraesophageal Hernia

Computed Tomographic Evaluation of Paraesophageal Hernia
Vas W, Malpani AR, Singer J, Sundaram M, Chenoweth J (Univ Hosp; John Cochran VA Hosp, St Louis)
Gastrointest Radiol 14:291–294, Fall 1989   5-2

No more than 5% of operated hiatal hernias are paraesophageal hernias (PEH). Small hernias of this type may produce few symptoms, but if left untreated they may enlarge and produce significant or even catastrophic complications. A total of 2,400 chest and abdominal CT scans obtained for adults in a 1-year period were reviewed for the presence of PEH. Both oral and intravenous contrast were used routinely.

Four patients with a mean age of 64 years had PEH. Three of them had omentum as well as part of the stomach within the thoracic cavity (Fig 5–1). All patients had a large amount of intra-abdominal fat. None had symptoms from the hernia, and in no case was there a predisposing cause other than marked obesity. A barium study within a month of the CT examinations demonstrated the PEH in 3 of the 4 patients. Three other patients who had a large amount of fat in a paraesophageal location received a presumptive diagnosis of paraesophageal omental hernia; all had normal findings on barium studies.

In PEH the gastroesophageal junction usually is located in its normal position beneath the diaphragm, and reflux is lacking. The initial abnormality is protrusion of the gastric fundus through the esophageal hiatus and into the

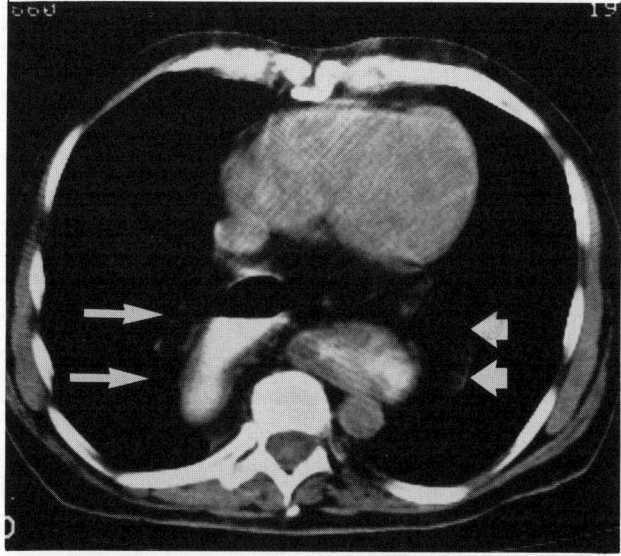

Fig 5–1.—Large PEH straddling midline. Air-fluid level is seen in upside-down intrathoracic stomach *(long arrows)*. Omental component is seen in left side of hernia *(short arrow)*. (Courtesy of Vas W, Malpani AR, Singer J, et al: *Gastrointest Radiol* 14:291–294, Fall 1989.)

posterior mediastinum. Patients have been seen with incarceration and obstruction; torsion, perforation, and gangrene are possible complications of this true anatomical hernia. Elective surgery is the best approach; the repair is straightforward even for elderly patients.

▶ Because it represents a true hernia, with a fundus of the stomach extending up through the diaphragmatic hiatus, PEH can be associated with a number of complications that may require emergency repair, which carries a high morbidity and mortality. The benign course with elective surgery makes an early diagnosis beneficial. This study illustrates the CT findings of PEH on routine abdominal and thoracic examinations that allow early recognition of this potentially serious condition.—P.B. Miner, Jr., M.D.

The Stomach and Duodenum

Chapter 6. Physiology and Pathophysiology
  Alcohol Metabolism
  Gastric pH After Cholecystectomy

Chapter 7. Peptic Ulcer Disease
  Medical Therapy for Duodenal Ulcer
  Medical Therapy for Gastric Ulcer
  Recurrent Ulcer and Maintenance Therapy
  Nonoperative Therapy for Perforated Ulcer

Chapter 8. Surgical Therapy for Peptic Ulcer Disease

Chapter 9. Zollinger-Ellison Syndrome

Chapter 10. Postgastric Surgery Syndromes

Chapter 11. Gastric Surgery for Morbid Obesity

Chapter 12. Upper Gastrointestinal Bleeding

Chapter 13. Gastric and Duodenal Neoplasms
  Gastric Cancer
  Leiomyosarcoma
  Carcinoids

Chapter 14. *Helicobacter (Campylobacter) pylori*

Chapter 15. Gastric Emptying Problems

Chapter 16. Miscellaneous

6 Physiology and Pathophysiology

Alcohol Metabolism

Gastric Origin of the First-Pass Metabolism of Ethanol in Humans: Effect of Gastrectomy
Caballeria J, Frezza M, Hernandez-Muñoz R, DiPadova C, Korsten MA, Baraona E, Lieber CS (Bronx VA Med Ctr; Mt Sinai School of Medicine, New York; Univ School of Medicine, Trieste, Italy)
Gastroenterology 97:1205–1209, November 1989   6–1

The areas under the curve (AUCs) of blood ethanol concentrations are much smaller after oral than after intravenous administration of small doses of ethanol. To determine whether this difference is caused by gastric or intestinal ethanol oxidation, hepatic first-pass metabolism of ethanol, or a combination of these mechanisms, the AUCs of blood ethanol levels were compared after random administration of the same ethanol dose (0.15 gm/kg) via intravenous, oral, and intraduodenal routes to 5 abstaining alcoholic persons and via intravenous and oral routes to 10 persons with Billroth II subtotal gastrectomy. Ethanol was given after a standard meal.

In the nongastrectomized patients, blood alcohol levels were much lower after oral administration than after intravenous administration, although virtually the entire dose had disappeared from the stomach at the completion of the AUC. In contrast, the AUCs after the intraduodenal route did not differ significantly from those achieved with intravenous administration, indicating that neither the intestine nor the liver contributed appreciably to this first-pass metabolism. In the gastrectomized patients, the AUCs did not differ between oral or intravenous administration (Fig 6–1).

These findings indicate that gastrectomy completely abolishes the first-pass metabolism of alcohol. Gastric metabolism decreases the bioavailability of ingested alcohol and, thus, attenuates its systemic toxicity. The abolition of this "protective barrier" may increase the vulnerability to alcohol of gastrectomized patients.

▶ This article explains the frequently noted clinical observation that patients who have undergone subtotal gastric resection are often intolerant of alcohol, even if only modest doses are ingested. The following article indicates there are important differences in the gastric metabolism of alcohol between men and women, especially chronically alcoholic women.—N.J. Greenberger, M.D.

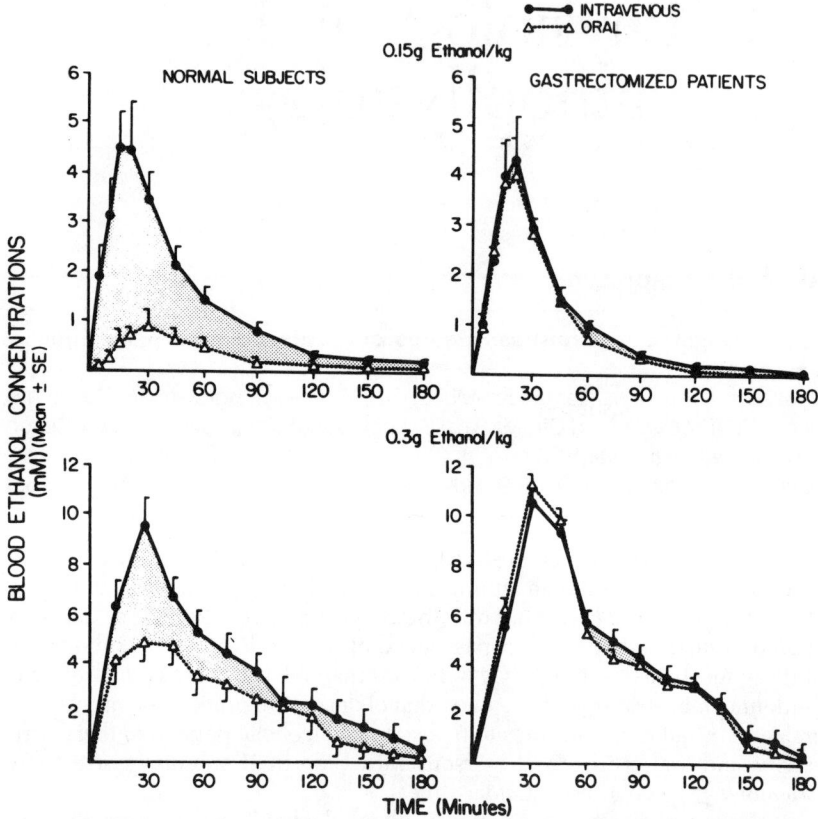

Fig 6–1.—Abolition of the differences in blood ethanol levels between oral and intravenous administration of either 0.15 or 0.3 g/kg body weight of ethanol in patients with Billroth II subtotal gastrectomy. (Courtesy of Caballeria J, Frezza M, Hernández-Muñoz R, et al: *Gastroenterology* 97:1205–1209, November 1989.)

High Blood Alcohol Levels in Women: The Role of Decreased Gastric Alcohol Dehydrogenase Activity and First-Pass Metabolism

Frezza M, di Padova C, Pozzato G, Terpin M, Baraona E, Lieber CS (Univ School of Medicine, Trieste, Italy; VA Med Ctr, Bronx, NY; Mt Sinai School of Medicine, New York)

N Engl J Med 322:95–99, Jan 11, 1990   6–2

Alcoholic liver disease develops more readily in women than in men, and women have higher blood ethanol levels after ingesting an equivalent oral dose of alcohol. A smaller distribution volume has been postulated as the reason but men and women have comparable blood ethanol levels after intravenous administration. The possibility of sex-related differences in gastric ethanol oxidation was examined in 20 men and 23 women; 6 in each group were alcoholic. Pharmacokinetic studies were done after oral and intravenous administration of ethanol, 0.3 gm/kg.

Both alcoholic and nonalcoholic women had higher blood ethanol levels than men after taking equivalent doses of ethanol (Fig 6–2). The mean area under the curve of blood ethanol concentrations was larger for women after oral, but not after intravenous administration. Among nonalcoholic persons, first-pass metabolism in women was 23% of that in men and gastric alcohol dehydrogenase activity was 59%. Alcoholic men had metabolism and enzyme activity levels about half those of nonalcoholic men. Alcoholic women had even lower enzyme activities, and their first-pass metabolism was virtually absent. Gastric alcohol dehydrogenase activity correlated significantly with the degree of first-pass metabolism.

The authors conclude that decreased gastric oxidation of ethanol in women may lead to increased bioavailability, and therefore promotes vulnerability to the acute and chronic complications of alcoholism. This situation may be worsened by other factors that impede ethanol oxidation, such as prolonged alcohol abuse and fasting.

▶ For an excellent brief review of the risk of alcohol intake in men and women, see the editorial by Schenker and Speeg (1). What follows has been abstracted from that paper.

The concentration of alcohol in the blood and other tissues is the result of its intake

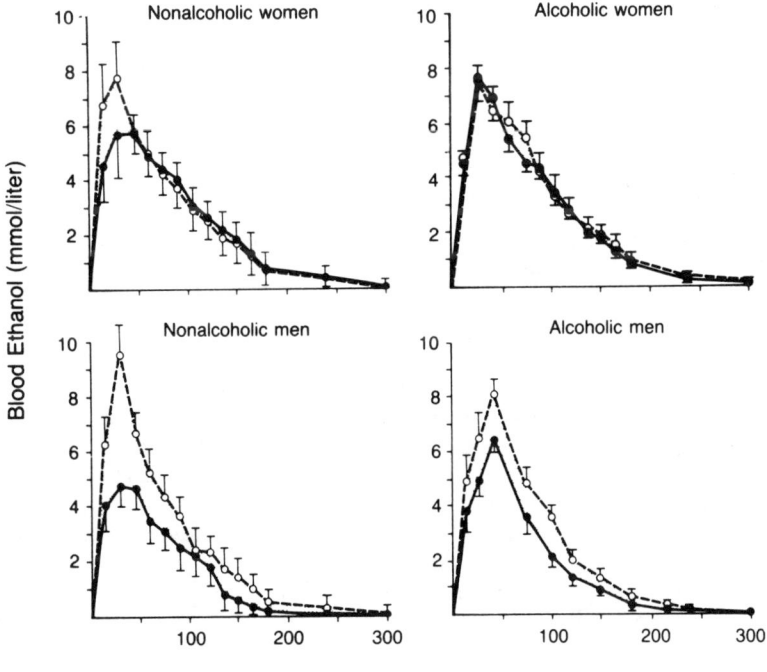

Fig 6–2.—Effects of sex and chronic alcohol abuse on blood ethanol concentrations. Ethanol was administered orally *(solid lines)* or intravenously *(dashed lines)* in a dose of 0.3 g/kg. The *shaded area* represents the difference between the curves for the 2 routes of administration (the first-pass metabolism). (Courtesy of Frezza M, di Padova C, Pozzato G, et al: *N Engl J Med* 322:95–99, Jan 11, 1990.)

route, usually oral; its distribution and its rate of elimination. Although the enzymes primarily responsible for alcohol metabolism, the alcohol dehydrogenases, are present in many tissues, the liver traditionally has been considered the principal site of alcohol metabolism. The paper by Frezza and co-workers indicates that alcohol dehydrogenase in the gastric mucosa may contribute substantially to alcohol metabolism, that this effect varies with sex, and that the gastric metabolism of alcohol is decreased in women and men with chronic alcoholism.

Early studies may have underestimated the usual importance of the gastric metabolism of alcohol, possibly because fasting persons were studied and large amounts of alcohol were ingested. More recent research showed that blood alcohol levels were significantly lower after oral than after intravenous administration of alcohol in doses of 0.15 or 0.3 g/kg of body weight in normal men studied after having eaten. (The latter dose is about 1.5 "standard" drinks for a man weighing 70 kg.) This decrease in the bioavailability of alcohol after alcohol ingestion appears to result from gastric alcohol metabolism and has been termed *gastric first-pass metabolism.* It may be considered a protective mechanism because it decreases the influx of alcohol into the liver and systemic circulation.

Reference

1. Schenker S, Speeg KV: The risk of alcohol intake in men and women: All may not be equal. *N Engl J Med* 322:127–130, 1990.

Gastric pH After Cholecystectomy

The Alkaline Shift in Gastric pH After Cholecystectomy
Brown TH, Walton G, Cheadle WG, Larson GM (Univ of Louisville)
Am J Surg 157:58–65, January 1989   6–3

It has been proposed that duodenogastric reflux is increased after cholecystectomy, especially in symptomatic patients, but the clinical status of primary duodenogastric reflux is controversial. Continuous ambulatory pH monitoring was used to assess 5 patients with cholelithiasis before cholecystectomy and 14 others who had undergone cholecystectomy at least 6 weeks before; 5 of the latter patients were symptomatic. In addition, 20 healthy persons were studied.

Postcholecystectomy patients had less time with the gastric pH less than 2 and more time when it was greater than 4 or 6. Symptomatic patients were especially likely to have more alkaline pH values. The precholecystectomy patients had pH tracings similar to those of the healthy persons.

Cholecystectomy is associated with an alkaline shift in the 24-hour gastric pH profile. This shift is most evident in symptomatic patients. It is possible that episodes of gastric alkalinity are related to some postcholecystectomy symptoms. The alkaline episodes may represent duodenogastric reflux, but this correlation remains to be proved.

▶ The authors ask a simple question that their study does not answer: does cholecystectomy lead to an alkalinization of the gastric lumen? The results of 24-hour pH monitoring of the stomach does show, however, that the postcholecystectomy patients studied have more gastric alkalinity than the 20 healthy controls who were studied in a similar manner. Furthermore, the stomachs of patients with upper gastrointestinal symptoms were more consistently alkaline. Patients who previously have had pyloroplasty or gastric resection are especially prone to symptomatic alkaline gastritis after cholecystectomy, possibly because of the continuous delivery of bile into the duodenum during the long interdigestive period of sleep. Recumbency in this situation would favor duodenogastric and esophageal reflux.—F.G.Moody, M.D.

7 Peptic Ulcer Disease

Medical Therapy for Duodenal Ulcer

Famotidine Therapy for Active Duodenal Ulcers: A Multivariate Analysis of Factors Affecting Early Healing
Reynolds JC (Univ of Pennsylvania)
Ann Intern Med 111:7–14, July 1, 1989   7–1

Characteristics affecting the healing rate of duodenal ulcers are of interest for guiding the duration of treatment with H_2 antagonists. A multicenter, prospective study examined possible factors with stepwise, multivariate analysis of 135 adult patients, all of whom were given famotidine, 40 mg orally at bedtime for 4 or 8 weeks.

Endoscopy showed complete healing in 78% after 4 weeks' treatment and in 94% by 8 weeks. Four factors at the time of diagnosis independently increased the odds of not healing: use of alcohol, ulcer diameter, upper gastrointestinal bleeding symptoms, and previous duodenal ulcer (table). The use of nonsteroidal anti-inflammatory drugs or salicylates before treament improved the odds of healing. No patient with all 5 risk factors healed, but all 23 patients who had no or only 1 risk factor healed. The other factors tested, including smoking, drinking coffee, and age, did not significantly affect the healing rate.

Alcohol consumption, symptomatic bleeding, ulcer size, history of duodenal ulcer, and previous use of nonsteroidal anti-inflammatory drugs or salicylates independently affect the rate of ulcer healing with famotidine. If the significance of these factors in choosing the duration of therapy is confirmed, such knowledge could have far-reaching clinical and economic implications.

▶ For comparison purposes, the efficacy of famotidine therapy for gastric ulcer is discussed here. The multicenter United States trial (1) compared the effect of a once-daily nighttime dose of H_2-receptor antagonist with placebo on the healing of gastric ulcer and relief of associated symptoms. The series included 157 patients with endoscopically verified benign gastric ulcers who were randomized in a double-blind fashion to either famotidine (40 mg at bedtime) or placebo. Antacid tablets were allowed as needed. The healing rates for famotidine were 45%, 66%, and 78% at weeks 4, 6, and 8, respectively. In comparison, placebo healing rates were 39%, 44%, and 64%. These differences were statistically significant in favor of famotidine at weeks 6 and 8, as well as in a life-table analysis. Nocturnal famotidine also was significantly better than placebo with respect to time to complete relief of pain and to the percentage of patients with complete relief of pain. It is interesting that no concomitant factor (including ulcer size, ulcer location, smoking history, or regular

Five Independent Factors Associated With Nonhealing Duodenal Ulcer After 4 Weeks of Treatment

Variable	Crude Odds Ratio (CI)*	Adjusted Odds Ratio (CI)*	P Value
Intercept			
Daily alcohol use	3.9 (1.6–9.8)	6.5 (2.0–20.7)	0.002
Maximal ulcer diameter > 10 mm	3.3 (1.4–7.6)	4.2 (1.5–11.6)	0.005
Symptoms of upper gastrointestinal bleeding	1.9 (0.8–4.4)	3.5 (1.2–10.2)	0.03
Previous duodenal ulcer	2.1 (0.9–4.8)	3.1 (1.05–9.0)	0.04
Use of NSAIDs or salicylates before initiating therapy†	0.5 (0.2–1.3)	0.2 (0.1–0.9)	0.04

*CI, 95% confidence limits.
†NSAIDs, nonsteroidal anti-inflammatory drugs.
(Courtesy of Reynolds JC: *Ann Intern Med* 111:7–14, July 1, 1989.)

alcohol use) affected healing rates in this study. Thus suppression of nocturnal acid secretion with famotidine (40 mg at bedtime) was more effective than placebo in promoting the healing of acute benign gastric ulcer and its associated symptoms. The results of this study suggest that suppression of nocturnal acid secretion alone is as effective as around-the-clock acid suppression in the healing of benign gastric ulcer.—N.J. Greenberger, M.D.

Reference

1. McCullough AJ, et al: Suppression of nocturnal acid secretion with famotidine accelerates gastric ulcer healing. *Gastroenterology* 97:860, 1989.

Medical Therapy for Gastric Ulcer

Suppression of Nocturnal Acid Secretion With Famotidine Accelerates Gastric Ulcer Healing

McCullough AJ, Graham DY, Knuff TE, Lanza FL, Levenson HL, Lyon DT, Munsell WP, Perozza J, Roufail WM, Sinar DR, Smith JL, Berman RS, Root JK, Worley WE, Humphries TJ (Case Western Reserve Univ; Metropolitan Gen Hosp, Cleveland; Nine Additional United States Study Sites)
Gastroenterology 97:860–866, October 1989   7–2

Nocturnal acid secretion has been emphasized in the pathophysiology and treatment of duodenal ulcer, but its role in gastric ulcer disease is less clear. The hypothesis that suppression of nocturnal acid secretion alone would accelerate gastric ulcer healing was tested in a United States multicenter, double-blind, placebo-controlled trial.

One hundred fifty-seven patients with endoscopically verified benign gastric ulcers were randomly assigned to receive a nighttime dose (40 mg) of famotidine, a recently developed H_2-receptor antagonist, or placebo. Antacids were allowed as needed. Endoscopy was performed at baseline and repeated at 4 weeks, and again at 6 and 8 weeks, if necessary.

Healing Rate for Ulcers

	Healing rates	
	Famotidine (n = 74)	Placebo (n = 75)
Week 4		
Cumulative rate	45%	39%
95% Confidence interval	(34%–56%)	(18%–40%)
Life-table analysis	45%	39%
95% Confidence interval	(34%–56%)	(18%–40%)
Dropouts	6	10
Week 6		
Cumulative rate	66%*	44%
95% Confidence interval	(55%–77%)	(33%–55%)
Life-table analysis	70% †	46%
95% Confidence interval	(59%–81%)	(35%–57%)
Dropouts	0	1
Week 8		
Cumulative rate	78% ‡	64%
95% Confidence interval	(69%–87%)	(53%–75%)
Life-table analysis	84% †	72%
95% Confidence interval	(75%–93%)	(61%–83%)
Dropouts	0	1

*Significantly different from placebo, $P < .01$.
†In life-table analysis famotidine group was significantly better than placebo, $P < .05$.
‡Significantly different from placebo, $P < .05$.
(Courtesy of McCullough AJ, Graham DY, Knuff TE, et al: *Gastroenterology* 97:860–866, October 1989.)

Both the cumulative ulcer healing rate method and life-table analysis (table) showed the ulcer healing rate was accelerated by famotidine. The difference in healing rates significantly favored famotidine at weeks 6 and 8. The percentage of patients with complete relief of pain was significantly higher for the famotidine group. Likewise, the time to complete relief of pain was significantly shorter for that group.

None of the concomitant factors, such as size of ulcer, location, smoking history, and regular use of alcohol, affected healing rates in this study. Famotidine was well tolerated, and no serious clinical or laboratory adverse effects were attributed to the dosing regimen used.

Suppression of nocturnal acid secretion with a nighttime dose of famotidine accelerates healing of gastric ulcers and relief of pain. This dosing regimen is well tolerated and may improve patient compliance. It appears that suppression of nocturnal acid secretion alone is as effective as around-the-clock acid suppression in the healing of benign gastric ulcer.

▶ Podolsky and his colleagues (1) have reexamined the important topic of gastric adenocarcinoma masquerading endoscopically as benign gastric ulcer. They reviewed retrospectively all cases of gastric adenocarcinoma in 3 hospitals for a 5-year period. Of 266 patients with gastric adenocarcinoma, 169 (63.5%) had endoscopy with biopsy before their diagnoses of cancer. In 159 (94%) of these 169 patients, the endoscopic findings suggested cancer; in the remaining 10 patients (6%) the endoscopic appearance suggested benign ulcer. *In six of these 10 patients the initial endoscopic biopsies did not reveal cancer, and correct diagnosis was delayed for as long as 14 months.* Three of the 10 patients had "early gastric cancer" by pathologic criteria at gastrectomy, although 1 had lymph node metastasis. The other 7 patients had pathologic criteria for advanced gastric cancer, and 3 had lymph node metastasis. In spite of advanced cancer, lymph node metastasis, or both in 8 of the 10 patients, five-year survival among these patients with benign-appearing ulcers was 70%, as compared with 17% among patients whose gastric lesions appeared malignant at endoscopy.

Podolsky reviewed several prospective, controlled clinical trials in which patients with benign-appearing gastric ulcers were given cimetidine, ranitidine, antacid, or placebo and found that 3% of 680 patients with endoscopically benign-appearing gastric ulcers were later found to have adenocarcinoma.

Reference

1. Podolsky I, Storms PR, Richardson CT, et al: Gastric adenocarcinoma masquerading endoscopically as benign gastric ulcer: A five-year experience. *Dig Dis Sci* 33:1057–1063, 1988.

Effect of Omeprazole and Ranitidine on Ulcer Healing and Relapse Rates in Patients With Benign Gastric Ulcer
Walan A, Bader J-P, Classen M, Lamers CBHW, Piper DW, Rutgersson K, Eriksson S (AB Hässle, Gastrointestinal Research, Mölndal, Sweden)
N Engl J Med 320:69–75, Jan 12, 1989

Cumulative Proportion of Patients With Healed Ulcers

	AT 4 WEEKS	AT 8 WEEKS
	no. healed/total (%; 95% confidence interval)	
Omeprazole, 20 mg (O_{20})	117/170 (69; 62 to 76)	153/172 (89; 84 to 94)
Omeprazole, 40 mg (O_{40})	131/164 (80; 73 to 87)	164/171 (96; 93 to 99)
Ranitidine (R)	103/175 (59; 51 to 67)	144/169 (85; 79 to 91)
	95% confidence interval	
Difference (O_{20} − R)	0 to 20	−3 to 11
Difference (O_{40} − R)	12 to 31	5 to 17
Difference (O_{40} − O_{20})	2 to 20	2 to 13

(Courtesy of Walan A, Bader J-P, Classen M, et al: *N Engl J Med* 320:69–75, Jan 12, 1989.)

Omeprazole is an effective inhibitor of gastric acid secretion that acts by blocking the final step in formation of hydrochloric acid involving the enzyme H^+,K^+-ATPase. A comparison was made of omeprazole in daily doses of 20 mg or 40 mg and ranitidine, 150 mg twice daily, in a double-blind, multicenter study enrolling 602 patients with gastric or prepyloric ulcers. Most patients had gastric ulcers measuring 5 mm to 10 mm.

Rates of ulcer healing at 4 weeks and 8 weeks clearly favored treatment with 40 mg of omeprazole (table). After 6 months, 59% of omeprazole-treated patients and 53% of those given ranitidine remained in remission. No ulcer symptoms were seen during follow-up in 52% of the patients given omeprazole and 48% of those given ranitidine.

Omeprazole is believed to be demonstrably superior to ranitidine in the treatment of benign gastric ulcer. Both ordinary ulcers and those induced by nonsteroidal anti-inflammatory drugs heal more rapidly with omeprazole therapy, and symptoms are relieved in a shorter time. More omeprazole-treated patients were in remission 6 months after treatment was withdrawn.

▶ In this study the healing rate of gastric ulcers in patients receiving concurrent nonsteroidal anti-inflammatory drugs (NSAIDs) also was assessed, with the following results: the healing rates at 4 weeks were 81% in the group receiving 40 mg of omeprazole, 61% in the group receiving 20 mg of omeprazole, and 32% in the group receiving ranitidine. Thus treatment with omeprazole, 40 mg/day, was superior to omeprazole, 20 mg/day, in the healing of gastric ulcers, with or without concurrent therapy with NSAIDs.

That treatment with omeprazole, 20 mg/day, is equivalent to ranitidine, 150 mg twice daily, in patients with resistant duodenal ulcer disease was also indicated in a recent report (1). Delchier and associates compared omeprazole, 20 mg once daily, and ranitidine, 150 mg twice daily, in healing duodenal ulcers unhealed by previous treatment with cimetidine, 0.3 g or more daily, for at least 6 weeks. In a double-blind, multicenter trial, 151 patients were randomly assigned to either omeprazole or ranitidine. Clinical assessments and endoscopies were carried out at 2 weeks and 4 weeks. Patient characteristics were similar in both groups. Statistical analysis showed no significant difference in healing rate, irrespective of the method of calculation. On an "intent-to-treat" analysis (151 patients), the healing rates were 46.6% with omeprazole, and 43.3% with ranitidine at day l5; and 70.7% with omeprazole, and 68.4% with ranitidine at day 29. After a further 4 weeks' treatment with omeprazole, healing occurred in 16 (80%) of 20 patients who still had active disease at day 29. Patients taking omeprazole and those taking ranitidine have similar decreases in daytime and nighttime epigastric pain and heartburn. Multivariate analysis (logistic regression) did not indicate any influence of age, sex, smoking, or alcohol habits, previous drug administered, duodenitis, or duodenal erosions on the healing rate. In this model, healing rate was not significantly influenced by previous treatment duration but was significantly influenced by ulcer size. Forty-one patients complained of adverse events: 19 taking omeprazole and 22 taking ranitidine.—N.J. Greenberger, M.D.

Reference

1. Delchier JC, et al: Double blind multicentre comparison of omeprazole 20 mg once daily versus ranitidine 150 mg twice daily in the treatment of cimetidine or ranitidine resistant duodenal ulcers. *Gut* 30:1173, 1989.

Recurrent Ulcer and Maintenance Therapy

A Randomized Study of Maintenance Therapy With Ranitidine to Prevent the Recurrence of Duodenal Ulcer
Van Deventer GM, Elashoff JD, Reedy TJ, Schneidman D, Walsh JH (VA Med Ctr, Los Angeles; Univ of California, Los Angeles)
N Engl J Med 320:1113–1119, Apr 27, 1989   7–4

There is a high rate of recurrence during the year after an active duodenal ulcer has healed. In a 2-year, double-blind trial, 140 patients with documented healed duodenal ulcers were randomized to receive prophylactic therapy with ranitidine, 150 mg nightly, or placebo to prevent recurrent duodenal ulceration. Endoscopy was performed annually and when symptoms suggested the recurrence of ulcers. In both groups, verified recurrent ulcers were treated for 4 or 8 weeks with open-label ranitidine, 150 mg twice a day, and patients whose ulcers healed within 8 weeks resumed randomized treatment.

The rate of ulcer recurrence decreased significantly from 63% in those given placebo to 37% in those given ranitidine (table). The length of time to the first visible recurrent ulcer was significantly longer in the ranitidine-treated group, extending the median ulcer-free interval by 1–2 years. The first recurrences of ulcer were asymptomatic in half of the ranitidine-treated group and in one fourth of those given placebo. Patients who had a relapse while receiving maintenance therapy with ranitidine were not as responsive to open ranitidine therapy as the placebo-treated patients were. Alcohol consumption, smoking, early or repeated ulcers, and duodenal scarring or erosion were associated with a poor outcome, and patients with these risks benefited most from prophylactic ranitidine.

Prophylactic therapy with ranitidine is effective in preventing the recurrence of duodenal ulceration. Patients who consume alcohol, smoke, have a

Outcome	Outcome of 2-Year Trial	
	TREATMENT GROUP	
	RANITIDINE (N = 70)	PLACEBO (N = 70)
	no. of patients (%)	
Treatment success	41 (59)	26 (37)
No ulcer recurrence	31	14
Ulcer recurrence by 2 yr	10	12
Treatment failure	15 (21)	30 (43)
2 Duodenal ulcers in 6 mo	2	21
Unhealed duodenal ulcer	8	5
Gastric ulcer	4	4
Bleeding ulcer	1	0
Dropped from study	14 (20)	14 (20)
Death	1	0
Medical reason	3	4
Adverse event	1	1
Noncompliance	9	9
Total with ulcer recurrence	26 (37)*	44 (63)†

*Ten in whom treatment succeeded, 15 in whom it failed, 1 with an adverse event.
†Twelve in whom treatment succeeded, 30 in whom it failed, and 2 who did not return (dropped because of noncompliance).
(Courtesy of Van Deventer GM, Elashoff JD, Reedy TJ, et al: N Engl J Med 320:1113–1119, Apr 27, 1989.)

history of ulcer disease, or duodenal scarring or erosion are most likely to benefit from prophylactic therapy with ranitidine.

▶ The key finding in this study is that prophylactic treatment with ranitidine is effective in reducing the recurrence rate of duodenal ulceration. However, the recurrence rates of 37% for the ranitidine treatment group and 63% for the placebo group are, in essence, only point prevalence rates; the actual recurrence rates for both groups may well be higher. This is because endoscopic evaluations were carried out at only 12 and 24 months and when symptoms suggested the recurrence of ulceration. As half of the recurrences in the ranitidine group and one fourth in the placebo group were asymptomatic, it is highly likely that some ulcer recurrences were missed. In this regard, Boyd et al. (1) assessed the recurrence of duodenal ulcers in patients during maintenance therapy by carrying out endoscopic examinations at monthly intervals for 1–13 months; they noted an annual ulcer recurrence rate of 48%. Asymptomatic recurrent ulcers heal, and it was emphasized that examination of asymptomatic persons at 6-month intervals would have failed to detect nearly half of all recurrences.

The role of smoking as a risk factor for duodenal ulcer recurrence remains somewhat controversial. It was noted as a risk factor in the study by VanDeventer et al. but was not associated with ulcer recurrence in other studies (2,3). Further, it has not been found to be a risk factor in the initial healing of duodenal ulcers (see Abstract 33-3).—N.J. Greenberger, M.D.

References

1. Boyd EJS, et al: Does maintenance therapy keep duodenal ulcer healed? *Lancet* 1:1324, 1988.

2. Penston JG, Wormsley KG: Long-term treatment of duodenal ulcers. *Gastroenterology* 94:A349, 1988.
3. Marks IN, Wright JP, Denver M, et al: Ranitidine heals duodenal ulcers. *S Afr Med J* 61:152, 1982.

Nonoperative Therapy for Perforated Ulcer

A Randomized Trial of Nonoperative Treatment for Perforated Peptic Ulcer
Crofts TJ, Park KGM, Steele RJC, Chung SSC, Li AKC (Chinese Univ of Hong Kong, Shatin)
N Engl J Med 320:970–973, Apr 13, 1989

The conservative management of perforated peptic ulcer is not widely accepted. The role of nonsurgical management of perforated peptic ulcer was investigated in a 13-month prospective randomized trial involving 83 patients with clinical diagnoses of perforated peptic ulcer. Forty patients were assigned to conservative management, consisting of resuscitation, nasogastric suction, and intravenously administered antibiotics (cefuroxime, ampicillin, and metronidazole) and ranitidine. The other 43 patients underwent immediate laparotomy and repair of the perforation.

In the nonsurgical group, 11 patients (28%) had no improvement after conservative management and underwent surgery. Three of these patients had perforated gastric carcinoma or sigmoid cancer and showed no improvement after 12 hours. One patient in the surgically treated group had perforated gastric carcinoma. There were 4 (4.8%) deaths, 2 in each group. The incidence of morbidity, such as infection, cardiac failure, or renal failure, was similar in both groups. The hospital stay was significantly longer in the nonsurgically treated groups. Patients aged more than 70 years were significantly less likely to respond to conservative treatment than were younger patients (table).

Except for patients aged more than 70 years, an initial period of nonoperative treatment with careful observation may be safe in patients with perforated peptic ulcer. This treatment regimen may obviate the need for emergency surgery in more than 70% of patients. Also, the delay does not cause additional morbidity in those patients who do not improve with nonoperative treatment and eventually require surgery.

Outcome of Nonoperative Treatment According to Age Group

Age	Success	Failure	Total
		no. of patients	
<40	8	0	8
40–70	18	5	23
>70	3	6*	9

*Significantly higher failure rate than in the other 2 age groups ($P < .05$ by χ^2 analysis).
(Courtesy of Crofts TJ, Park KGM, Steele RJC, et al: *N Engl J Med* 320:970–973, Apr 13, 1989.)

▶ Berne and Donovan (1) report a similar experience with the nonoperative treatment of perforated duodenal ulcer. Their paper concerns 35 adults in whom perforation of a duodenal or prepyloric ulcer was treated nonoperatively between July 1979 and April 1988 at the Los Angeles County–University of Southern California Medical Center. Each patient had pneumoperitoneum with clinical evidence of peritonitis, and a gastroduodenogram documented a sealed perforation. Ulcers were believed to be acute in 27 patients and chronic in 8. These 35 patients represented 12% of 294 patients with duodenal and prepyloric peptic ulcers with perforation treated during the same period. An intra-abdominal abscess developed in 1 of the 35 patients. Reperforation did not occur. Mortality for the 259 patients treated operatively during this period was 6.2%; mortality of the 35 patients treated nonoperatively was 3%. Berne and Donovan conclude that duodenal ulcer can be treated safely and nonoperatively when a gastroduodenogram documents self-sealing.—N.J. Greenberger, M.D.

Reference

1. Berne TV, Donovan AJ: Nonoperative treatment of perforated duodenal ulcer. Arch Surg 124:830, 1989.

8 Surgical Therapy for Peptic Ulcer Disease

The Need for Definitive Therapy in the Management of Perforated Gastric Ulcers: Review of 202 Cases
Hodnett RM, Gonzalez F, Lee WC, Nance FC, Deboisblanc R (Louisiana State Univ)
Ann Surg 109:36–39, January 1989   8–1

Perforation of a gastric ulcer is frequently a fatal complication. Because these lesions are often grouped with the less lethal duodenal ulcer perforations, the mortality associated with this condition is underestimated. To identify those factors relevant to diagnosis and survival (range, 2 days to 99 years) 202 patients with a mean age of 55 years with perforated gastric ulcers were retrospectively studied. Patients with "channel ulcers" or peptic ulcers were excluded from the study. Initial symptoms included abdominal pain in 93% of patients, nausea and vomiting in 42%, and hematemesis in 5%. Of 194 patients for whom a medical history was obtained, 57% had no identifiable ulcer symptoms. Chest and abdominal roentgenograms were the most helpful studies, showing pneumoperitoneum in 76% of those examined.

Definitive surgery was performed in 53 patients, and nondefinitive surgery was performed in the remaining 128 patients. Of 21 patients who received no surgery, 10 were treated medically, and diagnosis was made at autopsy in 11. Of the patients not treated surgically, there were 20 deaths, accounting for a mortality of 95%. The overall mortality was 26%; mortality with operation was 18%; mortality without operation was 95%. Mortality for the 128 patients treated with nondefinitive surgical procedures was 29%. Subsequent operative treatment was required in 25.7% of these patients. In the 53 patients treated with definitive procedures, the mortality was only 11.3%. It was 52.8% for patients with systolic blood pressure of 90 mm Hg or less; 10 were treated medically, and all died. Of 26 patients treated operatively, the mortality was 35%; 40% of all patients survived operation without complication. The most common complication was atelectasis; sepsis and postoperative myocardial infarction were the most lethal complications.

Immediate and aggressive surgical treatment is indicated by the high mortality among untreated and medically treated patients. The superiority of the definitive operative procedures for the patients with perforated gastric ulcer is shown by the higher mortality and need for reoperation in patients who were given nondefinitive operations.

▶ The message is clear; perforated gastric ulcers require aggressive, definitive treatment. Prepare the patient for surgery and do an appropriate resectional procedure. Distal gastrectomy is the procedure of choice for lesser curve ulcers; ulcers close to the esophagogastric junction can be treated effectively by excision, in conjunction with truncal vagotomy and drainage. All other temporizing approaches have a high failure rate, as experienced in this study from New Orleans.—F.G. Moody, M.D.

Costs of Medical and Surgical Treatment of Duodenal Ulcer
Sonnenberg A (VA Med Ctr, Milwaukee)
Gastroenterology 96:1445–1452, June 1989

Proximal gastric vagotomy and intermittent and maintenance therapy with H_2-antagonists are all effective in the long-term treatment of duodenal ulcer. Assuming that inclusion of costs may narrow the overlap of success rates among these 3 interventions and thus allow a clear-cut choice favoring one over the other, the model Markov chain was used to compare their costs by a medical decision analysis. Expenditures were based on the American health care system.

With maintenance therapy, the average costs per patient rose from $600 after 1 year to $7,600 after 15 years. Intermittent therapy cost as much as maintenance therapy, but the latter provided 8% and 4% more time spent free of ulcer relapse and pain, respectively. Although proximal gastric vagotomy was associated with less future costs of subsequent ulcer relapses, the high price of the initial procedure made it the most expensive therapy. In a sensitivity analysis, the order of the therapeutic options regarding their cost-effectiveness remained robust to changes in the assumption underlying the model. In the United States, the initial gastric operation cost as much as two thirds of the gross average annual income compared with only one seventh in European countries. Despite being initially expensive, proximal gastric vagotomy turned out to be the cheapest therapeutic strategy in European countries after 6 years.

In the United States, maintenance therapy provides the best long-term management of duodenal ulcer, whereas gastric surgery is a cost-effective therapeutic option in Europe.

▶ The author has analyzed the cost of duodenal ulcer therapy from the perspective of the health care system paying for it. Proximal gastric vagotomy emerged as the most cost-effective therapy in Europe. In America, the high initial cost detracted from the benefits of a reduction in future relapses. Maintenance therapy with H_2 blockers provided the cheapest long-term management. It would be interesting to see how the sensitivity analysis would rank proximal gastric vagotomy when performed in a managed care environment in our country. Elective proximal gastric vagotomy is a low morbidity procedure that should require only 3 or 4 days of hospitalization, or even less if a motel for convenient ambulatory care is adjacent to the operative facility.—F.G. Moody, M.D.

Changing Pattern of Admissions and Operations for Duodenal Ulcer
Bardhan KD, Cust G, Hinchliffe RFC, Williamson FM, Lyon C, Bose K (District Gen Hosp, Rotherham; Trent Regional Health Authority, Sheffield, England)
Br J Surg 76:230–236, March 1989

Hospital admissions for patients with duodenal ulcer, with or without complications, have been declining in the past 25 years. The effect of the increasing use of H_2-receptor antagonist (H_2RA) on admission rates of patients with duodenal ulcer in the Trent region of the United Kingdom was investigated.

Admission rates were expressed per million residents. There was a 3.7-fold increase in H_2RA use from 1978 to 1983. However, overall admission rates for perforation changed little: there were 99 between 1972 and 1976, before H_2RA use, and 103 between 1977 and 1984, during H_2RA use. Admission rates for hemorrhage rose by 8%. The overall rates concealed large increases in the admission rates for patients aged 65 years or more of 33% for perforation and 28% for hemorrhage. Emergency admission rates for uncomplicated duodenal ulcer were unchanged, but the proportions of patients with that condition operated on dropped by 58%. Waiting-list admissions for uncomplicated duodenal ulcer dropped by 43%, from 187 in the pre-H_2RA period to 106 in the H_2RA period, and the proportions of patients undergoing surgery fell from 162 to 76. The combined effect resulted in a decrease of 53% in the operation rates.

The use of H_2RA has not reduced emergency admissions for patients with duodenal ulcer but is associated with a reduction in waiting-list admissions and in the number undergoing surgery for uncomplicated duodenal ulcer. The reduction has been even more pronounced when the drugs have been used more intensively. Much of the decrease can be attributed to the changing natural history of the disease, but H_2RA has a significant additional effect.

▶ Many factors govern the prevalence of peptic ulcer disease in a community and the incidence of complications from it that require hospitalization and surgical therapy. This carefully performed study in the Trent region of the United Kingdom documents a positive influence on reducing the need for an operation for peptic ulcer, even though the incidence of perforation and hemorrhage remained unchanged or increased slightly since the pre-H_2 blocker era. Lack of change in these serious complications relates to the increase in the age of the population among whom they are more frequently experienced. It is heartening to know that H_2 blockade is making a difference in view of its frequent usage and high cost to society.—F.G. Moody, M.D.

9 Zollinger-Ellison Syndrome

Mechanism for Increase of Gastrin Release by Secretin in Zollinger-Ellison Syndrome
Chiba T, Yamatani T, Yamaguchi A, Morishita T, Nakamura A, Kadowaki S, Fujita T (Kobe Univ, Kobe; Awaji Hosp, Sumoto, Japan)
Gastroenterology 96:1439–1444, June 1989   9–1

Secretin normally inhibits gastrin release, but the serum gastrin is increased by secretin administration in patents with Zollinger-Ellison syndrome (ZES). Peptide effects on gastrinoma cells were examined using dispersed cells from an endocrine tumor of the pancreas in a patient with ZES.

Both secretin and 3-isobutyl-1-methylxanthine significantly increased the release of immunoreactive gastrin from human gastrinoma cells (Fig 9–1). The effect of secretin was inhibited by somatostatin. In the presence of guanosine 5′–triphosphate, secretin enhanced adenylate cyclase activation in cell membranes, and this effect was countered by somatostatin. Removal of guanosine 5′-triphosphate abolished both the stimulatory effect of secretin and the inhibitory effect of somatostatin on adenylate cyclase activation. Pretreatment of cells with pertussis toxin abolished the effects of somatostatin.

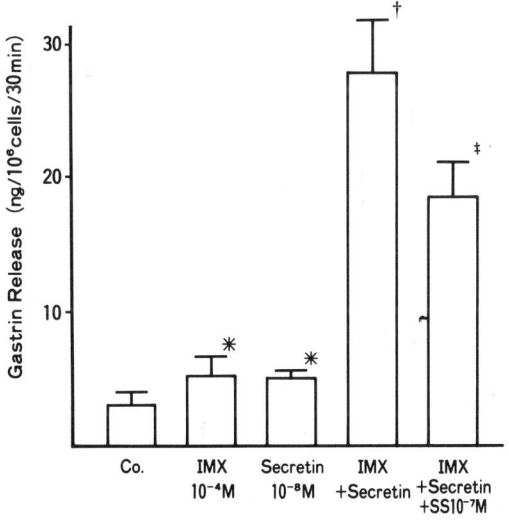

Fig 9–1.—Effects of various secretagogues on release of immunoreactive gastrin from human gastrinoma cells. Values represent mean ± SEM (no. = 6). *Significantly different from control ($P < .05$); †significantly different from IMX alone ($P < .01$); ‡significantly different from IMX + secretin ($P < .01$); SS, somatostatin. (Courtesy of Chiba T, Yamatani T, Yamaguchi A, et al: *Gastroenterology* 96:1439–1444, June 1989.)

60 / The Stomach and Duodenum

Secretin and somatostatin appear to act directly on gastrinoma cells to stimulate and inhibit gastrin secretion, respectively. Studies using isolated antral G cells will show whether secretin exerts a direct inhibitory action on these cells.

▶ To summarize briefly, these studies suggest that secretin and somatostatin act directly on gastrinoma cells to stimulate and inhibit gastrin secretion, respectively, by modulating adenylate cyclase activation, probably via guanine nucleotide-binding proteins.

For a concise, up-to-date review of diagnosis of gastrinoma, see the editorial by Wolfe (1).—N.J. Greenberger, M.D.

Reference

1. Wolfe MM: Diagnosis of gastrinoma: Much ado about nothing? Ann Intern Med 111:697–699, 1989.

Long-Term Efficacy and Safety of Omeprazole in Patients With Zollinger-Ellison Syndrome: A Prospective Study
Maton PN, Vinayek R, Frucht H, McArthur KA, Miller LS, Saeed ZA, Gardner JD, Jensen RT (Natl Inst of Diabetes and Digestive and Kidney Diseases, Bethesda, MD)
Gastroenterology 97:827–836, October 1989   9–2

The agent omeprazole is a substituted benzimidazole that markedly inhibits gastric acid secretion. Its efficacy was examined in 40 patients with Zollinger-

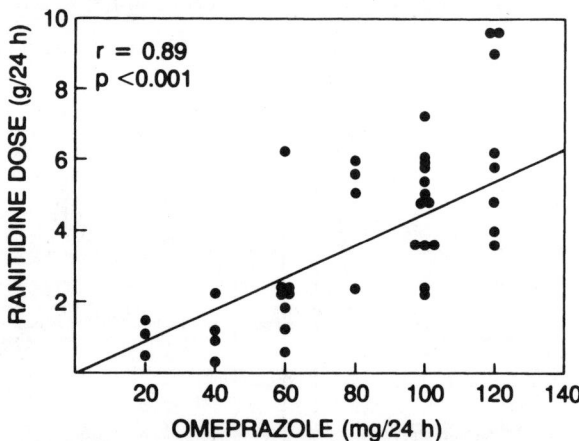

Fig 9–2.—Relationship between total daily dose of histamine H_2-receptor antagonists and total daily dose of omeprazole in 40 patients. The total daily dose of each H_2-receptor antagonist required before starting omeprazole to control acid secretion was expressed in ranitidine equivalents for patients taking cimetidine or famotidine. (Courtesy of Maton PN, Vinayek R, Frucht H, et al: *Gastroenterology* 97:827–836, October 1989.)

Ellison syndrome (ZES), 11 of whom had metastatic gastrinoma. In most patients once-daily treatment reduced acid to less than 10 mEq/hour in the hour before the next dose. The dose needed correlated with the dose of histamine H_2-receptor antagonist required (Fig 9–2), but not with the fasting serum gastrin level.

Treatment with omeprazole, 60 mg every 12 hours, consistently reduced gastric acid output to within the appropriate range. Most patients remained symptomatic when taking H_2-receptor antagonists, but they improved consistently when given omeprazole. Gastritis and duodenitis resolved when present, and no side effects attributable to omeprazole were observed. In addition, no significant laboratory abnormalities were ascribed to the drug. Treatment for longer than a year did not alter the intrinsic acid secretory capacity of the stomach.

Long-term omeprazole therapy is effective and safe in patients with ZES, although larger doses may be needed than for idiopathic duodenal ulcer or reflux esophagitis. The serum level of gastrin did not change, and no evidence of gastric carcinoid development was found during treatment.

▶ These studies support the view that omeprazole is now the drug of choice for patients with Zollinger-Ellison syndrome. Increased doses of omeprazole were required for only 11 of 40 patients, and for only 5 of these was the increase required because acid output increased to > 10 mEq/hour. It was noted that splitting the once-per-day dosage of omeprazole into two equal 12-hour doses increased the efficacy of the drug for those patients in whom 120 mg of omeprazole once per day failed to reduce acid output to < 10 mEq/hr. This is surprising in view of the long duration (> 24 hours) of omeprazole. Maton and co-workers found no evidence of the development of gastric carcinoid tumors during omeprazole therapy, in contrast to studies in rats in which long-term (2-year) omeprazole therapy did induce carcinoid tumors (1).

Lehy et al. studied patients with Zollinger-Ellison syndrome, who had long-standing hypergastrinemia and were committed to long-term antisecretory treatment with drugs such as omeprazole, to determine whether changes occur in the gastric endocrine cell behavior (2). They raised this question because proliferation of endocrine argyrophil cells, mainly the enterochromaffin-like type observed in these patients theoretically could lead to fundic carcinoid tumors. Lehy and associates demonstrated noticeable fundic argyrophil hyperplasia, whatever the antisecretory treatment, as well as significant increases in gastrin cell densities in the antral mucosa of omeprazole-treated patient.—N.J. Greenberger, M.D.

Reference

1. Ekman L, Hansson E, Havu N, et al: Toxicological studies on omeprazole. *Scand J Gastroenterol* 20 (Suppl 108):53, 1985.
2. Lehy T, Mignon M, Cadiot C, et al: Gastric endocrine cell behavior in Zollinger-Ellison patients upon long-term potent antisecretory treatment. *Gastroenterology* 96:1029,1989.

Microgastrinomas of the Duodenum: A Cause of Failed Operations for the Zollinger-Ellison Syndrome
Thompson NW, Vinik AI, Eckhauser FE (Univ of Michigan, Ann Arbor)
Ann Surg 209:396–404, April 1989   9–3

Zollinger-Ellison syndrome formerly was treated with total gastrectomy because of the assumption that gastrinomas would have metastasized by the time the correct diagnosis was made. However, gastrinomas in patients with Zollinger-Ellison syndrome now are being discovered at an earlier stage. Although controversy over the operative management of these patients still exists, it is generally agreed that patients with sporadic disease and no evidence of metastases should undergo surgical exploration to locate and excise an isolated gastrinoma. Accurate preoperative localization of the tumor therefore has taken on an important role. The usefulness of preoperative percutaneous transhepatic venous gastrin sampling to localize occult gastrinomas was discussed.

During a 10-year period, transhepatic venous gastrin sampling was perfomed in 46 patients with confirmed Zollinger-Ellison syndrome. None of the patients had evidence of metastatic gastrinoma by conventional diagnostic studies. A gastrinoma was found at operation in 45 patients; 1 patient was not operated on after a large duodenal ulcer became perforated on the day before exploration was scheduled. None of the patients had palpable tumors despite complete and careful mobilization of the duodenum and pancreas. In each case, the gastrinoma was found in an area corresponding to the region where preoperative gastrin sampling had identified a high level of gastrin. Most tumors had diameters, were no greater than 2 mm, and most were located in the duodenal wall. In 5 patients, the duodenal microgastrinomas were the only source of hypergastrinemia. In 4 of those 5 patients, tumors were detected only after duodenotomy with direct inspection and eversion of the mucosa (Fig 9–3). Although the tumor in the fifth patient could not be found, his postoperative course suggested complete tumor excision.

Transhepatic venous gastrin sampling in patients with confirmed Zollinger-Ellison syndrome has greatly improved the precision with which areas of suspected gastrinomas can be identified before exploratory surgery is undertaken. Duodenotomy, with eversion of the mucosa of those intraluminal regions identified as having high gastrin levels can increase greatly the number of patients with the syndrome who will be cured after localized tumor resection.

▶ This extraordinary report of an extraordinary experience with an extraordinary tumor, microgastrinomas of the duodenum, demonstrates again that what you carefully look for you will find. In my own experience, 2-mm bumps within the pancreatic facing wall of the duodenum are not uncommon in patients without peptic ulcer disease or hypergastrinemia. For example, the minor papilla is about this size, and as I palpate for it when exploring the inside of the duodenum, I often feel extraneous areas of firmness beneath the duodenal epithelium. I am persuaded by this report, however, that venous splanchnic sampling is a useful adjunct for patients in whom Zollinger-Ellison syndrome is suspected, and that careful exami-

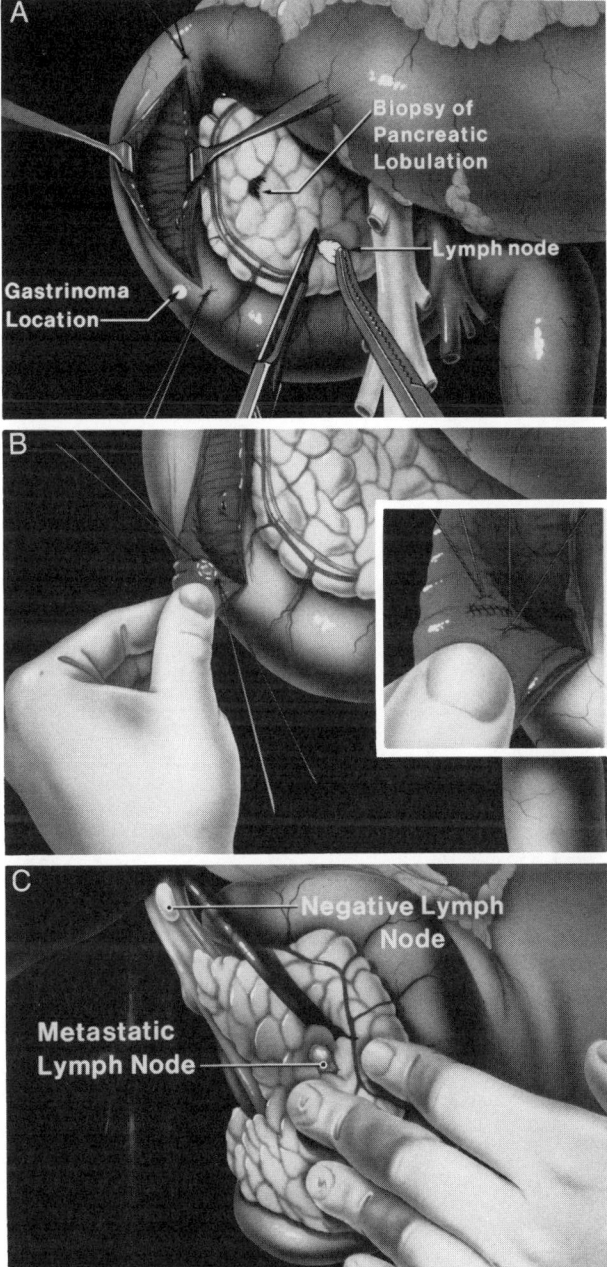

Fig 9–3.—A, duodenotomy, location of 2-mm gastrinomas in anterior duodenal wall, excision of small lymph node on pancreatic capsule. **B,** local excision of duodenal gastrinoma and mucosal closure. **C,** location of only involved node (posterior peripancreatic) with foci of metastatic gastrinoma. (Courtesy of Thompson NW, Vinik AI, Eckhauser FE: *Ann Surg* 209:396–404, April 1989.)

nation of the lumen of the duodenum by palpation in the absence of a pancreatic mass should be an integral part of the exploration. My only point is that not all minilumps are functioning endocrine tumors. The majority are clusters of Brunner's glands or a condensation of submucosal fibrous tissue.—F.G. Moody, M.D.

10 Postgastric Surgery Syndromes

Gastroscopic Screening of the Post-Gastrectomy Stomach: Relationship of Dysplasia to Remnant Cancer
Greene FL (Univ of South Carolina, Columbia)
Am Surg 55:12–15, January 1989

Aggressive endoscopic screening was instituted in 1980 to assess patients who had undergone gastrectomy in 1960–1975. A total of 233 patients with benign peptic ulcer disease had partial gastric resection in this period. In 1980–1985, 163 of these patients underwent contrast studies of the upper gastrointestinal tract and flexible fiberoptic gastroscopy with directed biopsy to identify early gastric-remnant cancer.

In 45 patients, who had a single screening examination, 3 remnant cancers were found at esophagogastroduodenostomy. Of 118 patients who underwent 2 or more assessments, 7 (5.8%) had mild to moderate dysplasia in the gastric remnant. Carcinoma developed in 2 of these patients, and 3 had progressive dysplastic changes on follow-up gastroscopic assessments; the mean postgastrectomy interval in these 7 patients was 21.5 years. None of the 7 patients had symptoms or signs of active gastrointestinal tract disease.

Dysplasia in the gastric remnant can be identified by repeated gastroscopy in patients undergoing partial gastric resection for ulcer disease. The finding of dysplasia is an indicator of associated adenocarcinoma, and calls for aggressive endoscopic screening.

▶ Patients with progressive dysplastic change in the mucosa of a gastric remnant are at high risk for gastric cancer. What I gleaned from this article is that patients who had gastric resection 10 or more years ago for peptic ulcer should have endoscopic examination of the remnant and multiple biopsies even if they are asymptomatic. If early gastric cancer is found, a completion gastrectomy should be performed. A finding of dysphasia presents a quandary, especially if the patient is asymptomatic. I would strongly consider offering an otherwise healthy person with a long life expectancy a complete gastrectomy if moderate-to-severe dysphasia is documented, either at the time of initial screen or on subsequent endoscopic examination. The interval between endoscopic examinations and biopsy should be governed by the appearance of the epithelium on gross inspection and histologic examination. Patients with gastric remnants clearly are at risk for gastric cancer if the remnants are long enough; however, numerous reports have established that the risk for clinical manifestations of cancer developing in a gastric remnant is slightly higher than the incidence of gastric cancer in general when considered for age.—F.G. Moody, M.D.

The Surgical Treatment of Chronic Gastric Atony Following Roux-Y Diversion for Alkaline Reflux Gastritis
Vogel SB, Woodward ER (Univ of Florida)
Ann Surg 209:756–762, June 1989

When gastric retention and its sequelae occur after Roux-en-Y biliary diversion for alkaline reflux gastritis, medical measures and prokinetic drugs are ineffective. To improve gastric emptying and to relieve symptoms, 37 patients who were late failures of Roux-en-Y diversion underwent further gastric resection. Either subtotal or more extensive gastrectomy was performed; 10 patients in whom initial revisional treatment failed later had near-total or total gastrectomy.

An excellent to good response was achieved with further resection in 20 patients, and 7 had a fair response; the resection failed in 10 patients. The patients with a fair response were quite pleased with the clinical outcome. Most of the failures responded to complete total gastrectomy with complete resolution of symptoms and resumed a relatively normal diet. There were no postoperative deaths and no anastomotic leaks. Gastric retention decreased after operation according to the technetium-99m-labeled solid-food emptying test (Fig 10–1).

After intensive medical treatment of patients who have gastric retention after Roux-en-Y diversion for alkaline reflux gastritis, extensive gastric resection with Roux-en-Y reconstruction offers the best chance of restoring a normal dietary life-style.

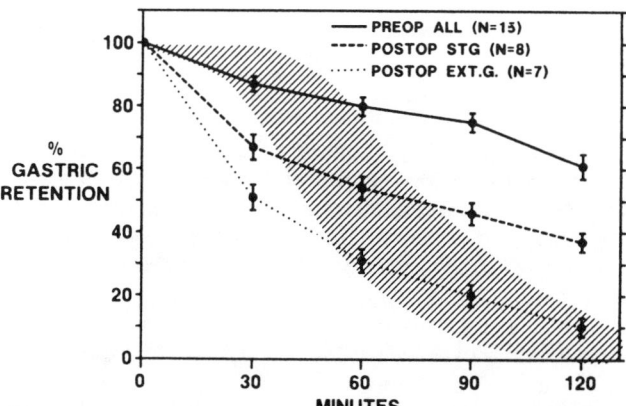

Fig 10–1.—Technetium 99 radionuclide solid-food gastric emptying test. Preoperative study in the entire group of 15 patients and postoperative results in 8 patients after 70% to 80% resection (*STG*) and 7 patients who underwent 85% to 95% resection (*EXT. G*). (Courtesy of Vogel SB, Woodward ER: *Ann Surg* 209:756–762, June 1989.)

➤ Vogel and Woodward make a good point: postgastrectomy patients with gastric retention after Roux-limb conversion for bile gastritis must have near total or total gastrectomy to restore normal feeding without symptoms. Whatever is wrong with such patients' stomachs probably is what led to their having gastric surgery in the first place. Because there is no way to predict who these unfortunate patients will be, I employ proximal gastric vagotomy whenever possible for the treatment of peptic ulcer. Curiously, patients who have gastrectomy for gastric cancer or gastric ulcer seem less prone to gastric emptying problems that first have the clinical and epithelial characteristics of alkaline gastritis. It is possible that, because these patients usually do not have a truncal vagotomy, they are absolved from the complication. The youth of the patient population (28 years) suggests that psychosocial factors also may be prominent in the chronic gastric disability experienced by these patients.—F.G. Moody, M.D.

11 Gastric Surgery for Morbid Obesity

Gastric Surgery for Morbid Obesity: Complications and Long-Term Weight Control
Yale CE (Univ of Wisconsin, Madison)
Arch Surg 124:941–946, August 1989   11–1

The value of gastric surgery for morbid obesity has been questioned because of the lack of complete long-term follow-up data. The results of bypass with Roux-en-Y gastrojejunostomy, unbanded gastrogastrostomy, and vertical banded gastroplasty were compared using data for 537 consecutive patients operated on for morbid obesity in 1977–1984. Follow-up was 5 years, after the Roux-en-Y and unbanded gastrogastrostomy operations and 3 years after vertical banded gastroplasty. All but 6% of patients were available for late follow-up.

Both the Roux-en-Y gastrojejunostomy and vertical banded gastroplasty provided effective weight control over the long term, whereas unbanded gastrogastrostomy did not. Weight control was somewhat better with the Roux-en-Y procedure, but the vertical banded gastroplasty is simpler and safer, as well as more physiologic. Staple-line disruption was least frequent with this operation, and the same was true for late stomal stenosis.

Both gastric bypass with Roux-en-Y gastrojejunostomy and vertical banded gastroplasty can promote weight loss in patients with morbid obesity, but only those who accept responsibility for their postoperative conduct. Most patients can benefit by trading slightly better weight control for the greater safety of the more physiologic gastroplasty procedure.

▶ Roux-en-Y gastrojejunostomy and vertical-banded gastroplasty, when employed as gastric reduction procedures for the treatment of morbid obesity, provided similar outcomes. In Yale's hands, the vertical-banded gastroplasty was safer and easier to perform. However, the follow-up was shorter and the weight loss containment less than the bypass procedure. The value of this paper is that only 6% of patients were lost to follow-up. Sequential rather than random design detracts from the value of the study with regard to true relative efficacy, but the outcomes are a good approximation of what can be accomplished by a senior bariatric surgeon.—F.G. Moody, M.D.

Gastric Restrictive Operations for Morbid Obesity
Benotti PN, Hollingshead J, Mascioli EA Bothe A Jr, Bistrian BR, Blackburn GL
(Harvard Med School; New England Deaconess Hosp, Boston)
Am J Surg 157:150–155; January 1989

Gastric restrictive surgery continues to evolve, its goals being to maximize weight loss and minimize treatment failures. Restrictive procedures for morbid obesity was performed in 1982–1988 in 289 patients after referral to a multidisciplinary obesity center because medical attempts had failed. Roux-en-Y bypass operations were done in the first 5 years, after which the vertical banded gastroplasty was introduced.

Of the 180 patients followed, 82% had Roux-en-Y gastric bypass, 12% had vertical banded gastroplasty, and 6% had revision of an unsatisfactory bypass procedure. Overall mortality was 1%, with no operative deaths. The most frequent perioperative complications were wound seroma and atelectasis–pneumonia. The most common late complications were vitamin B_{12} deficiency, iron deficiency, and dumping. An overall loss of 50% to 64% of excess weight was noted, despite a tendency for late weight gain (Fig 11–1). About 5% of patients were considered treatment failures 1 year after surgery.

Gastric restrictive surgery is an effective approach to morbid obesity when responses to medical measures fail. Further surgical modifications designed to promote weight loss must be viewed critically in relation to operative risk.

▶ The multidisciplinary obesity treatment group at the New England Deaconess Hospital reports a relatively high rate of early success with gastric restrictive procedures. I agree with the admonition that such procedures must be accomplished without operative mortality and with only minimal early and late morbidity. Their results suggest that the Roux-en-Y gastric bypass has worked well in their hands and might have been even more effective if a small pouch (15 mL) had been employed. The size of the pouch appears to be the key to inducing a consistent response to gastric restriction; the size of the opening of the Roux limb is probably

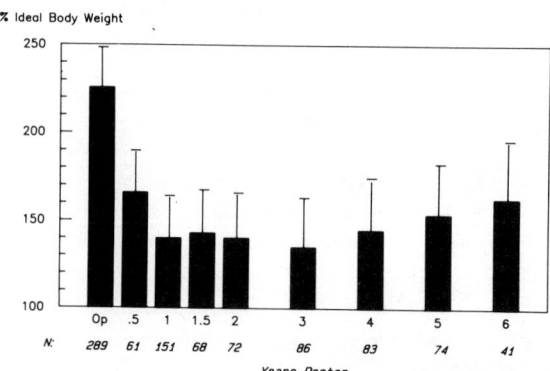

Fig 11–1.—Weight loss in morbidly obese patients undergoing gastric surgery. Percentage of ideal body weight expressed as mean ± SD. (Courtesy of Benotti PN, Hollingshead J, Mascioli EA, et al: Am J Surg 157:150–155, January 1989.)

of secondary importance, although I always make it a snug 1 cm in circumference. The Roux limb is essential, however, for a lasting effect because caloric wasting is a critical component of the long-term outcome. Unfortunately, as morbidly obese patients lose weight, they must consume fewer calories because they cannot dispose of the excess by thermogenesis.—F.G. Moody, M.D.

Gastric Banding in the Treatment of Morbid Obesity
Kirby RM, Ismail T, Crowson M, Baddeley RM (Gen Hosp, Birmingham, England)
Br J Surg 76:490–492, May 1989   11–3

Gastroplasty has revolutionized the surgical management of morbid obesity. Separation of the stomach into 2 compartments by a band passed about its upper part has been reported to be a simple and effective form of gastroplasty. Gastric banding was performed in 30 patients with morbid obesity. The patients, most of them women, had a mean age of 38 years and a mean weight of 135 kg. A Dacron or Teflon band was used to provide a 50-mL proximal compartment and a 1.2-cm stoma into the distal stomach. The 2 compartments were sutured to one another lateral to the band.

During follow-up for 6–24 months, 2 patients had banding reversed and in 7 others conversion to vertical gastroplasty was performed. The loss of excess weight was 33% at 3 months and 70% at 2 years. Fifteen patients required a total of 22 procedures for technical complications, but no deaths resulted from surgery and there were no late deaths. Most patients eventually were able to take meals of reasonable size.

Although gastric banding promotes weight loss, its complication and reoperation rates are unacceptable. The vertical Silastic ring gastroplasty now is preferred.

▶ Gastric banding would appear to be the least morbid way to produce a small proximal gastric pouch, but such is not the case. This report from Birmingham, England, reveals the need for a high rate of reoperation primarily to relieve intractable vomiting. I hope this report will encourage others who use this procedure to publish their results. If it is a morbid procedure, then it should be dropped from the surgical armamentarium.—F.G. Moody, M.D.

Anatomic, Motor, and Clinical Assessment of Vertical Banded Gastroplasty
Behrns KE, Soper NJ, Sarr MG, Kelly KA, Hughes RW (Mayo Med School, Rochester, Minn)
Gastroenterology 97:91–97, July 1989   11–4

Vertical banded gastroplasty is a widely used procedure for morbid obesity, but the mechanisms by which it and other gastric resective procedures lead to weight loss are uncertain. Gastric anatomy, motility, and emptying were evaluated in 11 patients at least 7 months after vertical banded gastroplasty, at

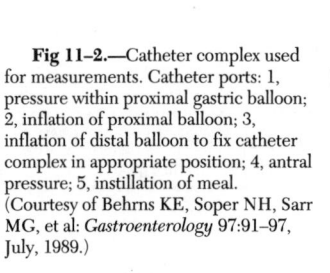
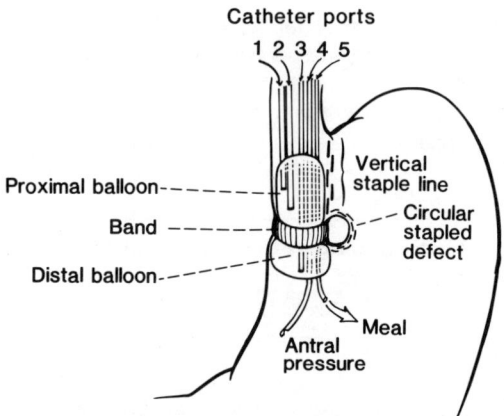

Fig 11-2.—Catheter complex used for measurements. Catheter ports: 1, pressure within proximal gastric balloon; 2, inflation of proximal balloon; 3, inflation of distal balloon to fix catheter complex in appropriate position; 4, antral pressure; 5, instillation of meal. (Courtesy of Behrns KE, Soper NH, Sarr MG, et al: *Gastroenterology* 97:91–97, July, 1989.)

which time they had lost a mean of 31% of excess body weight. Stomal diameter, volume, and the distensibility of the proximal pouch were determined by a balloon distention method (Fig 11-2). Gastric emptying was assessed by scintigraphy with and without distention of the proximal pouch.

All the patients had lost weight, with a mean loss of 28 kg. However, 7 patients regained 3–20 kg beginning 3–15 months after operation. Stomal diameters ranged from 10 to 15 mm, and pouch capacities, from 20 to 150 mL. The mean intrapouch pressure increased from 13 to 22 mm Hg on distention to half maximal capacity, but little more at full capacity. Nearly maximal pouch distention during emptying of a test meal decreased antral contractile activity and hastened emptying in the early but not the later phase. Weight loss did not correlate definitively with stomal diameter, pouch volume, or gastric emptying.

Proximal gastric distention did not substantially affect antral motility or gastric emptying in these patients. Weight loss after vertical banded gastroplasty could not be related to any of the factors studied.

▶ Why gastric reduction and stomach restrictive procedures succeed, or fail, for that matter, to induce long-term weight reduction in patients with morbid obesity, is not known. The digestive surgeons at the Mayo Clinic have clearly documented that weight loss is not related to a disturbance in gastric motility or to stomal size after ventral-banded gastroplasty. Pouch size appears to be an important factor in the ventral-banded as well as the gastric bypass procedure. More studies of this type and quality are needed to provide an intellectual base to this promising empiric approach to an otherwise untreatable disease.—F.G. Moody, M.D.

12 Upper Gastrointestinal Bleeding

Multipolar Electrocoagulation in the Treatment of Peptic Ulcers With Nonbleeding Visible Vessels: A Prospective, Controlled Trial
Laine L (Univ of Southern California; Los Angeles County–Univ of Southern California Med Ctr, Los Angeles)
Ann Intern Med 110:510–514, April 1989   12–1

Patients with peptic ulcers in whom a nonbleeding visible vessel in an ulcer crater is found on endoscopy have a 45% chance of recurrent bleeding. The potential benefit of endoscopic multipolar electrocoagulation in the treatment of these patients was assessed in a prospective, randomized, sham-controlled trial. Seventy-five patients (mean age, 44 years) had a bloody nasogastric aspirate sample, melena, or hematochezia; unstable vital signs, a transfusion of at least 2 units of blood in 12 hours, or a decrease in the hematocrit of at least 0.06 in 12 hours; and endoscopic evidence of an ulcer with a nonbleeding visible vessel. All underwent either sham or real multipolar electrocoagulation at the time of diagnostic endoscopy.

Patients given the multipolar electrocoagulation treatment had marked improvement in their hospital course compared with the patients given the sham treatment (table). The rate of recurrent bleeding and mean requirement for transfusion were approximately half those in controls. The need for emergency surgery, length of hospital stay, and cost of hospitalization were significantly less in the treatment group. The overall mortality was 1%. Bleeding was

Results of Endoscopic Multipolar Electrocoagulation Compared With Sham Treatment in Patients Who Have Peptic Ulcers With Nonbleeding Visible Vessels*

Characteristic	Sham Treatment ($n = 37$)	Multipolar Electrocoagulation ($n = 38$)	Difference (95% CI)
Patients with rebleeding, %	41†	18	23 (3 to 43)
Blood transfusions, *units*	3.0 ± 0.6	1.6 ± 0.3	1.4 (0 to 2.8)
Patients with emergency surgery, %	30†	8	22 (5 to 39)
Hospital stay, *d*	6.2 ± 0.7 †	4.3 ± 0.4	1.9 (0.4 to 3.4)
Hospital cost, *$*	5730 ± 650†	3790 ± 410	1940 (400 to 3480)
Deaths, %	0	3	3 (...)‡

*Where appropriate, values are mean ± SE.
†$P < .05$ for sham treatment compared with multipolar electrocoagulation.
‡Data do not allow use of normal approximation to calculate 95% confidence interval for the difference in proportions of deaths between the 2 groups.
(Courtesy of Laine L: Ann Intern Med 110:510–514, April 1989.)

induced in 7 (18%) of the 38 patients treated with electrocoagulation. Hemorrhage was controlled with continued multipolar electrocoagulation in 6 patients, but 1 required urgent surgery. No perforations were observed.

Endoscopic treatment with multipolar electrocoagulation is effective in patients who have major upper gastrointestinal tract hemorrhage and ulcers with a nonbleeding visible vessel.

➤ A recent NIH consensus development conference on therapeutic endoscopy and bleeding ulcers has been reported[1], and I would like to summarize the conclusion and recommendations of that conference:

1. In the United States, more than 100,000 patients a year have bleeding from peptic ulcers.

2. Despite advances in diagnosis and treatment, the mortality associated with bleeding ulcers has remained largely unchanged, averaging between 6% and 10% during the past 30 years.

3. Bleeding from peptic ulcers stops spontaneously in 70% to 80% of patients.

4. A surgeon should be involved from the outset as part of the team caring for the patient with a bleeding peptic ulcer.

5. Patients at high risk for persistent or recurrent bleeding are those with large initial blood losses and active bleeding, or pigmented protuberances (visible vessels) at endoscopy.

6. Patients at low risk for subsequent bleeding are those with clean ulcer bases or those that contain flat pigmented spots at endoscopy.

7. The heater probe and multipolar (also known as bipolar) electrocoagulation are the most promising modalities for endoscopic hemostatic therapy.

8. In the hands of the qualified therapeutic endoscopist, the rate of complications of endoscopic hemostatic therapy is acceptably low, considering the natural history of bleeding peptic ulcers.

9. Endoscopic hemostatic therapy should be used only for patients who are at high risk for persistent or recurrent bleeding and death.

10. Clinical efficacy and safety of endoscopic hemostatic therapy should be assessed by multicenter, randomized, controlled trials.—N.J. Greenberger, M.D.

Reference

1. NIH Consensus Conference on Therapeutic Endoscopy and Bleeding Ulcers. JAMA 262:1369, 1989.

13 Gastric and Duodenal Neoplasms

Gastric Cancer

Total Versus Subtotal Gastrectomy for Adenocarcinoma of the Gastric Antrum: A French Prospective Controlled Study
Gouzi JL, Huguier M, Fagniez PL, Launois B, Flamant Y, Lacaine F, Paquet JC, Hay JM (French Assocs for Surgical Research, Toulouse, France)
Ann Surg 209:162–166, February 1989   13–1

Considerations of both postoperative mortality and long-term survival enter into the choice between elective total gastrectomy (TG) and subtotal gastrectomy (SG) for cancer of the lower third of the stomach. A multicenter trial in 1980–1985 enrolled 201 patients with antral adenocarcinoma. Of the 169 evaluable patients, 93 underwent TG and 76 had SG. Total gastrectomy usually did not extend to the spleen; repair was done with a standard Roux-en-Y esophagojejunostomy. Subtotal gastrectomy consisted of a subtotal distal gastrectomy with reconstruction by a Billroth II gastrojejunostomy.

The proximal margin of clearance was 10 cm in patients having TG and 7.5 cm in those having SG. Postoperative deaths included 3 after SG and 1 after TG. No difference in 5-year survival was found. Survival related closely to both node involvement and serosal extension. The extent of resection did not influence survival in groups matched for node involvement and serosal extension.

This, the first prospective randomized trial comparing TG and SG for adenocarcinoma of the gastric antrum, showed no difference in 5-year survival. Both the risk of cancer in the gastric remnant and the functional and nutritional sequelae of TG are relevant considerations.

▶ The French Associations for Surgical Research are to be congratulated for carrying out this controlled trial on the relative merits of subtotal versus total gastrectomy for adenocarcinoma of the antrum of the stomach. It is surprising that the mortality for total gastrectomy was less than that for subtotal gastrectomy (1% versus 4%). It is possible that the former procedure was done by the more senior surgeons. Even if that were the case, one cannot escape the conclusions that total gastrectomy does not enhance survival over what, in the hands of most surgeons, would be a less morbid procedure. This is a "must" article for the resident's file.—F.G. Moody, M.D.

A Long-Term Follow-Up Study of Patients With Gastric Cancer Detected by Mass Screening
Yamazaki H, Oshima A, Murakami R, Endoh S, Ubukata T (Osaka Cancer Detection and Prevention Ctr; Ctr for Adult Diseases, Osaka, Japan)
Cancer 63:613–617, Feb 15, 1989   13–2

Mass screening for gastric cancer has been done for more than 25 years in Japan, chiefly with photofluorographic radiography. A total of 1,139 patients with cancer detected by mass screening in 1961–1985 were reviewed. About two thirds of the patients were men. The series included 527 cases of early gastric cancer and 612 of advanced cancer.

Curative resection was carried out in 859 patients. Patients with screening-detected cancer had relative survival rates of 69% to 70%, which were virtually constant from 5 years after diagnosis and surgery. Hazard rates of screening-detected gastric cancer declined rapidly within 7 years and remained low subsequently. About two thirds of all patients with cancer detected by screening were cured.

Mass radiographic screening for gastric cancer in Japan has substantially improved the prognosis.

▶ Res ipse loquitur! The thing speaks for itself. I am often asked why we do not do mass screening in the United States, and the answer is apparent: the incidence of gastric cancer is too low for such screening to be time- or cost-effective. Clearly, high-risk groups—those with a family history of gastric cancer or pernicious anemia (although this is open to challenge), and those who have recently immigrated to America from high-risk areas—should have endoscopy at an early age. That early detection increases the chances for cure severalfold should encourage early endoscopic examination of the stomachs of patients who are first seen with even mild but persistent upper gastrointestinal complaints.—F.G. Moody, M.D.

Leiomyosarcoma

Advanced Gastric Leiomyosarcoma
Estes NC, Cherian G, Haller CC, Jewell WR, Hermreck AS, Thomas JH, Hardin CA (Univ of Kansas Med Ctr, Kansas City)
Am Surg 55:353–355, June 1989   13–3

Twenty-two patients with a mean age of 63 years were operated on for gastric leiomyosarcoma from 1952 to 1986. Patients most often had upper gastrointestinal bleeding, abdominal pain, or a mass upon admission. Five patients had bled massively, and 10 had hematocrits of less than 30%. Upper gastrointestinal contrast studies showed an extrinsic mass or abnormality in 8 of 10 patients. Mucosal ulceration often was missed at endoscopy. All patients but 2 had advanced disease at first examination.

Ten patients had subtotal gastrectomy, 4 had total gastrectomy, and 4 underwent wedge resection of the stomach. Four patients had biopsy only. Gastric resection for cure was carried out in 15 patients. There was 1 postoperative death. Three patients were alive with disease after 2 years, and 1, after 5 years. Survival was 35% at 3 years and remained the same at 5 years. The extent of resection was not a factor as long as a tumor-free margin was achieved. Chemotherapy and radiotherapy were used only for metastatic disease and were not beneficial.

If complete resection of advanced gastric leiomyosarcoma is possible, the patient has a reasonable chance for cure, even if adjacent organs are involved. In addition, long-term palliation is a definite possibility.

▶ This is a timely paper with a clear message for gastroenterologists and surgeons. Large, bulky gastric leiomyosarcomas can and should be resected along with involved adjacent organs. As documented in this report, senior surgeons with extensive clinical experience can perform such procedures with an acceptable mortality. Adjuvant therapy is of no value and should not be employed in this lesion.—F.G. Moody, M.D.

Carcinoids

Carcinoids of the Duodenum: A Histologic and Immunohistochemical Study of 65 Tumors

Burke AP, Federspiel BH, Sobin LH, Shekitka KM, Helwig EB (Armed Forces Inst of Pathology, Washington, DC)
Am J Surg Pathol 13:828–837, October 1989   13–4

Carcinoid tumors of the duodenum usually are sporadic, but also may be associated with von Recklinghausen's disease, Zollinger-Ellison syndrome, and multiple endocrine neoplasia. Thirty-one of the 65 tumors studied were histologically separate from the pancreas. Eleven others were close to pancreatic ducts or acini.

Eighty-five percent of the tumors were argyrophilic, and 15% were argentaffin tumors. The nonspecific neuroendocrine markers chromagranin, Leu-7, and neuron-specific enolase were positive in more than 80% of the tumors. Nearly half of the tumors were positive for somatostatin and more than half were positive for gastrin. Serotonin was identified in 39% of tumors, calcitonin in 19%, insulin in 5%, and pancreatic polypeptide in 3%. None of the tumors contained adrenocorticotropic hormone or glucagon. Two thirds of tumors had gastrin-cholecystokinin-like reactivity.

Duodenal carcinoids elaborate nonspecific endocrine markers in most instances, and frequently produce multiple hormones. A few of the tumors suggest a correlation among an ampullary location, psammoma bodies, and somatostatin production.

▶ The carcinoid cell or cells have an amazing capacity to synthesize polypeptides. Fortunately, not all are secreted in sufficient quantity to cause troublesome symptoms; in fact, most are not. Less than half the tumors contained serotonin, an amine often implicated in the gastrointestinal component of the carcinoid syndrome. Duodenal carcinoids usually are not associated with neuroendocrine symptoms to suggest their presence, but first appear with upper gastrointestinal hemorrhage or peptic ulcer type pain. It is likely that all carcinoids are capable of producing a variety of substances, depending on the external signals that regulate their genetic machinery.—F.G. Moody, M.D.

14 Helicobacter (Campylobacter) pylori

Campylobacter Associated Gastritis in Patients With Non-Ulcer Dyspepsia: A Double Blind Placebo Controlled Trial With Colloidal Bismuth Subcitrate
Loffeld RJLF, Potters HVJP, Stobberingh E, Flendrig JA, Van Spreeuwel JP, Arends JW (Univ Hosp Maastricht; Bleuland Hosp, Gouda, The Netherlands)
Gut 30:1206–1212, 1989

Campylobacter pylori is susceptible to colloidal bismuth subcitrate (CBS). To verify the pathogenetic significance of *C. pylori* for gastritis and nonulcer dyspepsia, 50 consecutively seen patients with nonulcer dyspepsia and a *Campylobacter*-associated gastritis (CAG) were randomly assigned in a double-blind fashion: 26 to treatment with CBS, 240 mg, twice daily; 24 to placebo. After the blind treatment, an "open" treatment with CBS was started in both groups.

Treatment with CBS resulted in a significant reduction in colonization with *C. pylori* and a significant improvement in the Whitehead gastritis score. In contrast, no significant changes occurred in the 24 placebo-treated patients. Eighteen patients in the CBS group and 17 patients in the placebo group received additional open treatment with CBS. No further improvement in gastritis score was noted in these patients, but a further reduction in *C. pylori* colonization was observed. No significant difference in the overall assessment of subjective complaints was found between the CBS- and placebo-treated patients. Subjective complaints were improved in both treatment groups, except for nausea and meteorism, which improved more with CBS.

These data question the clinical significance of gastritis in relation to dyspeptic complaints and cast doubts on the clinical relevance of therapeutic measures aimed at eradication of *C. pylori*.

▶ The authors conclude that colloidal bismuth subcitrate appears to be effective in the elimination of *Helicobacter pylori* and diminishes the degree of gastritis, but has a positive effect on dyspeptic complaints, which are largely the result of a placebo effect. They also question the clinical significance of gastritis in relation to dyspeptic complaints. The following article, which documents the presence of *Helicobacter pylori* and gastritis in an appreciable number of asymptomatic persons, provides additional support for this concept.—N.J. Greenberger, M.D.

Prevalence of *Helicobacter pylori* Infection and Histologic Gastritis in Asymptomatic Persons

Dooley CP, Cohen H, Fitzgibbons PL, Bauer M, Appleman MD, Perez-Perez GI, Blaser MJ (Los Angeles County–Univ of Southern California Med Ctr; VA Med Ctr, Denver)
N Engl J Med 321:1562–1566, Dec 7, 1989   14–2

Infection of the stomach and duodenum with *Helicobacter pylori*, formerly known as *Campylobacter pylori*, is closely associated with gastritis and duodenal ulcer disease in patients with upper (gastrointestinal) symptoms. The prevalence of *H. pylori* infection was examined in 113 asymptomatic healthy adults by endoscopic biopsy of the gastric antrum and corpus.

Unsuspected lesions were found in 14% of the study group, most often in the form of mucosal erosions. Usually there were 3 or fewer erosions, which were confined to the gastric antrum. Abnormalities did not occur in those aged less than 40 years. *Helicobacter pylori* infection was identified in 32% of subjects, with its prevalence rising with advancing age (Fig 14–1). Erosions were equally frequent in those with and those without *H. pylori* infection.

Chronic gastritis was diagnosed in 42 cases, and there was *H. pylori* infection in 86%. Recent use of antibiotics was associated with *H. pylori* infection, but the use of bismuth was protective. Active chronic gastritis occurred only in those with *H. pylori*.

Both histologic gastritis and *H. pylori* infection are frequent in healthy persons and become more so with advancing age. This organism may have an etiologic

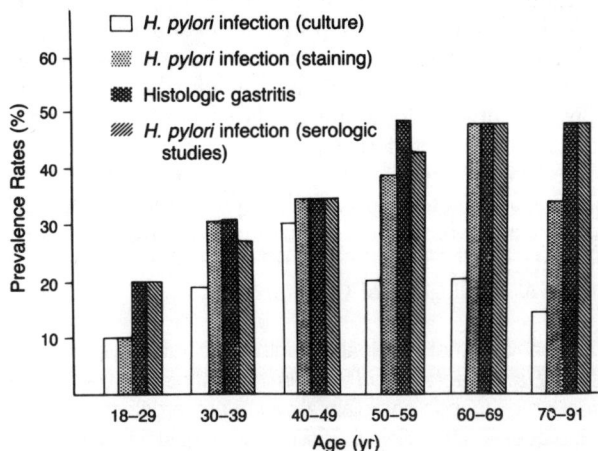

Fig 14–1.—Age-specific prevalence rates for *H. pylori* infection, according to results of cultures (no. = 108), staining (no. = 113), and serologic studies (IgA and IgG assay; no. = 98), and for histologic gastritis (no. = 113) in the study sample. Twenty stains, 20 cultures, and 15 serum samples were available for the subjects aged between 18 and 29 years; 22 stains, 19 cultures, and 15 serum samples for those between 30 and 39 years; 20 stains, 20 cultures, and 18 serum samples for those aged between 40 and 49 years; 21 stains, 19 cultures, and 21 serum samples for those aged between 50 and 59 years; 15 stains, 15 cultures, and 14 serum samples for those aged between 60 and 69 years; and 15 stains, 15 cultures, and 15 serum samples for those aged between 70 and 91 years. (Courtesy of Dooley CP, Cohen H, Fitzgibbons PL, et al: *N Engl J Med* 321:1562–1566, Dec 7, 1989.)

role in the development of gastritis. The findings are especially important in view of the possibility that gastritis is a precursor of gastric carcinoma.

► As the authors point out, the clinical importance of the carefully documented histologic abnormalities in macroscopically normal stomachs is uncertain. However, their data, as well as other accumulating evidence, suggest that histologic inflammation is not a cause of symptoms. Much remains to be learned about the pathogenesis of *H. pylori* infection, its adherence and virulence factors, and its effects on the stomach and duodenum. The bacterium is especially common in developing countries (1), where gastric carcinoma is more common than in industrialized countries. Gastritis may be a precursor lesion in the development of gastric carcinoma. Therefore, *H. pylori* infection may be of potential importance in the asymptomatic population. Studies of the prevalence of this infection in populations at high risk for gastric carcinoma need to be performed.—N.J. Greenberger, M.D.

Reference

1. Dwyer B, Kaldor JTW, Rauws K: The prevalence of *Campylobacter pylori* in human populations, in Ruthbone BJ, Pleatley RV (eds): *Campylobacter Pylori and Gastroduodenal Disease*. Oxford, England, Blackwell, 1989 pp 190–196.

Enlarged Gastric Folds in Association With *Campylobacter pylori* Gastritis
Morrison S, Dahms BB, Hoffenberg E, Czinn SJ (Case Western Reserve Univ; Univ Hosps of Cleveland; Rainbow Babies' and Children's Hosp, Cleveland)
Radiology 171:819–821, June 1989   14–3

Fifteen patients with symptoms in their upper gastrointestinal (GI) tracts were found to have *Campylobacter pylori* gastritis at endoscopic biopsy. At radiologic upper GI barium studies, enlarged gastric folds were seen in 7 of the 15. The 6 girls and 1 boy were aged 9 to 16 years.

All but 1 of the 15 children had chronic epigastric pain. Nine had vomited, and 3 had hematemesis. Symptoms were similar in those with and those without thickened gastric folds. The patients with abnormal findings on radiographs had normal serum levels of protein and albumin and lacked evidence of edema or anemia. Seven of the 8 patients without thickened gastric folds had gastritis at endoscopy, and 4 had ulcers. The histopathologic findings were comparable in the 2 patient groups.

Pathologic states that may produce thickened gastric folds in children include tumors, inflammatory and infectious disorders, and eosinophilic gastroenteritis. Diffuse chronic gastritis was the usual finding in children in this study. Endoscopy is necessary to definitively diagnose *C. pylori* gastritis.

► Thickened gastric folds in the body of the stomach are found in Ménétrier's disease, eosinophilic gastroenteritis, lymphoma, Zollinger-Ellison syndrome, and some gastric infections. In the antrum of the stomach, thickened gastric folds often indicate gastritis. It is not surprising that *Campylobacter pylori* should cause thickened gastric folds because it has been reported to be commonly associated with gastritis. This important diagnostic consideration for pediatric patients with gastritis will contribute to patient care, as patients may not require endoscopic studies to verify the presence of *Campylobacter pylori*. In the future, urea breath tests or serum antibody tests may clarify these issues for pediatric patients, but in the presence of increased gastric folds associated with clinical symptoms, it may be pragmatic to treat *Campylobacter pylori,* then await resolution of the symptoms before proceeding with additional tests.—P.B. Miner, Jr., M.D.

Effect of Roux-en-Y Biliary Diversion on *Campylobacter pylori*
O'Connor HJ, Newbold KM, Alexander-Williams J, Thompson H, Drumm J, Donovan IA (Gen Hosp; Dudley Road Hosp, Birmingham, England)
Gastroenterology 97:958–964, October 1989   14–4

Gastric mucosa from patients undergoing peptic ulcer operations that increase enterogastric reflux may change from being *Campylobacter pylori*-positive to *C. pylori*-negative and from a *C. pylori*-associated chronic gastritis to that associated with bile reflux. The effect of Roux-en-Y (RY) biliary diversion on *C. pylori* status and on associated mucosal abnormalities in the stomach was studied in 24 patients with symptomatic bile reflux after peptic ulcer operations. A retrospective histologic study of the gastric biopsies performed before and after RY diversion was undertaken. Mean time interval between the preoperative and postoperative endoscopic examinations was 4.7 years (range, 0.8–9.8 years). Using a histologic grading system, biopsy specimens were assessed for the presence of *C. pylori* and scored for severity of reflux gastritis.

Partial gastrectomy specimens resected at the initial operation, were available in 12 patients. Of these, 10 (83%) were positive for *C. pylori*. In the group of 24 patients studied, 13 (54%) were *C. pylori*-positive before RY diversion; this rose to 22 (92%) after biliary diversion. The median reflux score rose from 6 in the partial gastrectomy specimens to 11 before RY diversion, falling again significantly to 6 after biliary diversion. High reflux scores correlated strongly with the absence of *C. pylori.*

These data indicate that *C. pylori,* apparently eradicated after peptic ulcer operations that increase enterogastric reflux, may recolonize the gastric remnant after biliary diversion. Associated with these changes in *C. pylori* status is a change from type B gastritis in some peptic ulcer patients to reflux gastritis after gastric surgery and back to type B gastritis after biliary diversion.

▶ Roux-en-Y diversion generally has been accepted as an effective means of preventing reflux of small bowel contents into the stomach. As O'Connor and associates point out in the discussion of their paper, a curious feature of several previous studies on the outcome of diversionary surgery has been the failure to demonstrate a decrease in the degree of histologic gastritis, despite improvement in symptoms and virtual elimination of reflux as documented by biochemical analysis or scintigraphy, or both.

O'Connor and co-workers postulate that enterogastric reflux gives rise to an essentially "chemical" injury to the gastric mucosa that evokes a predominantly epithelial response where activity is reflected in the degree of compensatory foveolar hyperplasia. The mucosal response includes vasodilatation, congestion, and interstitial edema, but the inflammatory cell response seems to be unimportant. The findings indicate that these mucosal changes are reversible and that *C. pylori*, apparently eradicated after peptic ulcer operations that increase enterogastric reflux, may reappear in the gastric remnant after effective biliary diversion. Furthermore, the results suggest that, associated with changes in *C. pylori* status and enterogastric reflux, the predominant pattern of chronic gastritis in some peptic ulcer patients may change first from type B gastritis to reflux gastritis after gastric surgery and then back to type B gastritis after biliary diversion.

Thus, *recolonization* by *C. pylori* may account for the type B gastritis noted after Roux-en-Y diversion.—N.J. Greenberger, M.D.

15 Gastric Emptying Problems

Effect of Six Weeks of Treatment With Cisapride in Gastroparesis and Intestinal Pseudoobstruction
Camilleri M, Malagelada JR, Abell TL, Brown ML, Hench V, Zinsmeister AR (Mayo Clinic and Mayo Found, Rochester, Minn)
Gastroenterology 96:704–712, March 1989   15–1

The efficacy of cisapride in patients with upper gut dysmotility was investigated in a 6-week randomized, double-blind placebo-controlled trial. Eleven patients with gastroparesis and 15 patients with chronic idiopathic intestinal pseudo-obstruction were evaluated at entry into and at the end of the study by upper gastrointestinal manometry, scintigraphic evaluation of gastric emptying of solids and liquids, measurement of body weight, and scoring of symptoms: abdominal pain, nausea, vomiting, early satiety, bloating, and distention. Cisapride was given orally in a dosage of 10 mg 3 times daily.

Patients in the cisapride-treatment and placebo-treatment groups were strictly comparable for all parameters assessed at the beginning of the study. In the cisapride group, a significant increase in gastric emptying of solids was found compared with the placebo group (Fig 15–1). Additionally, cisapride

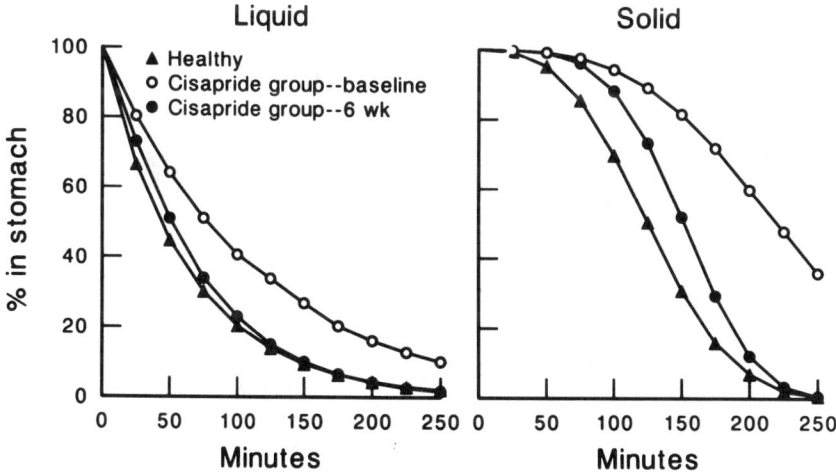

Fig 15–1.—Median liquid and solid gastric emptying curves of all patients in the cisapride group at baseline and at the end of the study. Note the normalization of liquid emptying and the improvement in solid emptying relative to healthy persons shown for comparison. (Courtesy of Camilleri M, Malagelada JR, Abell TL, et al: *Gastroenterology* 96:704–712, March 1989.)

tended to increase the postcibal antral motility and ameliorate the abnormal manometric features in patients with intestinal dysmotility, particularly the characteristics of fasting interdigestive motor complexes and the fed motor pattern. Total symptom scores improved with both cisapride and placebo. No significant difference was found in overall symptom response between the two groups, except for the marked improvement in abdominal pain in cisapride-treated patients.

These data confirm the effectiveness of cisapride in improving delayed gastric emptying in patients with upper gut dysmotility. However, the overall symptomatic benefit from cisapride was not significantly different from that of placebo. Longer term trials and dose-response studies are necessary to determine the clinical efficacy of cisapride.

▶ In their discussion, the authors emphasize several points. To observe a positive symptomatic response in these chronic diseases, it may be necessary to perform more prolonged therapeutic trials. The high placebo responsiveness may have been predictable for patients with symptoms of upper gut dysfunction characteristic of the syndromes studied. The duration of the trial may have been too short to overcome the initial placebo response, and this may also explain the lack of differences in weight gain between placebo and cisapride groups. Nevertheless, the sustained improvement of gastric emptying after 6 weeks of treatment with cisapride provides objective evidence that prolonged treatment would be a promising form of therapy. Camillari and colleagues emphasize that the long-term effects of this medication will need to be further evaluated by future studies.

The same investigators also have reported on another disorder of gastrointestinal motility, that is, idiopathic cyclic nausea and vomiting (1). They describe 8 patients (5 men and 3 women) with previously unexplained recurrent cyclic episodes of nausea and vomiting. In these patients, the symptoms developed a mean of once every 3.2 months and persisted a mean of 3.5 days. For no patient could a cause of symptoms be identified on conventional diagnostic tests. A detailed investigation of the gastrointestinal motility during an asymptomatic period revealed abnormal findings in all 8 patients. Gastric hypomotility was substantiated in 5 patients; small bowel dysmotility, in 6; delayed gastric emptying, in 2; and gastric dysrhythmia, in 2. The data demonstrate that abnormal gastrointestinal motility occurs during an asymptomatic state in patients with cyclic episodes of nausea and vomiting. Because all patients with this syndrome had abnormal gastrointestinal motility but normal results of other gastrointestinal studies, idiopathic cyclic nausea and vomiting may be related to altered gastrointestinal motility.—N.J. Greenberger, M.D.

Reference

1. Abell TL, Kim CH, Malageloda JR: Idiopathic cyclic nausea and vomiting: A disorder of gastrointestinal motility. *Mayo Clinic Proc* 63:1169–1175, 1988.

16 Miscellaneous

The Gastric Air–Fluid Sign: Aid in CT Assessment of Gastric Wall Thickening
Hammerman AM, Mirowitz SA, Susman N (Washington Univ)
Gastrointest Radiol 14:109–112, 1989   16–1

Computed tomography is of limited value in detecting a thickened gastric wall, especially if the stomach is incompletely distended. A transition in gastric wall thickness often is noted at or slightly above the gastric air–fluid or air–contrast level. Abdominal CT scans of 259 consecutively seen patients who had no known or clinically suspected gastrointestinal pathology were reviewed.

In 22% of cases there was apparent thickening, with an abrupt transition to normal wall thickness at or immediately above an air–fluid or air–contrast level (Fig 16–1). In several cases administration of additional contrast or effervescent granules, or both, led to disappearance of the air–fluid sign and thinning of the entire gastric wall (Fig 16–2).

Apparent thickening of the stomach wall often selectively affects the dependent part of the stomach, accounting for this "gastric air–fluid sign." This finding can be expected in perhaps one fifth of persons with a normal stomach.

▶ This paper is an important contribution to CT evaluation of gastric abnormalities. The determination of gastric wall thickening with CT is difficult because of the

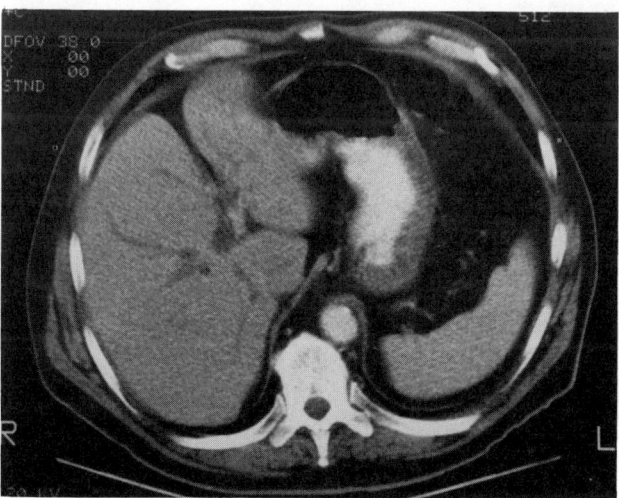

Fig 16–1.—Abrupt transition in wall thickness (gastric air–fluid sign) is noted on greater curvature *(arrow)* in patient with endoscopically proved normal stomach. (Courtesy of Hammerman AM, Mirowitz SA, Susman N: *Gastrointest Radiol* 14:109–112, 1989.)

88 / The Stomach and Duodenum

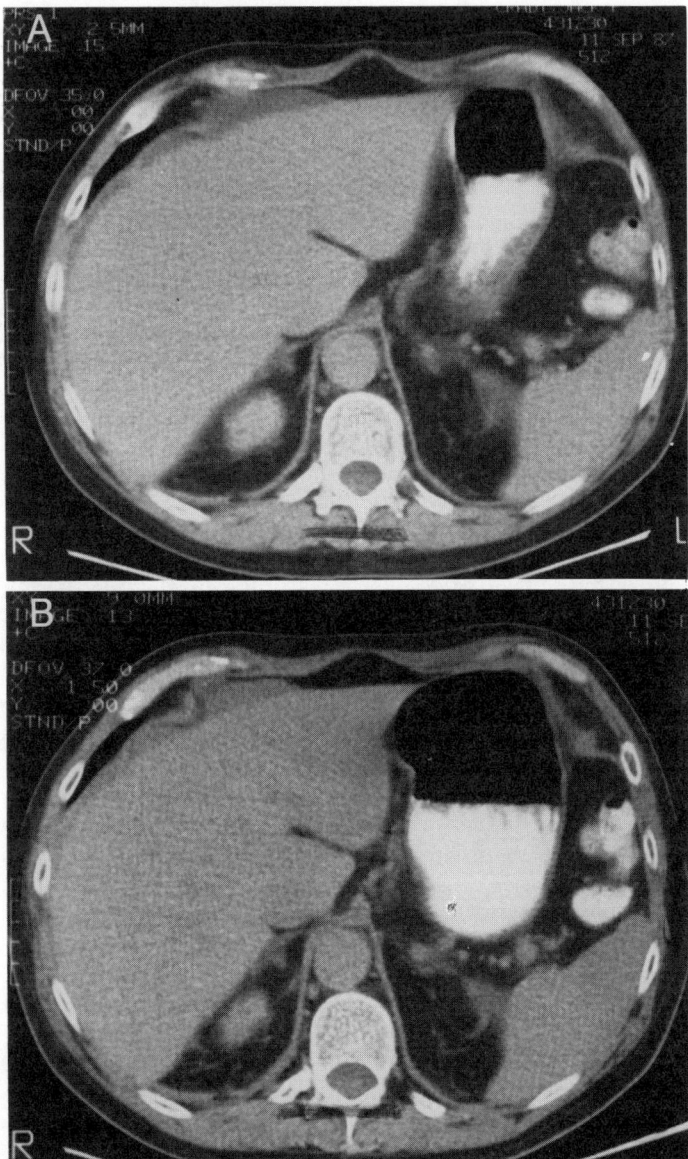

Fig 16–2.—**A,** contrast material and air in partially distended sotmach, with apparent gastric wall thickening below air–contrast level. Gastric wall above this level is of normal thickness. **B,** after administration of effervescent granules and additional oral contrast material there is increased distention of gastric lumen with uniform effacement of gastric wall. (Courtesy of Hammerman AM, Mirowitz SA, Susman N: *Gastrointest Radiol* 14:109–112, 1989.)

attenuation abnormalities associated with gastric mucus and fluid. The gastric wall often appears thickened on a CT scan. The gastric air–fluid sign will give the radiologist greater confidence in suggesting that the apparent thickening of the gastric wall is indeed normal. Miyake and co-workers (1) describe another CT finding of low attenuation that was useful in identifying mucinous adenocarcinoma. They believed the mucin was responsible for this low attenuation. These 2 findings should help in distinguishing some of the abnormalities of apparent gastric wall thickening seen with CT scans.—P.B. Miner, Jr., M.D.

Reference

1. Miyake H et al: *J Comput Assist Tomogr* 13:253, 1989.

The Small Intestine

Chapter 17. Pathophysiologic and Radiographic Considerations
    Food Hypersensitivity and Histamine
    Segmental Dilatation of the Small Bowel
    Intestinal Defect in Hemochromatosis
    The "Ileal Brake"

Chapter 18. Microvillus Inclusions Disease

Chapter 19. AIDS and Related Problems in Homosexual Men

Chapter 20. Short Bowel Syndrome
    In Neonates
    Somatostatin Analogues

Chapter 21. Alimentary Tract Duplications and Atresia

Chapter 22. Ileal Bypass for Hypercholesterolemia

Chapter 23. Neoplasms
    Inpatients With Familial Polyposis
    Recognition at Emergent Laparotomy

Chapter 24. Small Bowel Obstruction
    Diagnosis by Enteroclysis
    Postoperative

Chapter 25. Mesenteric Infarction

Chapter 26. Crohn's Disease and Related Topics
    Radiologic Considerations
    Immunosuppressive Therapy
    Strictureplasty
    Recurrence and Reoperation
    Cancer

Chapter 27. Nutrition
    Enteral and Parenteral Nutrition; Tube Feedings
    Percutaneous Endoscopic Gastrostomy and Jejunostomy
    Miscellaneous Considerations

17 Pathophysiologic and Radiographic Considerations

Food Hypersensitivity and Histamine

Spontaneous Release of Histamine From Basophils and Histamine-Releasing Factor in Patients With Atopic Dermatitis and Food Hypersensitivity
Sampson HA, Broadbent KR, Bernhisel-Broadbent J (Johns Hopkins Univ)
N Engl J Med 321:228–232, July 27, 1989   17–1

An earlier controlled clinical trial reported high rates of spontaneous histamine release in the basophils of children with proven food hypersensitivity, but not in the basophils of children who had no food allergies. Whether patients with atopic dermatitis and food hypersensitivity had similar high rates of spontaneous histamine release in vitro, whether elimination diets would affect the release rate, and whether a cytokine histamine-releasing factor mediates the spontaneous release of histamine from basophils were studied in 25 patients who had not yet started an allergen-avoidance diet (group 1); also included were 38 such patients who had been following an allergen-avoidance diet for at least 1 year (group 2), 20 patients with atopic dermatitis but no food allergies (group 3), and 18 normal controls who had no food allergies (group 4).

Group 1 patients had significantly higher spontaneous release rates of histamine from basophils than controls. Group 2 patients had significantly lower release rates of histamine than their untreated counterparts (Fig 17–1). Patients in group 3 had histamine release rates similar to those observed in normal controls (group 4).

Mononuclear cells from group 1 patients spontaneously produced a histamine-releasing cytokine in vitro that provoked the histamine release from basophils from other food-sensitive patients but not from basophils from normal controls. Adherence to the elimination diet significantly decreased the cytokine generation rate in basophils. The ability of the histamine-releasing cytokine to induce histamine release in basophils of other patients with food allergies was linked to the type of immunoglobulin E bound to the basophils' surface.

Patients with food allergies who are exposed to the relevant antigens pro-

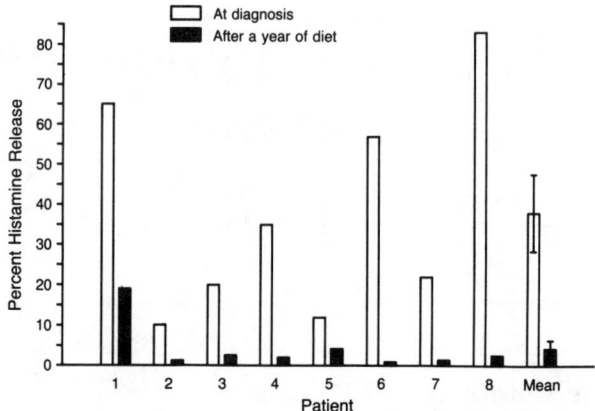

Fig 17–1.—Rates of spontaneous histamine release in 8 patients. Rates were determined at diagnosis and after 1 year of an appropriate allergen-avoidance diet (4 months for patient 1). (Courtesy of Sampson HA, Broadbent KR, Bernhisel-Broadbent J: *N Engl J Med* 321:228–232, July 27, 1989.)

duce a histamine-releasing factor that interacts with the immunoglobulin E bound to the surface of basophils.

Segmental Dilatation of the Small Bowel

Segmental Dilatation of the Small Bowel: Report of Three Cases and Literature Review
Ratcliffe J, Tait J, Lisle D, Leditschke JF, Bell J (Mater Children's Hosp; Royal Children's Hosp; Mater Misericordiae Hosp, Brisbane, Australia)
Radiology 171:827–830, June 1989   17–2

Segmental small bowel dilatation is a rare congenital disorder in which the caliber of the bowel lumen increases locally in the absence of obstruction and thickening of the muscle coat. The disorder may coexist with other serious abdominal conditions. Surgical removal of the dilated segment is curative. Thirty-three cases have been reported in the literature. In 3 new cases the lesion was demonstrated on radiographs obtained before laparotomy.

All but 2 of the 36 patients have been aged less than 16 years; most were aged less than 10. Seventeen patients had 19 midgut abnormalities including exomphalos, malrotation without exomphalos, and Meckel's diverticulum. The condition may arise from prolonged bowel obstruction in fetal life, which produces "cystic" or local segmental dilatation (Fig 17–2). A fluid level may be found in the dilated segment, prompting a small bowel study.

Some patients have had symptoms and signs of obstruction in the neonatal period. Anemia is frequent. Older infants and children may have features of intermittent obstruction. Vomiting of bile calls for urgent barium examination of the small bowel.

▶ The authors of this paper illustrate a rare congenital abnormality of the intestine consisting of numerous dilated bowel loops without apparent abnormalities of the intestinal muscle or focal luminal obstruction. Symptoms of intermittent obstruction

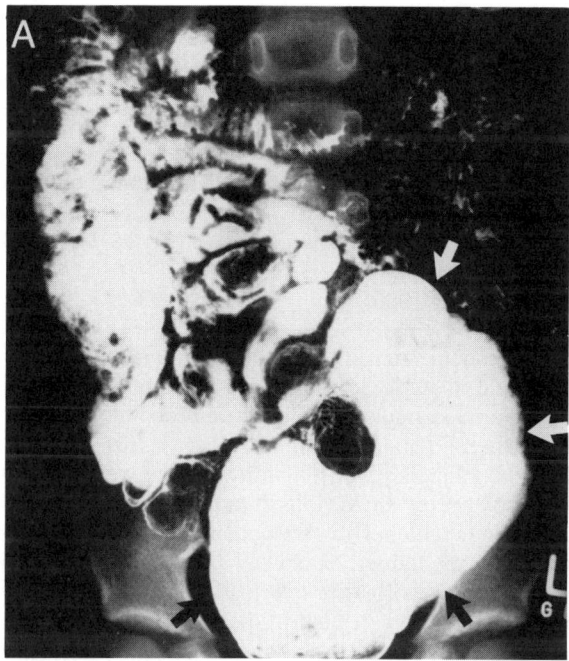

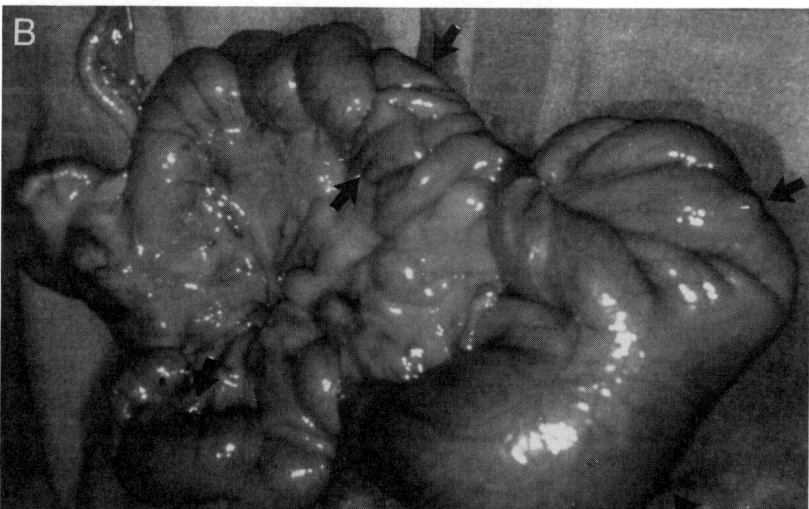

Fig 17–2.—A, 40-minute spot radiograph of barium study of whole abdomen of infant girl shows dilated segment in lower ileum *(arrows).* **B,** intraoperative photograph demonstrates dilated segment of bowel *(thick arrows)* and normal small bowel *(thin arrows).* (Courtesy of Ratcliffe J, Tait J, Lisle D, et al: *Radiology* 171:827–830, June 1989.)

or anemia may lead the physician to diagnose Crohn's disease in an older patient. Surgical resection is important in long-term management because it relieves the symptoms.—P.B. Miner, Jr., M.D.

Intestinal Defect in Hemochromatosis

Immunohistochemical Evidence for a Lack of Ferritin in Duodenal Absorptive Epithelial Cells in Idiopathic Hemochromatosis
Fracanzani AL, Fargion S, Romano R, Piperno A, Arosio P, Ruggeri G, Ronchi G, Fiorelli G (Univ of Milan; Univ of Brescia, Italy)
Gastroenterology 96:1071–1078, April 1989   17–3

Patients with idiopathic hemochromatosis (IH) have increased intestinal iron absorption for reasons that are not clear. In this study, gastroduodenal ferritin distribution was examined in duodenal and antral mucosal specimens from 24 patients with established IH. In addition, 10 patients with secondary hemochromatosis, 13 with iron deficiency, and 6 healthy persons were studied.

Any histologic differences between the various groups were not marked. Most patients with IH lacked detectable ferritin staining in duodenal epithelial cells, but interstitial macrophages stained positively (table). Hemosiderin granules were seen only in patients with iron overload. L-type ferritin was twofold to threefold higher in IH than in healthy persons when duodenal mucosal homogenates were analyzed. Levels of H-type ferritin were similar in the 2 groups.

In IH, the expression of ferritin in the duodenal absorptive epithelial cells is altered. Ferritin may have a regulatory role in iron absorption by these cells. The ferritin deficiency observed may be directly related to the inability to regulate iron absorption among patients with IH.

▶ I would like to cite a key paragraph from the discussion of this paper, as it highlights the key findings.

"The present findings have some implications for the mechanism of iron absorption and for the genetics of idiopathic hemochromatosis (IH). The observed lack of ferritin in absorptive cells may be directly related to the incapacity of IH patients to regulate iron absorption. It has been suggested that ferritin in these cells has the

Ferritin in Absorptive Epithelial Duodenal Cells (Immunohistochemical Stain)*

Subjects	n	Positive staining n	Percent
Normal	6	6	100
Iron deficiency	13	13	100
Secondary hemochromatosis	10	10	100
Idiopathic hemochromatosis	24	3	12.5

* In no case did absorptive epithelial cells contain hemosiderin.
Courtesy of Fracanzani AL, Fargion S, Romano R, et al: *Gastroenterolgy* 96:1071–1078, April 1989.

function of storing the unwanted iron that will be lost when epithelial cells are sloughed into the lumen; alternatively, it has been proposed that iron absorption is regulated by a balance between intracellular ferritin and transferrin. In both models ferritin has a regulatory/inhibitory role in iron absorption, and it may be expected that when it is absent, or present in a lower amount, the transfer of iron to the plasma is increased."—N.J. Greenberger, M.D.

Food Iron Absorption in Idiopathic Hemochromatosis
Lynch SR, Skikne BS, Cook JD (Univ of Kansas Med Ctr, Kansas City)
Blood 74:2187–2193, November 1989   17–4

The effect of the form of dietary iron on phenotypic expression of hemochromatosis was studied by evaluating the magnitude of the defect in both heme and nonheme iron absorption from a representative Western meal in patients with treated and untreated idiopathic hemochromatosis (IH). Iron absorption measurements, using double extrinsic radioiron tags to label independently the nonheme and heme iron components of a hamburger meal, were done with 75 healthy volunteers, 15 patients with IH, and 22 heterozygous relatives.

In healthy persons, absorption of both nonheme and heme iron stores was correlated inversely with iron stores as measured by the serum ferritin concentration. In patients with IH, absorption of both nonheme and heme iron was far greater than would be predicted from the relationship between absorption and serum ferritin observed in healthy persons (Fig 17–3). Nonheme iron absorption and serum ferritin were significantly inversely correlated, whereas heme iron absorption was independent of body iron stores. In heterozygous

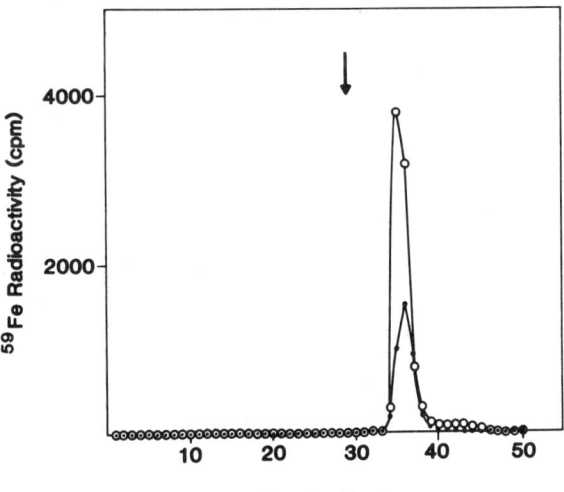

Fig 17–3.—Ion-exchange chromatography of human placental receptor. Pooled fractions from AcA34 were applied to DEAE Sephacel column. *Arrow* indicates start of gradient elution. (Courtesy of Lynch SR, Skikne BS, Cook JD: *Blood* 74:2187–2193, Nov 1, 1989.)

relatives, nonheme iron absorption did not differ significantly from that of healthy persons. However, when the meal was fortified with 20 mg of iron and 100 mg of vitamin C, nonheme iron absorption was significantly greater than that of the healthy persons.

Excessive nonheme absorption in patients with IH was confirmed, even with nonfortified meals. Such patients are particularly susceptible to significant iron overload from diets containing a high proportion of heme iron. Impaired nonheme absorption is also present in heterozygous persons, but this is demonstrable only when the test meal contains a large, highly bioavailable iron supplement.

▶ This interesting paper provides further documentation of the excessive absorption of dietary iron in homozygous patients with idiopathic hemochromatosis. However, additional observations indicate that, although the difference in absorption of nonheme iron from a normal diet in heterozygotes is negligible, *exaggerated absorption* of nonheme iron occurs from an iron-supplemented meal. Thus, impaired regulation of nonheme iron absorption can occur in heterozygotes under certain conditions.—N.J. Greenberger, M.D.

The "Ileal Brake"

The "Ileal Brake" After Ileal Pouch–Anal Anastomosis
Soper NJ, Chapman NJ, Kelly KA, Brown ML, Phillips SF, Go VLW (Mayo Clinic and Mayo Found, Rochester, Minn)
Gastroenterology 98:111–116, January 1990   17–5

In recent years many patients with chronic ulcerative colitis have been treated with colectomy, mucosal rectectomy, and ileal pouch–anal anastomosis (IPAA). This procedure generally is well accepted, but frequent stooling may cause distress and about half of these patients use antidiarrheal medications chronically. Infusion of nutrients into the normal ileum provides an "ileal brake" that slows gastric emptying and small bowel transport and augments intestinal absorption of carbohydrate. Oleic acid was infused into the ileal pouch in the hope of delaying defecation in 8 patients who had the IPAA procedure for ulcerative colitis.

Infusion of isotonic oleic acid emulsion was well tolerated by most patients. Gastric emptying of the liquid component of a test meal, assessed with ^{99m}Tc-diethylenetriamine pentaacetic acid (DTPA), was slowed by infusion of oleic acid into the ileal pouch. Small bowel transit, as estimated with ^{111}In-DTPA, also was slowed. Plasma levels of enteroglucagon, neurotensin, and peptide YY rose sharply 1 hour after eating on the day oleic acid was infused.

The ability to activate the ileal brake by infusing oleic acid into the ileal pouch may have clinical value for patients with rapid bowel transit and frequent stooling after the IPAA operation.

▶ Read and his associates recently described the effects of an "ileal brake" on upper gastrointestinal transit (1). Infusion of nutrients into the ileum of healthy persons slows gastric emptying and small bowel transit and augments intestinal absorption of carbohydrate. Details of the receptor and effector pathways of the ileal brake are unknown, but accumulating evidence suggests that the mechanism mediating the ileal brake is in part hormonal. Soper and associates showed that neither the ileal pouch infusion alone nor the meal alone altered plasma levels of enteroglucagon, neurotensin, or peptide YY, but the combination of the oleic acid infusion and the meal increased the levels of all 3 hormones.—N.J. Greenberger, M.D.

Reference

1. Holgate AM, Read NW: Effect of ileal infusion of intra-lipid on gastrointestinal transit, ileal flow rates, and carbohydrate absorption in humans after ingestion of a liquid meal. *Gastroenterology* 88:1005–1011, 1985.

18 Microvillus Inclusions Disease

Microvillus Inclusion Disease: An Inherited Defect of Brush-Border Assembly and Differentiation
Cutz E, Rhoads JM, Drumm B, Sherman PM, Durie PR, Forstner GG (Hosp for Sick Children, Toronto; Univ of Toronto)
N Engl J Med 320:646–651, March 9, 1989   18–1

Microvillus inclusion disease is a familial, severe enteropathy characterized by protracted diarrhea from birth and hypoplastic villous atrophy. Electron microscopic studies of surface enterocytes in a jejunal biopsy specimen show peculiar intracytoplasmic inclusions composed of neatly arranged brush-border microvilli. The clinical and pathologic features of 9 cases of microvillus inclusion disease are described.

Characteristically, all infants had severe watery diarrhea within 72 hours of birth. The pattern of inheritance was characteristic of autosomal recessive transmission. In spite of restrictive oral intake, stool volume was large during the course of the disease. Mean levels of stool electrolytes resembled those of jejunal fluid. No treatment was effective, although the use of somatostatin showed promise in controlling the diarrhea of 1 patient. Eight patients died before the age of 18 months. Jejunal biopsy specimens from all patients showed diffuse villous atrophy, crypt hypoplasia, normal or decreased number of inflammatory cells in the lamina propria, and absence of well-defined brush border on surface enterocytes (Fig 18–1). Transmission electron micrographs of the surface enterocytes confirmed the absence of surface microvilli or markedly shortened and disorganized microvilli, as well as the presence of numerous vesicular bodies and the characteristic intracytoplasmic microvillus inclusions often containing complete brush borders facing inward (Fig 18–2). Microvillus inclusions also were found in rectal biopsy specimens from all 3 infants studied.

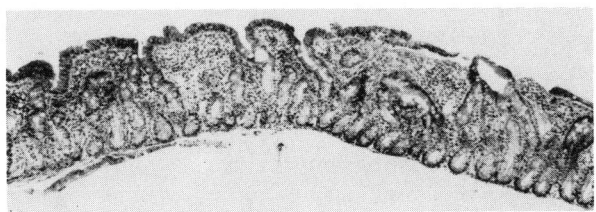

Fig 18–1.—Specimen of small intestine on light microscopy. Low magnification of histologic section shows total villous atrophy with short hypoplastic crypts. Hematoxylin and eosin; original magnification, ×40. (Courtesy of Cutz E, Rhoads JM, Drumm B, et al: N Engl J Med 320:646–651, March 9, 1989.)

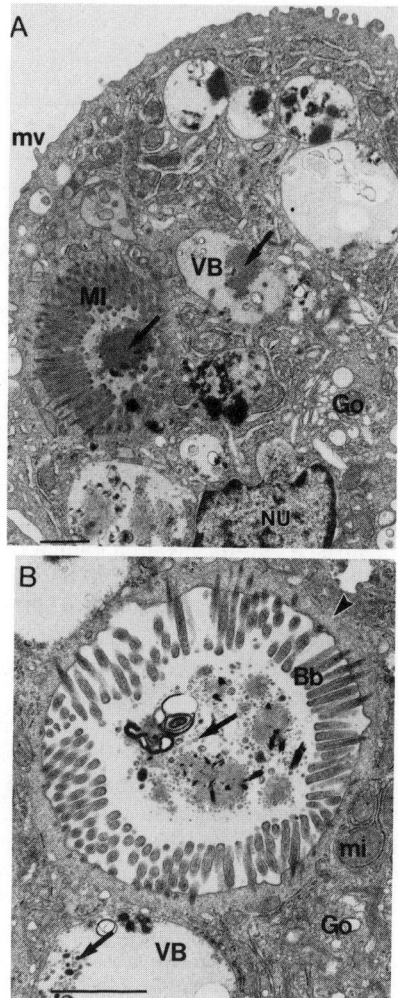

Fig 18–2.—Transmission electron micrographs of surface enterocytes. *Bars* represent 1 µm. **A,** the apical plasma membrane with absence of the brush border and few rudimentary microvilli *(mv)*. The supranuclear cytoplasm *(NU)* contains the Golgi complex *(Go)*, numerous vesicular bodies *(VB)* of different sizes and varying luminal content, as well as a characteristic microvillus inclusion *(MI)* with well-formed brush-border microvilli. Note the similar appearance of the moderately electron-dense material within the lumen of the microvillus inclusions and vesicular bodies *(arrows)*. **B,** a microvillus inclusion with inwardly facing brush-border *(Bb)* microvilli. Core filaments and the terminal web appear to be well developed *(arrowhead)*. The lumen of the inclusion has an aggregate of small vesicles, patches of moderately electron-dense floccular material, and myelin-like figures. Small vesicular structures *(arrow)* in the lumen of the vesicular body *(VB)* are similar to those seen within the microvillus inclusion *(arrow)*. *mi,* mitochondria. (Courtesy of Cutz E, Rhoads JM, Drumm B, et al: *N Engl J Med* 320:646–651, March 9, 1989.)

Microvillus inclusion disease has emerged as a new, distinct, clinicopathologic entity that needs to be differentiated from other enteropathies within the spectrum of intractable diarrhea. Its uniformly grave prognosis and autosomal recessive mode of inheritance make genetic counseling imperative.

▶ As the authors point out, the importance of the rectal and colonic lesions should not be overlooked. Microvillus inclusions were found in rectal biopsy specimens from 3 of 3 infants. In patient 9, a rectal suction biopsy indicated the diagnosis of microvillus inclusion disease at 2 weeks of age, 10 months before the diagnosis was confirmed with jejunal biopsy. This disease, with its high early mortality, probably is overlooked often because of the difficulties encountered in performing small bowel biopsies for very young and sick infants and because electron microscopic examination of such specimens is not performed routinely. No effective treatment for this disorder is available currently, although somatostatin may be transiently effective in controlling diarrhea.—N.J. Greenberger, M.D.

19 AIDS and Related Problems in Homosexual Men

Small Intestinal Structure and Function in Patients Infected With Human Immunodeficiency Virus (HIV): Evidence for HIV-Induced Enteropathy
Ullrich R, Zeitz M, Heise W, L'age M, Höffken G, Riecken EO (Free Univ of Berlin; Auguste-Viktoria Hosp, Berlin)
Ann Intern Med 111:15–21, July 1, 1989

Patients infected with HIV often have gastrointestinal symptoms. The cause of these symptoms is unclear, as a causative enteric pathogen often is not identified. To pinpoint the origin of gastrointestinal symptoms in HIV-infected patients, 44 men and 1 woman aged 22–57 years with confirmed HIV infection underwent diagnostic esophagogastroduodenoscopy. Symptoms included weight loss, diarrhea, epigastric and abdominal pain, nausea, vomiting, and dysphagia.

At the time of study, 13 patients were being treated with zidovudine; 5, with ganciclovir; and 3, with cotrimoxazole. All were evaluated for malabsorption. Biopsy and stool samples were examined for enteric pathogens. Distal duodenal biopsy samples obtained from 19 patients were examined morphometrically and by quantitative enzyme histochemical techniques. In addition, immunohistologic studies were done to ascertain the presence of HIV antigen p24.

Enteric pathogens, including *Candida albicans*, atypical mycobacteria, cytomegalovirus, *Giardia lamblia*, *Chlamydia trachomatis*, *Salmonella*, and *Shigella*, were found in 21 of the 40 patients. Two patients had Kaposi's sarcoma of the duodenum. Fifteen of 38 patients had HIV antigen p24 detected in mononuclear cells from the intestinal mucosa (table). However, the presence of HIV-infected mucosal cells did not correlate with CD4+ cell counts in peripheral blood.

Fifteen of 25 patients had no detectable lactase activity in the duodenal brush-border membrane, and when it was measurable, activity was significantly decreased. Patients infected with HIV but no intestinal infection and patients with HIV antigen p24 in their mucosa had decreased numbers of mitotic figures per crypt, but normal crypt depths. On the other hand, HIV-infected patients with additional enteric infections had a normal number of mitotic figures per crypt, but crypt depths were increased.

Infection with HIV may cause structural and functional damage to the

Laboratory Findings for Patients With HIV Infection Correlated With Stage of Disease, Intestinal Pathogens, and Mucosal HIV Antigen p24

	Normal Values[†]	Values for HIV-Infected Patients[‡]	HIV-Infected Patients with Abnormal Values	Stage of Disease		Mucosal HIV Antigen p24		Intestinal Infection	
				II/III	IV	Negative	Positive	Negative	Positive
Protein, g/L	76(65-87)	73(46-88)	7/40§	0/7	7/33	3/21	1/15	3/28	4/12
Albumin, g/L	40(33-49)	38(25-52)	7/40	1/7	6/33	3/21	2/15	4/28	3/12
Folic acid, nmol/L	22(9-34)	15.4(3.6-37.6)	11/28	2/4	9/24	5/13	5/11	5/18	6/10
Vitamin B$_{12}$, pmol/L	148-738	251(105-610)	4/28	1/4	3/24	1/13	2/11	2/18	2/10
Calcium, mmol/L	2.48(2.24-2.78)	2.12(1.62-2.57)	23/32	4/6	19/26	11/17	9/12	15/22	8/10
Zinc, μmol/L	16.7(14.5-19.9)	14.6(12.2-19.6)	4/8	0/1	4/7	2/4	1/2	3/6	1/2
H$_2$ exhalation (lactose)			7/12	0	7/12	5/8	2/4	6/8	1/4
D-Xylose absorption			2/7	0	2/7	1/5	1/2	1/5	1/2

*Serum phosphate concentrations were normal in 32 investigated cases.
†Median (2nd-98th percentile).
‡Median (minimum-maximum).
§Patients with abnormal values/patients studied.
(Courtesy of Ullrich R, Zeitz M, Heise W, et al: *Ann Intern Med* 111:15-21, July 1, 1989.)

mucosa in the small intestine. However, the presence of an opportunistic intestinal infection may mask the mucosal atrophy.

▶ Miller et al. (1) also have provided evidence indicating that the jejunal mucosal architecture is often abnormal in patients infected with HIV, and that such abnormalities can be masked by an opportunistic infection. These investigators measured fat absorption, using the ^{14}C triolein breath test in stages of HIV disease. Enteropathogens were not detected in the stool or jejunal mucosa of any subject at the time of jejunal biopsy. Partial villous atrophy, the sole histologic abnormality, was detected at any clinical stage of HIV disease. The ^{14}C triolein breath test was correlated quantitatively with the degree of jejunal villous atrophy.

The cause of chronic diarrhea and malabsorption in HIV disease is multifactorial. Opportunistic chronic enteric infection is undoubtedly a major cause of intestinal dysfunction. In a group of patients without demonstrable enteropathogens, however, there is clearly an epithelial morphological abnormality, partial villous atrophy, that may contribute to fat malabsorption. The etiology of such partial villous atrophy is unknown, but may be related to direct infection of epithelial cells by HIV, immunologic mechanisms, or both.—N.J. Greenberger, M.D.

Reference

1. Miller ARO, et al: Jejunal mucosal architecture and fat absorption in male homosexuals infected with human immunodeficiency virus. *Q J Med* 69:1009, 1988.

Treatment and Prophylaxis of *Isospora belli* Infection in Patients With the Acquired Immunodeficiency Syndrome
Pape JW, Verdier R-I, Johnson WD Jr (Haitian Study Group on Kaposi's Sarcoma and Opportunistic Infection, Port-au-Prince, Haiti; Cornell Univ)
N Engl J Med 320:1044–1047, April 20, 1989   19–2

Isospora belli is a common opportunistic enteric pathogen in patients with AIDS. It responds promptly to treatment with trimethoprim-sulfamethoxazole, but the incidence of recurrence is high. A total of 32 Haitian patients with AIDS complicated by *I. belli* infection and chronic diarrhea were studied to investigate the effect of long-term prophylaxis. Initially, all patients were treated with trimethoprim, 160 mg and sulfamethoxazole 800 mg administered orally 4 times daily for 10 days. Thereafter, 12 patients were randomized to receive sulfadoxine 500 mg and pyrimethamine, 25 mg, weekly; 10 patients received trimethoprim, 160 mg, and sulfamethoxazole, 800 mg, 3 times a week; and 10 patients received a placebo.

All stool specimens were negative for *I. belli* after 2 days of the initial 10-day course of treatment with trimethoprim-sulfamethoxazole. None of the 22 patients who received prophylactic therapy with either trimethoprim-sulfamethoxazole or sulfadoxine-pyrimethamine had a recurrence of symptomatic isosporiasis. In contrast, half of the placebo-treated patients had recurrent, symptomatic isosporiasis within a mean of 1.6 months after the initial treatment. *Isospora belli* was detected in the stool of only 1 patient who received trimethoprim-sulfamethoxazole, compared with 5 of 10 placebo-treated patients. Except for severe pruritus requiring discontinuation of the drugs in 2 patients, both drug combinations were well tolerated. Ten patients continued to receive the prophylactic regimen for a mean of 16 months without recurrent isosporiasis.

Isosporiasis in patients with AIDS can be treated effectively with a 10-day course of trimethoprim-sulfamethoxazole. Recurrent isosporiasis can be prevented by ongoing prophylaxis with either trimethoprim-sulfamethoxazole or sulfadoxine-pyrimethamine.

➤ Isosporiasis is an uncommon, but important diarrheal disease of human beings that, like cryptosporidiosis, is life-threatening in patients with AIDS. *Isospora belli* infection responds rapidly to therapy with trimethoprim-sulfamethoxazole, but patients with AIDS have a high rate of adverse reactions to this therapy. Weiss and colleagues (1) reported 2 patients with AIDS, sulfonamide allergy, and *I. belli* infection. Treatment with pyrimethamine alone, 75 mg/day, was successful, and recurrence was prevented with daily pyrimethamine therapy, 25 mg. Weiss and co-workers conclude that in patients with AIDS and sulfonamide allergy or intolerance, pyrimethamine, 75 mg/day, with folinic acid, 10 µg/day, seems a reasonable alternative therapy for *I. belli* infection.—N.J. Greenberger, M.D.

Reference

1. Weiss LM et al: *Isospora belli* infection: Treatment with pyrimethamine. *Ann Intern Med* 109:474–475, 1988.

20 Short Bowel Syndrome

In Neonates

Extensive Short-Bowel Syndrome in Neonates: Outcome in the 1980s
Caniano DA, Starr J, Ginn-Pease ME (Ohio State Univ; Children's Hosp, Columbus, Ohio)
Surgery 105:119–124, February 1989   20-1

The clinical courses, operative requirements, achievement of enteral alimentation, morbidity, and mortality of 14 infants with extensive short-bowel syndrome (SBS) treated from 1978 to 1987 were studied. Extensive SBS is defined as a residual jejunoileal length of 25% or less than the normal expected length for each infant's gestational age. Most of the SBS was a result of congenital abdominal wall or midgut anomalies, (e.g., gastroschisis, jejunal atresia, midgut volvulus, and congenital SBS); 2 of the cases were caused by necrotizing enterocolitis.

Mean residual jejunoileal length was 32 cm (range, 15–53 cm), which represented an average 16% of normal expected jejunoileal length for gestational age. Problems related to total parenteral nutrition (TPN) accounted for the greatest morbidity, and included catheter sepsis in 13 infants, cholestasis in 8, central venous thrombosis in 4, and cholelithiasis in 3. The survival rate was 86%. Two infants died of end-stage liver disease. Of the 12 survivors, 8 have achieved intestinal adaptation and had discontinued TPN, 3 were maintained with combined TPN-enteral feeding, and 1 received TPN only. An intact ileocecal valve, as compared with the absence of such a valve, allowed intestinal adaptation and enteral alimentation in patients with shorter jejunoileal length. The mean cost of the initial hospitalization was $315,000, with an average stay of 450 days.

Survival and eventual enteral alimentation can be anticipated for most neonates with extensive SBS. However, morbidity remains a problem, and methods to decrease the morbidity of prolonged TPN and to enhance the adaptive process of the residual intestine must be developed. Home-based TPN and enteral feeding for infants with SBS may lessen significantly the economic impact of this condition.

▶ The capacity for the small bowel to adapt to shortening of its length has been known in experimental animals for decades. Parenteral nutrition has allowed not only an increased survival from extensive enterectomy in infants, but also documentation that adaptation of the developing gut of man can lead ultimately to normal enteral feeding. However, it takes time, is costly, and is associated with a significant morbidity. We must study the adaptive process to learn how it might be accelerated. An average hospital stay of 450 days at a cost of more than $300,000 should provide a strong stimulus for more research in this important area.—F.G. Moody, M.D.

Somatostatin Analogues

Effect of a Long Acting Somatostatin Analogue SMS 201-995 on Jejunostomy Effluents on Patients With Severe Short Bowel Syndrome
Ladefoged K, Christensen KC, Hegnhøj J, Jarnum S (Rigshospitalet, Copenhagen)
Gut 30:943–949, July 1989

Patients with ileostomy and jejunostomy and severe short-bowel syndrome have excessive losses of sodium and water in stomal effluents. Permanent parenteral nutrition, which may be administered at home, is necessary for some patients. However, this procedure makes heavy demands on patients. Finding a way to reduce stomal effluents that would increase intestinal net absorption enough to make parenteral nutrition unnecessary would be clinically significant.

Five patients with Crohn's disease and 1 with radiation enteropathy were studied. One patient with Crohn's disease had an ileostomy; the rest had jejunostomies. Patients had normal food intake but, because of severe malabsorption, had required home-based parenteral nutrition for a mean of 35 months. Patients ate a constant diet with fixed daily amounts of all nutrients, including sodium and water, for 12 days, and continued with their usual daily parenteral programs. After a 2-day basal period, they were randomized to receive intravenous infusion of either placebo or a long-acting somatostatin analogue, SMS 201-295, 25µg/hr for 2 days. The treatment was reversed for the next 2 days, with patients acting as their own controls. After a new 2-day basal period, patients were again randomized to receive subcutaneous administration of either placebo or SMS for 2 days and vice versa for the next 2 days. The SMS was given in a dose of 50µg every 12 hours. Five patients continued with subcutaneous administration of SMS at home for a median of 22 weeks after the balance study was completed.

Fecal mass was reduced, and net intestinal sodium absorption was increased by intravenous infusion of SMS 25 µg/hr; however, net absorptions of potassium, magnesium, calcium, phosphate, zinc, nitrogen, and fat were unaffected. Subcutaneous injections of SMS had a similar effect on net intestinal absorption of sodium and water. In patients who continued the protocol at home, the effect on fecal sodium loss persisted. However, in 1 patient, fecal mass was increased to the point at which it exceeded pretreatment values.

It may be that SMS increases net absorption of sodium and water because of reduced secretion of digestive juices, rather than by increasing absorptive capacity. Although SMS may be useful as an antidiarrheal drug for patients with high-output jejunostomies or ileostomies, its effect is not significant enough to alter management for patients who require permanent parenteral nutrition.

▶ This is essentially a negative study in that, although somatostatin effected a net reduction in stomal fecal loss of water and sodium, the magnitude was not sufficient to affect the need for total parenteral nutrition. Furthermore, only the secretory limb of the process appeared to be involved. One would think that a decrease in intestinal motility would have provided a large resident time for absorption. The authors suggest that somatostatin therapy be used only for patients with severe stomal diarrheal symptoms.—F.G. Moody, M.D.

Somatostatin and Somatostatin Analogue (SMS 201-995) in Treatment of Hormone-Secreting Tumors of the Pituitary and Gastrointestinal Tract and Non-Neoplastic Diseases of the Gut
Gorden P, Comi RJ, Maton PN, Go VLW (Natl Inst of Diabetes and Digestive and Kidney Diseases, Bethesda, Md)
Ann Intern Med 110:35–50, Jan 1, 1989   20–3

Somatostatin, a peptide that can act as a neurotransmitter, a systemic hormone, or a local hormone, can inhibit the secretion of hormones and other cell products. The synthetic somatostatin analogue SMS 201–995 is given subcutaneously and can be administered 2 or 3 times a day. Its biologic half-life is 90–120 minutes. The analogue is generally well tolerated.

The analogue SMS 201–995 can lower plasma growth hormone and somatomedin-C levels in patients with pituitary acromegaly. In those with pituitary thyrotropin-producing pituitary tumors, the analogue has produced clinical and biochemical responses and is especially helpful when tumor resection is not feasible. Symptoms are controlled in some patients with gut neuroendocrine tumors (table), but optimal dosing and the possibility of drug resistance require further study. Diarrhea is controlled in patients with carcinoid syndrome and in most of those with pancreatic isletcell tumor producing vasoactive intestinal peptide.

Some nonmalignant disorders of the gut such as secretory diarrhea and fistulation of unknown cause can respond to treatment with somatostatin. Some success with the treatment in patients who have significant gastrointestinal bleeding is reported.

▶ For another review article on the therapeutic potential of the long-acting somatostatin analogue (octreotide) in gastrointestinal diseases, see the paper by O'Donnell and Farthing.(1). These authors critically review the use of octreotide in gut endocrine tumors as well as in the following disorders:

1. Upper gastrointestinal bleeding caused by esophageal varices: octreotide has been reported to be as effective as vasopressin.

2. Pancreatic and enterocutaneous fistulas: closure in 50% to 80% of patients has been reported.

3. Short bowel syndrome: improvement in fluid and electrolyte balance and reduced requirement for total parenteral nutrition has been noted.

4. Dumping syndrome: short-term benefits have been reported, but some patients are unable to handle the drug because of the occurrence of diarrhea.

Relative Usefulness of SMS 201–995 in Treating Symptoms of Gut Neuroendocrine Tumors

Syndrome	Usefulness of SMS 201-995	Other Available Therapy
Carcinoid syndrome	Very useful for flushing and diarrhea. The most effective drug available. Also useful in carcinoid crisis.	Parachlorophenylalanine, methyl dopa, phenoxybenzamine, chlorpromazine, cyproheptadine, methysergide, H_1 plus H_2 antagonists, steroids, tamoxifen—variably effective, mainly on diarrhea. Hepatic embolization and interferon effective but significant side effects.
Benign insulinoma	Not useful.	Surgery curative.
Malignant or nonresectable insulinoma	Uncertain. May make symptoms worse.	Diazoxide is treatment of choice. Also verapamil, diphenylhydantoin. Hepatic embolization and chemotherapy (streptozotocin, 5-fluorouracil) effective but significant side effects.

Gastrinoma	Not as useful as alternatives.	Cimetidine, ranitidine, famotidine, omeprazole—all can control symptoms.
VIPoma	Very useful—the most effective drug available.	Steroids, indomethacin, lithium carbonate, opiates, propranolol, phenothiazines, calcium chanel blockers—variably effective. Debulking surgery, hepatic embolization, chemotherapy (streptozotocin, chlorozotoxin) useful but significant side effects.
Glucagonoma	Uncertain—may help rash.	Oral and systemic zinc probably help rash. Nutritional supplements. Hepatic embolization, debulking surgery, and chemotherapy (streptozotocin, fluorouracil, or dacarbazine) effective but significant side effects.
GHRHoma	Useful second line therapy.	Pituitary surgery. Hepatic embolization.

Abbreviations: VIPoma, vasoactive intestinal peptide-producing tumor; GHRHoma, growth hormone releasing hormone-producing tumor. (Courtesy of Gorden P, Comi RJ, Maton PN, et al: *Ann Intern Med* 110:35–50, Jan 1, 1989.)

5. Irritable bowel syndrome: only anecdotal reports are available.
6. Pancreatitis: controlled trials are in progress.
7. Post-endoscopic retrograde cholangiopancreatography sequelae, i.e., pain, hyperamylasemia, and so on: studies are in progress.—N.J. Greenberger, M.D.

Reference

1. O'Donnell LJD, Farthing MJW: Therapeutic potential of a long-acting somatostatin analogue in gastrointestinal disease. *Gut* 30:1165, 1989.

21 Alimentary Tract Duplications and Atresia

Jejunal Atresia With "Apple Peel" Deformity: A Report of Eight Survivors
Manning C, Strauss A, Gyepes MT (Mem Hosp Med Ctr, Long Beach, Calif)
J Perinatol 9:281–286, September 1989   21–1

Until recently, few infants with apple peel atresia (APA) survived. The deformity, one of the most severe forms of intestinal atresia, now has a rapidly improving prognosis as a result of early detection, improved surgical techniques, and the development of total parenteral nutrition (TPN). Eight infants with APA, all of whom survived, were studied.

The 4 boys and 4 girls were born at 35 to 37 weeks' gestation. Birth weights varied considerably, from 1,760 g to 3,070 g. All but 1 of the mothers were multigravida and multipara; 5 had polyhydramnios. Prenatal ultrasound studies, obtained for 4 patients, showed polyhydramnios and dilatation of the fetal stomach and duodenum in 3 patients (Fig 21–1). Neonatal abdominal radio-

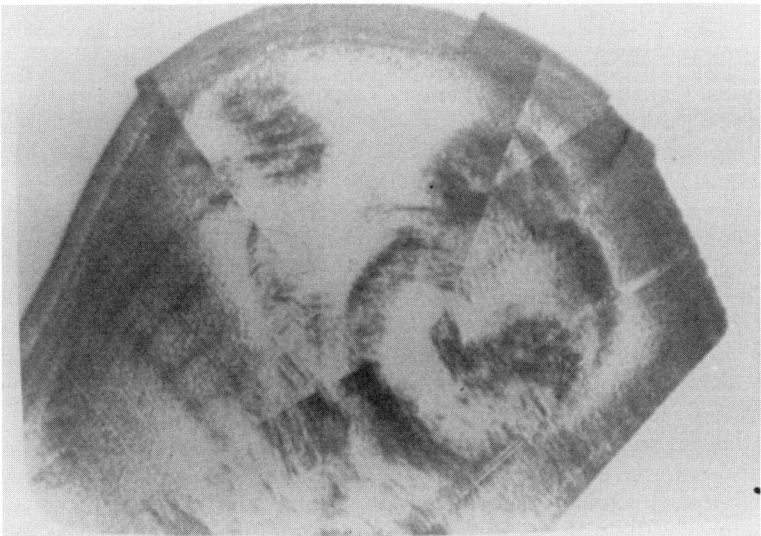

Fig 21–1.—Prenatal ultrasound scan of the fetal abdomen shows poyhydramnios, as well as a dilated stomach (S) and duodenal sweep (D). (Courtesy of Fletman D, McQuown D, Kanchanapoom V, et al: "Apple peel" atresia of the small bowel: prenatal diagnosis of the obstruction by ultrasound. *Pediatr Radiol* 9: 118, 1980. From Manning C, Strauss A, Gyepes MT: *J Perinatol* 9:281–286, September 1989.)

graphs revealed dilatation of the stomach and duodenal sweep in all but 1 infant.

Surgery was undertaken promptly and included resection of the atretic small bowel and appropriate anastomoses. Two infants required additional resections, and 1 was reoperated on for a rapidly developing stricture. All but 1 infant needed prolonged postoperative TPN. At discharge, ranging from 2 to 12 weeks, all were on oral feedings.

As part of APA, a substantial portion of the proximal embryonic jejunum disintegrates after vascular occlusion in the superior mesenteric artery. Pregnant women in whom polyhydramnios is suspected should undergo ultrasound scan so that gastric and duodenal dilatation can be detected. A definitive diagnosis of APA can be established only at surgery.

Between 1956 and 1986, the mortality associated with APA and multiple atresias dropped from 90% to 10%. In addition to early detection of such conditions and appropriate surgery, TPN has been a key factor in improving the survival rate. The short, postsurgical bowel can recover and grow while the infant is nourished parenterally for weeks or even months.

▶ The value of TPN in the treatment of neonatal gastrointestinal disorders that require resection of large segments of the gut is well illustrated in this report. Dudrick and his colleagues, in their pioneering work at the University of Pennsylvania, presciently chose to demonstrate the efficacy of TPN in weanling puppies. The positive results from their experiment and the subsequent application of TPN to children as well as adults have saved many lives. Finding a way to prevent such lesions as duodenal atresia or to treat them early in the course of a pregnancy before they contribute to loss of gut substance or function now remains.—F.G. Moody, M.D.

Surgical Management of Alimentary Tract Duplications
Holcomb GW III, Gheissari A, O'Neill JA Jr, Shorter NA, Bishop HC (Univ of Pennsylvania)
Ann Surg 209:167–174, February 1989

Duplications secondary to disordered embryonic development of the gut can occur anywhere from the mouth to the anus. Ninety-six infants and children seen since 1950 with 101 alimentary tract duplications were studied. About one third of the patients were seen before age 1 month. Seventy-five duplications were cystic, and 26 were tubular in form. In 19 patients, duplications were associated with atresia. Gastric mucosa was present in 21 duplications, and pancreatic tissue, in 5.

All of the thoracic duplications were cystic in form. These usually are found in the posterior mediastinum; most are in the lower half of the esophagus. Computed tomography demonstrates the relationship of the mass to adjacent structures without the invasiveness of barium esophagography. The gastric duplications also were cystic. Ileal duplications were relatively frequent, and in older patients often caused rectal bleeding and intussusception.

Isolated colonic duplications have widely varying presentations. The typical rectal duplication is cystic and presents itself as a gradually enlarging mass adjacent to the anal canal. Three of the study patients had combined thoracoabdominal duplications, and 5 had separate thoracic and intestinal duplications.

▶ Pediatricians and pediatric surgeons are quite aware of duplications of the gut and the clinical syndromes they produce. Many such lesions, however, are asymptomatic and escape detection until by chance an ultrasound or CT scan is obtained. This report documents the variety of such lesions that may affect the gut from esophagus to rectum.—F.G. Moody, M.D.

22 Ileal Bypass for Hypercholesterolemia

Reappraisal of Partial Ileal Bypass for the Treatment of Familial Hypercholesterolemia
Ohri SK, Keane PF, Swift I, Sackier JM, Williamson RCN, Thompson GR, Wood CB
(Hammersmith Hosp, London)
Am J Gastroenterol 84:740–743, July 1989   22-1

Familial hypercholesterolemia (FH) often is treated with partial ileal bypass (PIB). This treatment was evaluated in 11 patients with heterozygous FH, type IIa.

Six adult male and 5 adult female FH heterozygotes underwent PIB because serum cholesterol levels could not be controlled with conventional medical management. All patients underwent initial treatment with cholestyramine. Angiography established coronary artery disease in all but 1 patient. Six had undergone coronary artery bypass grafting, and 5 had had myocardial infarctions. After PIB, hypocholesterolemic drugs were discontinued for all patients, but they received vitamin B_{12} and remained on dietary restriction. Five patients with refractory hypercholesterolemia were given lovastatin. One of these was given both lovastatin and low-density lipoprotein-apheresis.

After PIB, mean total cholesterol levels declined by 26% at 1 month, and then rose steadily to 20% below preoperative levels over the next 20 to 24 months. All patients had postoperative diarrhea, but at 1 year, no patient had more than 5 bowel movements per day. Three patients had severe abdominal distention and postprandial flatus. Metronidazole was helpful for only 1 patient; reversal of the ileal bypass eventually was necessary in the other 2. After reversal, these patients were given lovastatin to control recrudescence of hypercholesterolemia. In the other patients given lovastatin, 2, who were on 40 mg/day, had 18% reduction in mean serum cholesterol levels, and the other, who received 20 mg/day, had a reduction of 16%. Ten patients remained alive and well; 1 patient died after a myocardial infarction 55 months after surgery.

Lovastatin acts synergistically with PIB to lower cholesterol levels, and also allows for reversal of bypass in symptomatic patients. The advent of lovastatin and other drugs inhibiting hydroxymethyl-glutaryl coenzyme A reductase may reduce the necessity for PIB in patients with FH; however, the long-term effects of these drugs has yet to be determined.

▶ Partial ileal bypass (PIB) lowers serum cholesterol by about 20% of its preoperative values. The small number of patients studied and the need for reversal of the procedure in 2 of 11 detracts from the effectiveness of the therapy. Furthermore, PIB appears to be no more effective in lowering cholesterol than HMG coA reductase lowering drugs. A better understanding of the pathogenesis of atherosclerosis possibly will provide a more specific therapy for its complications. Meanwhile, patients at high risk such as those reported here should receive treatment and be given a choice between the pill or the knife.—F.G. Moody, M.D.

23 Neoplasms

Inpatients With Familial Polyposis

Upper Gastrointestinal Cancer in Patients With Familial Adenomatous Polyposis
Spigelman AD, Williams CB, Talbot IC, Domizio P, Phillips RKS (St Mark's Hosp, London; St Bartholomew's Hosp, London)
Lancet 2:783–785, Sept 30, 1989   23-1

The risk of upper gastrointestinal cancer is increased in patients with familial adenomatous polyposis, and upper gastrointestinal cancer is a major cause of death in these patients. To determine the prevalence and natural history of polyps and identify patients at particular risk of duodenal cancer, 102 patients with familial adenomatous polyposis were screened.

Upper gastrointestinal endoscopy showed dysplasia in 94 patients and hyperplasia in 6. Ninety-one percent of these abnormalities involved the second and third parts of the duodenum only. The periampullary area was abnormal in 87 of 97 patients, with adenoma in 72, hyperplasia in 13, and inflammation in 2. In contrast, gastric dysplasia was found in only 6 of 73 patients who had gastric biopsy.

When the severity of duodenal polyposis was classified on a 5-grade scale (stages 0–IV) based on number of polyps, size, histology, and severity of dysplasia, most patients had stage II or III disease. Eleven patients with a mean age of 51 years had stage IV duodenal polyposis.

For most patients with familial adenomatous polyposis who have mild to moderate disease, an interval of 3 years between follow-up endoscopies seems appropriate. However, patients with severe (stage IV) disease who are at greatest risk of malignant change must have endoscopy at least yearly. Preventive surgery, such as duodenotomy or pancreaticoduodenectomy, may be indicated for patients with severe adenomatous polyposis who have rapid growth of polyps, polyp induration, or consistently severe dysplasia.

▶ This study, along with other similar reports, indicates that upper gastrointestinal cancer, related to adenomatous polyps, is a major cause of death among patients with familial adenomatous polyposis. Careful screening of the upper gastrointestinal tract of these patients should improve our knowledge of the natural history of these polyps and further define the most appropriate treatment at various stages of the disease. It is interesting to note that within the duodenum, the greatest concentration of adenomas is on or around the papilla. This distribution raises the question of whether adenoma formation is related to bile exposure and to some tumor-promoting substance in bile.

How should familial adenomatous polyposis be managed? Spigelman and colleagues suggest that patients have regular upper gastrointestinal endoscopy at which periampullary maps are drawn and video tapes and still photographs are taken to record the natural progress of their gastroduodenal polyps. However, the treatment of such upper gastrointestinal polyps remains controversial. As Spigelman et al. point out, endoscopic removal is often unpractical because sessile polyps cannot be snared and perforation may occur, whereas endoscopic electrocoagulation may cause periampullary scarring and bile duct obstruction. For patients with severe duodenal polyposis, rapid polyp growth, and severe dysplasia, the choices are duodenotomy with tumor removal (which is usually only of temporary benefit) or pancreaticoduodenectomy. The latter procedures have potential morbidity, which must be weighed against the uncertain natural history of these polyps. If both severe dysplasia and abnormal flow cytometry can be demonstrated in polyps, and especially if such polyps are recurrent, I believe pancreaticoduodenectomy is warranted.—N.J. Greenberger, M.D.

Recognition at Emergent Laparotomy

Primary Small Bowel Malignant Tumors: Unrecognized Until Emergent Laparotomy
Brophy C, Cahow CE (Yale Univ)
Am Surg 55:408–412, July 1989   23–2

Primary small bowel carcinomas comprise less than 1% of all gastrointestinal (GI) malignancies, but their clinical presentation is often ubiquitous. The Yale surgical experience with primary small bowel malignancies from 1969 to 1983 was reviewed.

Records of 45 primary small bowel carcinomas were included in the study. Data for clinical presentation, diagnostic work-up, surgical treatment, pathologic findings, and follow-up were evaluated. Patients included 26 females and 18 males, with age at presentation ranging from 6 to 77 years. The average age was 53 years.

The most common symptom was abdominal pain, followed by nausea, vomiting, or both, and weight loss. The average weight lost was 20 pounds. Two patients were asymptomatic. Sixty-four percent of patients had surgical emergencies. Fourteen patients had bowel obstruction, 11 had GI hemorrhage, and 4 had small bowel perforation. In the remaining 16 patients, surgical exploration was undertaken for persistent symptoms, a mass lesion on CT scan, or an abnormality on GI series.

Thirty-eight patients had surgical resection of the tumor, whereas 7 had palliative bypass procedures. At laparotomy, 70% of patients had distant metastases. Eighteen percent of patients had postoperative complications, and there was 1 postoperative death. The overall 5-year survival rate was 41%, but 83% of patients with carcinoid tumors had 5-year survival. Six living patients had known recurrence of their tumors more than 5 years after initial resection.

A high index of suspicion and early diagnostic procedures, including a small bowel series, are important to prevent many small bowel tumors presenting as surgical emergencies. Small bowel tumor should be suspected in patients with abdominal pain of unknown origin, occult GI bleeding, or unexplained weight loss.

➤ Brophy and Cahow provide a well-documented report of their experience with small bowel tumors. A unique feature of their series is that more than half of their patients were first seen as surgical emergencies, suggesting delay in diagnosis. That 70% had metastatic disease at the time of presentation adds further testimony to the difficulty in making an early diagnosis of these clinically silent lesions. Obtaining a small bowel follow-through as a component of an upper barium roentgenogram of the gastrointestinal tract is the key to early diagnosis.—F.G. Moody, M.D.

24 Small Bowel Obstruction

Diagnosis by Enteroclysis

Closed Loop Obstruction: Diagnosis by Enteroclysis
Price J, Nolan DJ (John Radcliffe Hosp, Oxford, England)
Gastrointest Radiol 14:251–254, 1989   24-1

Closed loop obstruction of the small bowel is an acute surgical emergency. Death may result from intestinal infarction, perforation, and peritonitis. Enteroclysis is an accurate means of demonstrating the site and degree of obstruction and often its cause. The enteroclysis tube may be left in place to promote decompression. Closed loop obstruction was diagnosed in 5 patients by using enteroclysis.

Closed loop obstruction often is caused by an adhesive band, but an internal hernia through a mesenteric or omental defect may be responsible. The loop fills with exudate to form a pseudotumor. Isolated gas-distended loops can produce the "coffee bean" sign on plain radiographs. Proximal obstruction may be accompanied by thickened valvulae conniventes.

Enteroclysis provides an accurate diagnosis of closed loop obstruction before gross dilation and formation of pseudotumor have taken place. Thickened valvulae conniventes in the closed loop may indicate impending strangulation.

▶ A closed loop obstruction is difficult to diagnose because the loop of bowel is obstructed at both ends and generally is filled with fluid. It may arise from adhesions or an internal hernia through the mesentery or omentum. The diagnosis by enteroclysis indicates the possibility of diagnosis before serious complications arise. Cho and co-workers (1) report two patients with closed loop obstruction identified with CT and sonographic findings of an isolated conglomerate of dilated fluid-filled loops fixed as U-shaped distended loops with thickened bowel wall and extraluminal fluid. Surgical intervention is necessary for this serious diagnosis before complications arise.—P.B. Miner, Jr., M.D.

Reference

1. Cho KC et al: *J Comput Assist Tomogr* 13:256, 1989.

Postoperative

The Management of Patients With Suspected Early Postoperative Small Bowel Obstruction
Pickleman J, Lee RM (Loyola Univ, Maywood, Ill)
Ann Surg 210:216–219, August 1989   24–2

Authorities disagree on appropriate management of early postoperative small bowel obstruction, possibly because few researchers have studied this presentation specifically, the condition has been variously defined, and the diagnosis is often difficult. A large series of patients with early postoperative small bowel obstruction was studied in an effort to formulate treatment guidelines.

Charts of all patients with early postoperative small bowel obstruction treated during a 10-year period were studied. Patients were included if signs and symptoms occurred within 30 days of surgery and lasted 1 week or more or if symptoms of small bowel obstruction of any duration appeared 7 to 30 days after surgery.

Of 53 males and 48 females, ranging in age from 4 to 87 years (mean, 58 years), 65 had undergone 1 or more prior celiotomies, and 26 had histories of small bowel obstruction, 22 of whom had required surgical intervention. Sixty-two patients had obstructive symptoms within the first week, with an average of 4 days.

Ninety-five patients underwent abdominal radiography, but only 73% of such studies were diagnostic of small bowel obstruction. An upper gastrointestinal study with small bowel follow-through identified a definite point of obstruction in 72% of patients for whom it was performed. Barium enema identified only 33% of obstructions. Obstruction was most often caused by adhesions and inflammatory processes.

Ninety-one patients were treated with nasogastric suction, and 10 were treated with a long intestinal tube. Neither tube had any advantage over the other in resolving the obstructions.

Twenty-three patients underwent reoperation an average of 7.7 days after nasogastric or long-tube suction. None of these patients had ischemic bowel at resection and in none was bowel resection required. When signs, symptoms, and laboratory data for patients who recovered without operation were compared with those for patients who were reoperated on, there were no significant differences between the groups. No patients in either group had bowel infarction. Three patients treated surgically died, as did 4 in the nonoperated-on group. No deaths were attributable to bowel infarction or intra-abdominal sepsis.

Because ischemic bowel is unlikely in patients with early postoperative small bowel obstruction, 1 to 2 weeks of nasogastric suction is recommended for initial treatment. After this period, improvement should not be expected without surgery.

▶ Pickleman and Lee provide evidence for what I have assumed was sound management of early postceliotomy intestinal obstruction, a 10- to 14-day period of nasogastric decompression. A nasojejunal tube usually is not required. The problem is usually one of procrastination and continued trials of suction beyond 2 weeks. This is clearly a mistake because surgical intervention will allow prompt resolution of the point of obstruction, which by that time will have declared that it is refractory to conservative management.—F.G. Moody, M.D.

25 Mesenteric Infarction

Comparison of Five Methods of Assessment of Intestinal Viability
Brolin RE, Semmlow JL, Sehonanda A, Koch RA, Reddell MT, Mast BA, Mackenzie JW (Univ of Medicine and Dentistry of New Jersey, New Brunswick)
Surg Gynecol Obstet 168:6–12, 1989   25–1

A major unsolved problem in surgical treatment of the gastrointestinal tract is the evaluation of viability of ischemic small intestine. A device consisting of a strain gauge probe was designed to be capable of quantitative measurement of intestinal ischemic damage. This device, the electronic contractility meter, is clipped on the serosal surface of the small intestine and delivers a precisely controlled electrical stimulus that produces a well-defined smooth muscle contraction over a 15-second response period. The minimal stimulus in milliamperes necessary to produce a smooth muscle contractile response was the threshold stimulus level (TSL). In 30 dogs resection and anastomosis in ischemic intestinal segments were carried out to relate TSL, intestinal color, peristalsis, Doppler ultrasound, and resection margin histologic findings to survival.

Five fatal anastomotic leaks occurred, all resulting from intestinal necrosis. At 4 of the 5 anastomoses that leaked, Doppler pulse in the marginal artery was absent compared with 8 of the 25 that healed. The mean TSL at the resection site was 51 mamp in nonsurvivors vs. 38 mamp in surviving dogs. In normal intestine the mean TSL was 22 mamp. Both Doppler ultrasound and TSL were correlated with resection margin histologic findings. No correlation was found between presence of peristalsis and histologic grade on survival rate. Intestinal color correlated with resection margin histologic findings but not survival. The TSL measured by the electronic contractility meter and marginal artery Doppler signal were the only 2 of the 5 methods of viability assessment that correlated with survival.

The quantitative measurements obtained with the electronic contractility meter were more sensitive indices of viability than the presence of pulsatile arterial flow as measured with Doppler ultrasound.

▶ The authors deal with 2 issues: the histologic characteristics of ischemic bowel and survival of the host as related to measurement of collateral blood flow and smooth muscle contractility. Doppler measurements of blood flow in the marginal artery were correlated with the healing potential of an anastomosis and survival of the animal with ischemic gut. The threshold electrical stimulus for muscle contraction was even more sensitive in this regard. This is certainly a more elegant way to test muscle inability than pinching the bowel wall with forceps, the usual clinical maneuver. I agree that the presence or absence of peristalsis and the color of the bowel is of little predictive value unless the gut is frankly gangrenous.—F.G. Moody, M.D.

Acute Mesenteric Infarction in Elderly Patients
Finucane PM, Arunachalam T, O'Dowd J, Pathy MSJ (Univ of Wales, Cardiff)
J Am Geriatr Soc 37:355–358, April 1989

Early surgical intervention can reduce the mortality associated with mesenteric insufficiency leading to acute bowel infarction. In elderly patients, however, bowel infarction can behave atypically. Death occurs quickly when this acute abdominal condition remains unrecognized. To identify clinical features in elderly patients and to compare outcome after admission to a surgical unit with that after assignment to a medical ward, data on 32 patients who met the criteria of ischemia secondary to primary vascular disease during the 8-year study period were reviewed. The patients' mean age was 78.5 years; 18 (56%) were women. Mesenteric thrombosis caused bowel infarction in 14 (44%) patients; 4 had a mesenteric embolus; 8 had mesenteric atherosclerosis; and in 6, mesenteric insufficiency was the presumed cause.

Eighteen patients were admitted to a surgical unit; 13, to a medical unit; and 1 died in transit to the hospital (Fig 25–1). Those in the surgical group were

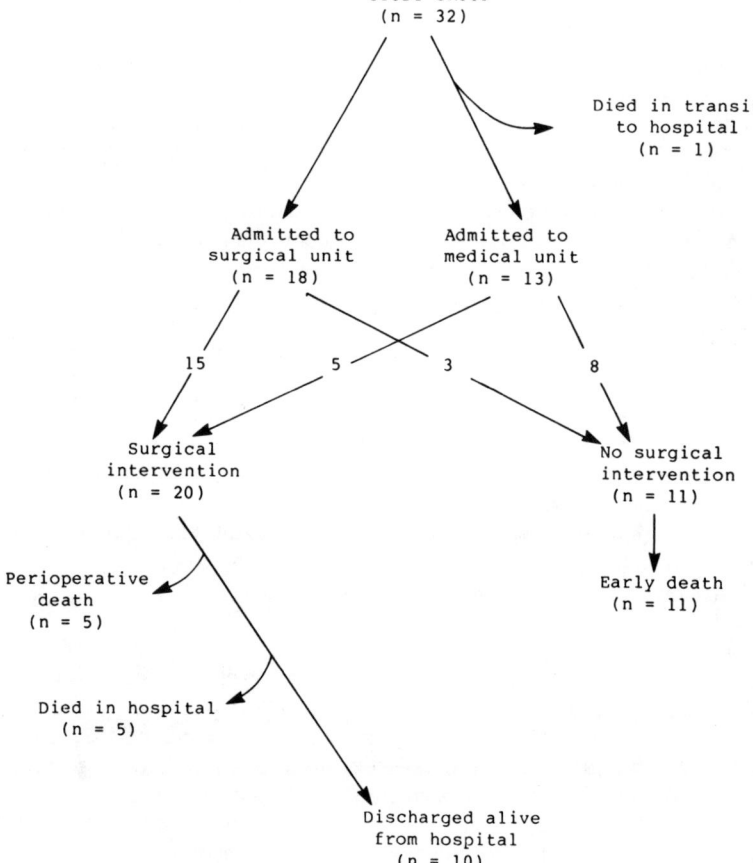

Fig 25–1.—Flow diagram showing the units to which patients were admitted and the outcome of hospitalization. (Courtesy of Finucane PM, Arunachalam T, O'Dowd J, et al: *J Am Geriatr Soc* 37:355–358, April 1989.)

more likely to have symptoms typical of bowel infarction, (e.g., abdominal tenderness and pain). Fifteen from the surgical group and 5 from the medical group underwent bowel resection. All 11 patients who did not undergo surgery died an average of 4 days after the onset of symptoms. Eight (44%) of the surgical group, but only 2 (15%) of the medical group survived to leave the hospital.

Mesenteric vascular disease is an uncommon condition and may go unrecognized, especially in elderly patients admitted to medical wards. Acute confusion was present in 29% of the patients. This sign should be a warning, whereas the absence of abdominal pain or tenderness should not rule out the possibility of bowel infarction.

▶ Bowel infarction from acute mesenteric ischemia in the elderly is a tough call. The only way to diagnose it is to perform a celiotomy and look at the bowel. The increasing use of the laparoscope by general surgeons possibly will provide more enthusiasm for an early look at the status of the small bowel in such patients.—F.G. Moody, M.D.

26 Crohn's Disease and Related Topics

Radiologic Considerations

Diagnosis of Fistulae and Sinus Tracts in Patients With Crohn Disease: Value of MR Imaging
Koelbel G, Schmiedl U, Majer MC, Weber P, Jenss H, Kueper K, Hess CF (Eberhard-Karls-Universität, West Germany)
AJR 152:999–1003, May 1989   26–1

The value of magnetic resonance (MR) imaging in assessing Crohn's disease was examined in 17 patients who had pelvic or abdominal fistulas or sinus tracts. Multislice spin-echo techniques were used. Fistulas and sinus tracts were confirmed by contrast-enhanced CT, sonography, sinography, or barium studies. An attempt was made to evaluate the levator ani on axial and coronal MR images.

Fistulas and sinus tracts appeared on T_1-weighted images as linear or tubular structures of low-signal intensity. Muscle inflammation associated with sinus tracts was hypointense on T_1 images and brighter on T_2-weighted images. Magnetic resonance imaging, as well as CT and sonography, failed to demonstrate fistulas encased by extensive inflammation in 2 cases. The origin of a fistula or sinus tract in the bowel wall was demonstrated in most patients. The MR findings correlated closely with the abnormalities seen on CT.

Fistulas may be mistaken for muscle inflammation on CT, and their enteric orifices may not be evident. Magnetic resonance imaging may overcome some of the limitations of CT in these cases. Coronal MR images effectively demonstrate the perirectal spread of fistulas and abscesses. However, neural and vascular structures in the perineum can be mistaken for fistulas on MR images.

▶ The usefulness of CT has been recognized for some time in evaluating fistulas and abscesses in patients with Crohn's disease. Magnetic resonance studies may provide better definition of pelvic floor musculature and identify the tract of a fistula better than CT because definition of muscle layers is improved with MR resolution. For the radiologist interested in MR and Crohn's disease the 11 figures in this paper are useful for review because they define numerous fistulas and areas of fluid accumulation in the pelvic floor, documenting the better resolution of MR than of CT.—P.B. Miner, Jr., M.D.

Immunosuppressive Therapy

Methotrexate Induces Clinical and Histologic Remission in Patients With Refractory Inflammatory Bowel Disease

Kozarek RA, Patterson DJ, Gelfand MD, Botoman VA, Ball TJ, Wilske KR (Virginia Mason Clinic, Seattle)
Ann Intern Med 110:353–356, March 1, 1989

Because of its anti-inflammatory properties methotrexate, an antimetabolite, may be useful in treating inflammatory bowel disease. In an open-label study 21 patients with refractory inflammatory disease, including 14 with Crohn's disease and 7 with chronic ulcerative colitis, received methotrexate, 25 mg intramuscularly weekly for 12 weeks, and were then switched to a tapering oral dose if clinical and objective improvement was noted. Azathioprine or 6-mercaptopurine trials previously had failed in 10 patients. Sulfasalazine and metronidazole therapy were continued while the prednisone dose was tapered.

Sixteen patients had significant clinical improvement as evidenced by the modified Crohn's Disease Activity Index, which fell significantly from a mean of 13.3 to 5.4, and the Ulcerative Colitis Activity Index, which fell from 13.3 to 6.3 (table).

Eleven of 14 patients with Crohn's disease and 5 of 7 patients with chronic ulcerative colitis had improvement. Steroid therapy was tapered in 14 of 17 patients and was withdrawn from 5. Five patients with Crohn's disease had colonoscopic healing, and 4 had normal histology at 12 weeks. In contrast, none of the 7 patients with ulcerative colitis had completely normal histologic findings on repeat biopsy specimens, despite histologic improvement in 5. Side effects included transient leukopenia, mild increases in levels of transaminase, nausea and diarrhea, brittle nails, and atypical pneumonitis.

Although the results of this pilot study are encouraging, further studies are necessary before methotrexate can be recommended for treatment of inflammatory bowel disease.

▶ Methotrexate is an antimetabolite and anti-inflammatory drug that has been applied to a heterogeneous group of illnesses, including rheumatoid arthritis, polymyositis, psoriasis, Reiter's syndrome, and refractory asthma. I would like to cite a key paragraph of the discussion section of this paper.

"Although there is a precedent in treating refractory chronic ulcerative colitis or Crohn's disease with immunosuppressive agents such as 6-mercaptopurine or azathioprine, methotrexate therapy differs in several ways. In the dosage used, immunosuppression does not appear to occur. In addition, whereas azathioprine and 6-mercaptopurine often require between 3 and 6 months to induce remission, methotrexate may work more quickly. Thus, several patients with inflammatory bowel disease improved dramatically in as little as 2 weeks, and most patients who responded improved markedly after 8 to 10 weeks. Because of the investigational nature of this treatment, we elected to discontinue methotrexate therapy if there was no significant clinical improvement after 12 weeks. It is possible, however, that a longer treatment course may have been beneficial in the nonresponding patients

Clinical Response and Corticosteroid Dosing of Administration of Methotrexate to 14 Patients With Refractory Crohn's Disease

Patient	Disease Site	Follow-up in Weeks	Response	Prednisone Dose		Modified Crohn's Activity Index		Ongoing Methotrexate Therapy
				at Onset	at 12 Weeks	at Onset	at 12 Weeks	
1	Colon	40	Yes	20	0	15	5	Yes
2	Colon	30	Yes	0	0	10	2	Yes
3	Small bowel	36	Yes	20	0	15	6	Yes
4	Colon	22	Yes	15	10	15	2	No
5	Colon	22	Yes	10	2.5	7	2	Yes
6	Colon	12	No	40	15	14	9	No
7	Small bowel	12	No	0	0	15	15	No
8	Small bowel	9	Yes	60	0	15	7	Yes
9	Small bowel, colon	18	Yes*	0	0	15	7	Yes
10	Small bowel	12	Yes	15	15	13	6	Yes
11	Small bowel	20	Yes	60	20	15	3	Yes
12	Colon	32	Yes	20	0	11	1	Yes
13	Small bowel, colon	12	No	40	15	12	10	No
14	Small bowel, colon	26	Yes	0	0	4	0	Yes
Mean†		22.5		21.4 ± 5.6	5.5 ± 2.0‡	13.3 ± 0.9	5.4 ± 1.5§	

*Patient relapsed off parenteral methotrexate.
†Mean is ± standard error where applicable.
‡P = .0006 determined by paired t-test.
§P = .0001 determined by paired t-test
(Courtesy of Kozarek RA, Patterson DJ, Gelfland MD, et al: Ann Intern Med 110:353–356, March 1, 1989.)

similar to the course sometimes required for response to 6-mercaptopurine or azathioprine."—N.J. Greenberger, M.D.

6-Mercaptopurine in the Management of Inflammatory Bowel Disease: Short- and Long-Term Toxicity

Present DH, Meltzer SJ, Krumholz MP, Wolke A, Korelitz BI (Lenox Hill Hosp, New York; New York Med College, Valhalla; Mount Sinai School of Medicine, New York)
Ann Intern Med 111:641–649, Oct 15, 1989

Despite its proved efficacy many physicians are reluctant to use 6-mercaptopurine to treat inflammatory bowel disease because of its potential side effects. Data were reviewed from 18 years of treating 120 patients with ulcerative colitis and 276 patients with Crohn's disease with 6-mercaptopurine. Data on follow-ups averaging 60.3 months were obtained for 90% of the patients.

Toxicity directly induced by 6-mercaptopurine included pancreatitis in 13 patients (3.3%), bone marrow depression in 8 (2%), allergic reactions in 8 (2%), and drug hepatitis in 1 (0.3%; Table 1). All these complications were reversible and no patient died. Most cases of marrow depression were related to dose and were quickly reversible when 6-mercaptopurine was stopped. Infectious complications occurred in 29 patients (7.4%); 7 (1.8%) were severe, including 1 case of herpes zoster encephalitis. All these infections also had been seen in patients with inflammatory disease who were not taking immunosuppressives. All infections resolved, and no deaths occurred.

Twelve neoplasms (3.1%) were recorded, but only 1 (0.3%), a diffuse histiocytic lymphoma of the brain, had a probable association with the use of 6-mercaptopurine (Table 2). One child had a Wilm's tumor at age 4 years, but no other tumors or congenital abnormalities were observed in infants born to mothers who took 6-mercaptopurine during pregnancy.

The low incidence of toxicity of 6-mercaptopurine and the potential toxicity of long-term steroid therapy make 6-mercaptopurine a reasonable alternative in the management of patients with intractable inflammatory bowel disease.

▶ The major findings in this study are summarized below. Of 396 patients with ulcerative colitis or Crohn's disease treated with 6-mercaptopurine, toxicity directly

Table 1.—Toxicity Directly Induced by 6-Mercaptopurine in 396 Patients With Inflammatory Bowel Disease

Toxicity	Number (Percent)
Pancreatitis	13 (3.3)
Bone marrow depression	8 (2.0)
Allergic reactions	8 (2.0)
Drug hepatitis	1 (0.3)
Total	30 (7.6)

All toxicities were reversible; no patients died.
(Courtesy of Present DH, Meltzer SJ, Krumholz MP, et al: *Ann Intern Med* 111:641–649, Oct 15, 1989.)

TABLE 2.—Neoplasms Observed in Patients Taking 6-Mercaptopurine

Type of Neoplasm	Type of Inflammatory Bowel Disease	Taking Drug at Diagnosis of Tumor	6-Mercaptopurine			Duration off Drug	Other Medications at Time of Tumor
			Duration	Mean Dose	Cumulative Dose		
			mo	mg	g	mo	
Histiocytic lymphoma	Crohn disease	No	9	100	27	11	Steroids, sulfa
Malignant melanoma	Ulcerative colitis	No	24	75	54	3	Steroids, sulfa, antibiotics
Islet-cell carcinoma	Crohn disease	No	7	100	21	30	Steroids, sulfa, antibiotics
Carcinoma, lung	Crohn disease	No	12	75	27	72	None
Carcinoma, colon	Ulcerative colitis	Yes	3	75	7	—	Steroids
Adenomatous polyps	Ulcerative colitis	Yes	58	60	100	—	Sulfa
Basal-cell carcinoma	Crohn disease	No	83	50	125	4	Steroids, sulfa
Basal-cell carcinoma	Crohn disease	Yes	14	75	32	—	Steroids
Prolactinoma	Ulcerative colitis	No	42	100	126	71	Sulfa, cholestyramine
Carcinoma, breast	Crohn disease	No	47	75	106	12	Sulfa
Papilloma, bladder	Crohn disease	Yes	17	50	26	—	Sulfa, antibiotics
Adenoma, thyroid	Ulcerative colitis	Yes	12	75	27	—	Sulfa

(Courtesy of Present DH, Meltzer SJ, Krumholz MP, et al: *Ann Intern Med* 111:641–649, Oct 15, 1989.)

attributable to the drug occurred in 7.6% and infectious complications occurred in 7.4%. No deaths occurred from either complication. Neoplasms were observed in 3.1%, a percentage similar to that seen in patients with inflammatory bowel disease not taking immunosuppressives. Therefore, contrasting the level of toxicity reported in this study with the potential toxicity of long-term steroid therapy, the authors consider 6-mercaptopurine to be a reasonable alternative in the management of intractable inflammatory bowel disease.

Present and associates reviewed 4 trials in which azathioprine was used to treat ulcerative colitis and 8 randomized controlled trials in which immunosuppressive drugs were used for Crohn's disease. Azathioprine showed significant steroid sparing in patients with ulcerative colitis, but the trials failed to demonstrate any consistent endoscopic or symptomatic improvement. Of 8 randomized controlled trials of immunosuppressive agents for Crohn's disease, 2 showed statistically significant efficacy in maintenance of remission, 1 showed significant steroid sparing, and 1 showed significant steroid sparing as well as clinical improvement. Four trials showed no statistically significant improvement, but 2 suggested subsets of patients who might have responded.—N.J. Greenberger, M.D.

A Placebo-Controlled, Double-Blind, Randomized Trial of Cyclosporine Therapy in Active Chronic Crohn's Disease
Brynskov J, Freund L, Rasmussen SN, Lauritsen K, Schaffalitzky de Muckadell O, Williams N, MacDonald AS, Tanton R, Molina F, Campanini MC, Bianchi P, Ranzi T, Quarto di Palo F, Malchow-Møller A, Østergaard Thomsen O, Tage-Jensen U, Binder V, Riis P (Herlev Univ Hosp, Copenhagen; Aalborg Hosp, Aalborg; Odense Univ Hosp, Odense, Denmark, Dalhousie Univ–Victoria Gen Hosp, Halifax, NS; Ospedale Maggiore, Milan, Italy; et al)
N Engl J Med 321:845–850, Sept 28, 1989   26–4

The pathogenesis of Crohn's disease is as yet unknown, but evidence suggests an autoimmune origin. Low-dose cyclosporine provides an acceptable therapeutic compromise in patients with active chronic Crohn's disease because the risk of cyclosporine associated nephropathy is offset by its potential for efficacy.

During a 19-month study period 71 patients with active chronic Crohn's disease were randomly assigned treatment with cyclosporine, 5–7.5 mg/kg/day orally, or placebo for 3 months. Thirty-seven patients aged 19–60 years received cyclosporine, and 34 patients aged 16–68 years received placebo. Of the 70 patients who had previously been given steroids, 44 (63%) had resistance, 21 (29%) had intolerance, and 5 (7%) had both resistance to and intolerance of steroid therapy. One patient had refused steroid therapy.

After 3 months of treatment 22 (59%) of the 37 cyclosporine-treated patients and 11 (32%) of the 34 placebo-treated patients had clinical improvement. The difference between the 2 groups was statistically significant (table). Improvement was substantial in nearly one third of the cyclosporine-treated patients. Plasma orosomucoid levels and the Crohn's Disease Activity Index values were significantly improved during cyclosporine treatment.

Improvement During the 3-Month Treatment Period		
	CYCLOSPORINE (N = 37)	PLACEBO (N = 34)
	no. with improvement (percent)	
Two weeks	19 (51)	7 (21)
One month	19 (51)	8 (24)
Two months	21 (57)	10 (29)
Three months (end point)	22 (59)	11 (32)
Therapeutic gain*	27 percent	
(95 percent confidence limits)	(5 and 49 percent)	
P value	0.032	
Six-month follow-up	14 (38)	5 (15)
Therapeutic gain*	23 percent	
(95 percent confidence limits)	(4 and 43 percent)	
P value	0.034	

*Difference between the percentage of patients with improvement during cyclosporine administration and the percentage with improvement during placebo administration.

(Courtesy of Brynskov J, Freund L, Rasmussen SN, et al: N Engl J Med 321:845–850, Sept 28, 1989.)

The 3-month treatment period was followed by a 3-month follow-up period during which the patients were gradually withdrawn from treatment; however, improvement continued in 14 cyclosporine-treated patients (38%) and in 5 placebo-treated patients (15%). Side effects were minor and included paresthesias or temperature intolerance in the limbs. Baseline characteristics prognostic for improvement or lack of improvement with cyclosporine therapy could not be identified.

Cyclosporine has a beneficial therapeutic effect in patients with active chronic Crohn's disease who are resistant to or intolerant of corticosteroids. However, long-term follow-up studies are required to determine the possible ultimate benefit of cyclosporine in Crohn's disease.

▶ Although the improvement rate for the cyclosporine-treated patients was 59%, it should be emphasized that this occurred at a trial end point of only 3 months. This figure is in agreement with an anecdotal report in the literature and also corresponds to a 67% response rate reported recently for 77 patients with inflammatory bowel disease, resistant to conventional therapy, who were treated with the immunosuppressive agents azathioprine or 6-mercaptopurine[1]. However, there are data suggesting that the recurrence rate rises greatly when cyclosporine is discontinued[2,3]. Accordingly, Brynskov and associates emphasize that (1) long-term follow-up data from their study clearly are needed, (2) further clinical trials would appear to be justified, and (3) because of the above mentioned issues the use of cyclosporine to treat Crohn's disease should be restricted to formal clinical research programs at centers experienced with this treatment.—N.J. Greenberger, M.D.

References

1. O'Brian J, Bayless T: Immunosuppression agents in the treatment of Crohn's disease including ileitis and ileocolitis. *Gastroenterology* 96:A370, 1989 (abstract).

2. Allison AC, Paunder RE: Cyclosporine for Crohn's disease; alimentary pharmacology and therapeutics, *Alimentary Pharmacol Ther* 1:39, 1987.
3. Pedtekian KM, William CN, MacDonald AS, et al: Open study of cyclosporine in patients with severe active Crohn's disease refractory to conventional therapy. *Can J Gastroenterol* 2:5, 1988.

Strictureplasty

Ten-Year Experience of Strictureplasty for Obstructive Crohn's Disease
Dehn TCB, Kettlewell MGW, Mortensen NJM, Lee ECG, Jewell DP (John Radcliffe Hosp, Oxford, England)
Br J Surg 76:339–341, April 1989   26–5

Although strictureplasty has gained acceptance in the treatment of Crohn's disease, the procedure remains controversial. In a study of 30 operations performed during a 10-year period, generally good results were found in carefully selected patients.

The 24 patients had a median age of 33 years and were followed up for a median period of 40 months. Eighty-six strictureplasties were performed at the 30 operations. Seventeen of the patients had previously undergone 36 operations for Crohn's disease. Fifteen patients had single strictureplasties, whereas 1 patient had 21 of the procedures.

No deaths occurred during the early postoperative period, and no fistulas or wounds were related to operative site. Parenteral nutrition was given to 77% of the patients for a median of 7 days postoperatively. Thirteen patients have been symptom free; 4 required additional surgery; 4 were readmitted for medical treatment; and 3 have had minor attacks of abdominal pain.

Repeated resections in patients with Crohn's disease are associated with short bowel syndrome and malnutrition. In selected patients, preservation of the intestine can be safe and effective. In this patient group, the median weight gain 3 months after surgery was 4 kg. The lesions that respond best to strictureplasty are short and fibrous. The procedure in conjunction with conventional excisional surgery is recommended as a means of preserving intestine and relieving obstructive symptoms.

▶ The surgeons at the Radcliffe Hospital confirm that strictureplasty as described by Williams in Birmingham, England, is effective in selected patients with Crohn's of the small intestine. The procedure offers a way to preserve bowel length in patients with the diffuse form of the disease. Furthermore, it confirms that involvement of the bowel wall does not preclude its healing properties when incised and reapproximated.—F.G. Moody, M.D.

Recurrence and Reoperation

Crohn's Disease: Risk of Recurrence and Reoperation in a Defined Population
Shivananda S, Hordijk ML, Pena AS, Mayberry JF (Univ Hosp, Leiden; Univ Hosp, Rotterdam, The Netherlands; City and Univ Hosps of Nottingham, England)
Gut 30:990–995, July 1989   26–6

Several studies based on selected populations have shown a significant recurrence of Crohn's disease (CD) after apparently curative resection, but evidence has been conflicting. The necessity for repeated surgical intervention in an unselected population of patients with CD in a defined area was recorded.

Two hundred ten patients with CD were identified in an epidemiologic study of inflammatory bowel disease between 1979 and 1983. Patients' records were studied for data on age, sex, year of disease onset and diagnosis, and follow-up to the end of 1983. Surgical and pathologic reports of resected specimens also were evaluated. Follow-up data were available for all but 2 patients who died at home.

Duration of the disease ranged from less than 1 year to 48 years. Fifty-six percent of patients underwent resection. Sixty-one patients underwent ileocecal resection, 14 had a proctocolectomy, 12 had a segmental colectomy with end-to-end anastomosis, and 8 had a subtotal colectomy with ileostomy. Half the proctocolectomies were 2-stage procedures. Eighteen percent of patients had recurrences requiring further surgery; 11 had recurrences at the anastomotic site. Life-table analysis showed that 17% of patients required further resection for recurrence, and 8%, for relapse, after 10 years. By 20 years, the rate of recurrence climbed to 56%. Patients aged more than 30 years had a 1.5 times greater risk of requiring reoperation than younger patients. The initial site of disease was not a factor in recurrence, nor was preoperative duration of disease, delay in diagnosis, or late surgery.

Surgery may not be permanently curative in patients with CD. However, the need for further resection may be less than has been previously thought.

▶ This encouraging report suggests that over a short interval of follow-up, Crohn's recurrence after resection is not as common as previously reported. A greater than 50% recurrence rate at 20 years means that 1 of 2 patients who live that long will have a recurrence, a relatively high number in my book. However, the principles of management of the complications of Crohn's are well defined: resect for complications (bleeding, perforation, obstruction or fistulas), with removal of as little bowel as is possible, and follow the patients carefully on a yearly basis.—F.G. Moody, M.D.

Cancer

Crohn's Disease With Adenocarcinoma and Dysplasia: Macroscopical, Histological, and Immunohistochemical Aspects of Two Cases
Cuvelier C, Bekaert E, De Potter C, Pauwels C, De Vos M, Roels H (Univ Hosp, Ghent Belgium)
Am J Surg Pathol 13:187–196, March 1989 26–7

Patients with chronic inflammatory bowel disease are at increased risk for cancer of the colon. Although patients with longstanding Crohn's disease seem to have an increased incidence of both large and small intestine cancer, authorities differ as to the increased risk for small bowel cancer in patients with Crohn's disease. Multifocal ileal and colonic adenocarcinomas were found in 2 patients with Crohn's disease of long duration.

One patient, a 52-year-old woman, had been treated for Crohn's disease for 10 years. The other, a 31-year-old man, had had ileocolonic Crohn's disease for more than 12 years. Both had been treated with sulfasalazine. The woman had refused surgery 3 years before she underwent resection of the terminal ilium, ileocecal valve, and cecum. The man was severely ill on admission. During surgery, 50 cm of terminal ileum, ileocecal valve, cecum, and a portion of colon were removed in 2 parts because of imminent perforation.

In the first case, dysplasia and cancer were found only in the terminal ileum (Fig 26-1), whereas in the second case, there were several cancers from the ileum toward the transverse colon. Both patients had a clinically unsuspected Dukes C1 mucinous adenocarcinoma (Fig 26-2, right) along with large foci of polypoid villous dysplasia (Fig 26-2, left) or with multifocal high-grade dysplasia and intramucosal carcinoma. Various diseased areas demonstrated different staining patterns for carcinoembryonic antigen (CEA), with the intensity of CEA staining paralleling the histologic degree of dysplasia and neoplasia. Cytokeratin expression was more pronounced in high-grade dysplasia and invasive carcinoma.

If dysplasia is found in an intestinal biopsy specimen from a patient with Crohn's disease, the pathologist should suspect carcinoma. Because the clinical symptoms of carcinoma might be masked by the symptoms of inflammatory bowel disease, it would be advisable to take multiple sections from strictures and polypoid lesions. Immunohistochemical staining with CEA and cytokeratin is also useful.

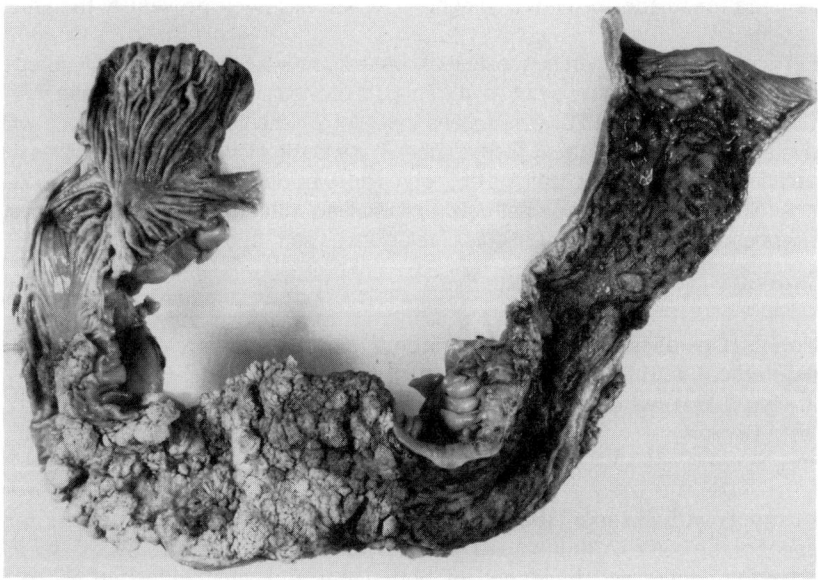

Fig 26-1.—Surgical specimen showing large area of inflamed mucosa interrupted by polypoid tissue. The ileocecal valve and cecum are uninvolved. (Courtesy of Cuvelier C, Bekaert E, De Potter C, et al: *Am J Surg Pathol* 13:187-196, March 1989.)

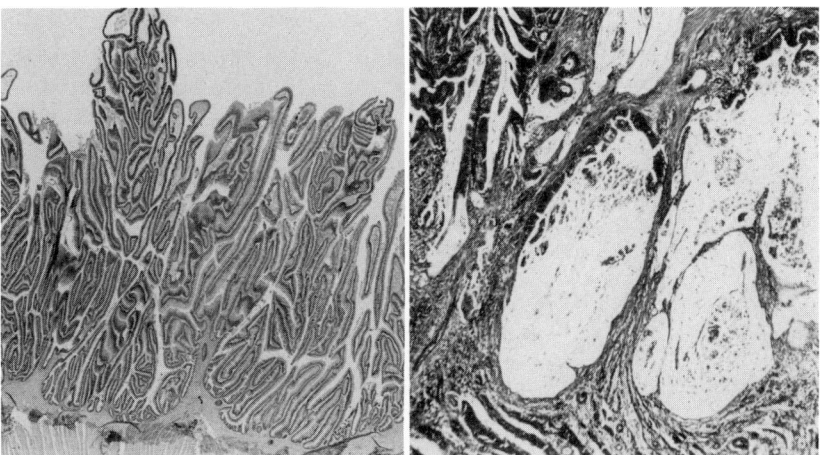

Fig 26–2.—Left, polypoid low-grade villous dysplasia adjacent to diseased mucosa. **Right,** mucinous adenocarcinoma invading the small bowel wall. (Courtesy of Cuvelier C, Bekaert E, De Potter C, et al: *Am J Surg Pathol* 13:187–196, March 1989.)

▶ Crohn's disease of the small as well as large intestine may have a malignant potential, but as pointed out by the authors, it is much less than that which confronts patients with ulcerative colitis. The problem of early detection is similar for the 2 conditions because the symptoms of the disease preclude detecting early signs of cancer. The finding of dysplasia on histologic examination of biopsies is an ominous sign.—F.G. Moody, M.D.

27 Nutrition

Enteral and Parenteral Nutrition; Tube Feedings

Five Years of Experience in Patients Receiving Home Nutrition Support With the Implanted Reservoir: A Comparison With the External Catheter
Howard L, Claunch C, McDowell R, Timchalk M (Albany Med Ctr, Albany, NY)
J Parenter Enteral Nutr 13:478–483, September–October 1989   27–1

Long-term venous access usually has been achieved with an externalized catheter in the superior vena cava, inserted via the subclavian or external jugular vein. Implanted subcutaneous reservoirs became available about 10 years ago for patients with malignancy. Because of a concern about possible complications, the newer technology has been used less frequently for patients with severe bowel dysfunction who are receiving home parenteral nutrition (HPN). The safety of implanted reservoirs in patients receiving HPN was assessed, and the device was compared with the external catheter.

The 27 patients using implanted reservoirs chose such a device over the external catheter after consultation with hospital staff. The decision is important because of its long-term implications and the differences in self-management associated with the two types of venous access. Those patients were compared with 2 control groups using the external catheter: 46 patients who started HPN in the same 5-year period and 17 patients who had experience with both types of venous access.

Common underlying diagnoses were Crohn's disease (25%), mesenteric thrombosis (20%), cancer (15%), and hyperemesis gravidarum (15%). The average infusion time for both types of venous access was 22 months; an average of 1 complication occurred every 2 years. Infection accounted for two thirds of the complications; one third were mechanical. Similar rates of infection were found for both devices. Skin erosion was seen only with the reservoir, whereas clotting was more common with the external catheter.

Of patients who used both types of venous access, 80% preferred the implanted reservoir. Patients without malignancy who are receiving HPN may have a life expectancy of several decades. Trouble-free functioning and patient acceptability are thus important considerations in the choice of venous access. An implanted catheter should be offered as an option to these patients.

▶ The external catheter compared favorably with an implanted device for the delivery of total parenteral nutrition (TPN), but patients preferred the catheter. I imagine that the enthusiasm of the TPN team had a great deal to do with this preference. Their conclusion that patients can survive for an indefinite period on self-administered TPN is correct, and it should be offered to patients who otherwise cannot sustain their nutrition orally.—F.G. Moody, M.D.

Differential Neutrophil Activation Before and After Endotoxin Infusion in Enterally Versus Parenterally Fed Volunteers

Meyer J, Yurt RW, Duhaney R, Hesse DG, Tracey KJ, Fong Y, Richardson D, Calvano S, Dineen P, Shires GT, Lowry SF, Davis JM (Cornell Univ, New York)
Surg Gynecol Obstet 167:501–509, December 1988   27–2

Nutritional support during the perioperative period is known to lower the rate of sepsis and other complications. Few studies, however, have compared the relative benefits of enteral feeding with those of parenteral feeding. The differential effects of the route of feeding on neutrophil (PMN) activation, a measure of increased susceptibility to infection, were investigated.

Nine healthy male volunteers were given a standard dose of endotoxin to promote a clinical condition similar to sepsis. A week before the infusions, 4 were fed a regular oral hospital diet and 5 received total parenteral nutrition (TPN). Before and after the infusion of endotoxin, measurements were made for plasma C3a levels, circulating PMN counts, PMN migration to leukotriene B4 (LTB4), the peptide, N-formyl-methionyl-leucyl-phenylalanine (FMLP), zymosan activated serum, and generation of LTB4.

At base line, volunteers who received TPN had a neutrophil count approximately twice that of the enterally fed group. Plasma C3a levels, absolute circulating PMN counts, and chemotaxis to LTB4 were elevated significantly in the enterally fed volunteers. The intravenously fed group had higher generation of LTB4 at base line. After 1 hour, enterally fed volunteers had a more rapid neutrophilia than those fed intravenously. Plasma C3a levels rose only in the enterally fed group. Chemotaxis to FMLP and zymosan activated serum did not differ between the 2 feeding groups.

The significant differences in numbers of circulating neutrophils, neutrophil function, and plasma complement levels persisted for 4 hours after the injection of endotoxin. The route of feeding can significantly affect neutrophil function, and parenteral feeding may impair host responsiveness.

▶ This unique study of healthy volunteers provides evidence that parenteral nutrition impairs host leucocyte and complement response to endotoxin. It is likely that even more impairment would occur in an already immunocompromised host. Whether that turns out to be the case or not, there is general agreement on clinical grounds that enteral feeding should be maintained or initiated as early as possible after its interruption in injured ill and postoperative patients.—F.G. Moody, M.D.

Effect of Albumin Supplementation During Parenteral Nutrition on Hospital Morbidity

Brown RO, Bradley JE, Bekemeyer WB, Luther RW (Univ of Tennessee, Memphis; Regional Med Ctr at Memphis)

Tests of serum levels of albumin in hospitalized patients have shown a significant correlation between lower concentrations of serum albumin and increased hospital morbidity. Patients with hypoalbuminemia frequently have normal serum albumin (NSA) added to their parenteral nutrition (TPN) formula in doses of 12.5 or 25 g/L. However, this form of supplementation has been controversial, because NSA is expensive and its therapeutic benefit has not been documented. The outcomes for 61 patients receiving TPN with or without NSA were compared.

The 31 patients in group 1 received TPN plus NSA until their measured serum albumin levels were >3 g/dL; 30 patients in group 2 received TPN alone. Group 2 patients weighed significantly more than those in group 1, but the 2 groups were well matched in age, sex, medical condition, and initial serum albumin concentrations.

The difference in total hospital days between the 2 groups—36 days for group 1 and 41.8 days for group 2—approached statistical significance. Patients in group 1, as expected, had a significant rise in serum albumin during TPN; the rise in group 2 was small and insignificant. Measurements of urinary urea nitrogen and nitrogen balance studies showed no significant differences between groups 1 and 2.

The number of complications after the initiation of TPN was significantly lower in group 1 (33) than in group 2 (80). Significantly more patients in group 2 had septicemia and pneumonia. There were no differences in mortality between the groups. The additional expense of NSA appears to be offset by the significant reduction of morbidity in patients receiving TPN with NSA.

▶ Albumin, as expected, elevated the serum albumin when it was added to parenteral nutrition. Although mortality was similar to that of matched controls, complications of parenteral nutrition and septic complications in general were fewer among those receiving exogenous albumin. Albumin possibly served as an additional protein supplement or in some way enhanced vascular perfusion. The authors should pursue the mechanism of this interesting finding, which has been alluded to by others in a variety of clinical settings.—F.G. Moody, M.D.

TEN Versus TPN Following Major Abdominal Trauma: Reduced Septic Morbidity
Moore FA, Moore EE, Jones TN, McCroskey BL, Peterson VM (Denver Gen Hosp; Univ of Colorado Health Sciences Ctr, Denver)

Nutritional support of seriously injured patients is an important part of critical care. Recent research on animals suggests that enteral feeding (TEN) is better than parenteral nutrition (TPN) at improving resistance to infection. The effects of early TEN and TPN in critically injured patients were compared.

Seventy-five patients with an abdominal trauma index between 15 and 40 were randomly assigned at initial laparotomy to either a TEN or a TPN group. All feedings contained 2.5% fat, 33% branched chain amino acids, and a calorie-to-nitrogen ratio of 150:1. Enteral feeding was given through a needle catheter jejunostomy. Feedings were begun within 12 hours of surgery in both groups and were infused at a rate sufficient to achieve positive nitrogen balances in the patients.

Eighty-six percent of the patients in the TEN group tolerated the jejunal feedings unconditionally. The nitrogen balance remained comparable throughout the study. The traditional markers of nutritional protein—albumin, transferrin, and retinol-binding protein—were better restored in patients receiving TEN feedings. Seventeen percent of the TEN group and 37% of the TPN group had infections. Major septic morbidity occurred in 3% of the TEN group, compared with 20% of the TPN group.

Enteral feeding is significantly better than parenteral nutrition in reducing major septic complications in critically injured patients, and it is also well tolerated.

▶ The power of a randomized trial lends strong support to the conclusion that TEN is associated with less septic complications in injured patients than TPN. It is surprising that most patients tolerated enteral feedings within 12 hours of laparotomy, suggesting that they had single-organ penetrating injury. I would recommend this approach, however, even for patients with multiple organ blunt injury because they can be tided over a period of ileus by parenteral nutrition. A complete return of small bowel propulsive function apparently is not necessary for judicious increments of enteral feeding. Furthermore, one should not defer because of delayed gastric or colonic function because their return is late in the postileus state.—F.G. Moody, M.D.

The Effects of an Anabolic Steroid and Peripherally Administered Intravenous Nutrition in the Early Postoperative Period
Hansell DT, Davies JWL, Shenkin A, Garden OJ, Burns HJG, Carter DC (Royal Infirmary, Glasgow, Scotland)
J Parenter Enteral Nutr 13:349–358, July–August 1989

Patients who have undergone surgery have an increase in urinary nitrogen excretion and loss of body protein. This metabolic response may result in a risk of increased morbidity and mortality among patients who are already in a weakened condition. The value of total parenteral nutrition (TPN), administered in an attempt to minimize postoperative nitrogen losses, has been questioned. One alternative treatment, an anabolic steroid, was evaluated in 60 surgical patients.

Twenty-four hours before surgery for colorectal cancer, patients were randomly assigned to receive a single intramuscular injection of 50 mg of stanozolol or to a control group with no injection. On the first 4 postoperative days, patients were further randomized to receive a fluid regimen consisting of dextrose-saline, amino acids, or glucose-amino acid-fat (GAF) via a peripheral vein. Indirect calorimetry was used to calculate preoperative and postoperative fat and carbohydrate oxidation rates.

Patients were well matched for age, body weight, percentage weight loss, and lean body mass. Preoperative urinary nitrogen excretion levels were similar for the 3 groups. The administration of stanozolol significantly improved postoperative nitrogen balance in patients receiving amino acids. Stanozolol did not significantly affect fat and carbohydrate oxidation rates. Patients in the stanozolol and control amino acid groups had a postoperative fall in carbohydrate oxidation and a rise in fat oxidation. The 2 dextrose-saline and 2 GAF groups, however, had no significant changes in fat and carbohydrate oxidation. Cumulative nitrogen balance was significantly better in the 2 GAF groups than in all the other groups.

Patients with cancer receiving amino acid infusions show improved postoperative nitrogen balance after preoperative administration of the anabolic steroid stanozolol. Patients receiving a more complete nutritional regimen, combining glucose, amino acids, and fat, have a positive postoperative nitrogen balance unaffected by stanozolol.

▶ Most trials suffer from lack of random design, but this study reflects the converse: a double randomization in a relatively small population. The results support the conclusions, however, because the study group was relatively homogeneous. An anabolic steroid enhances nitrogen balance when the 3 essential substrates—fat, carbohydrate, or amino acids—are not provided.—F.G. Moody, M.D.

Relative Importance of Amino Acid Infusion as a Means of Sparing Protein in Surgical Patients
Humberstone DA, Koea J, Shaw JHF (Auckland Hosp, Auckland, New Zealand)
J Parenter Enteral Nutr 13:223–227, May–June 1989

Surgical patients with compromised nutritional status are at increased risk for poor outcome. To meet energy demands and conserve protein, patients often are given enteral and parenteral nutritional support. The effects of glucose, lipid, and amino acid infusion on protein and glucose kinetics were assessed in 41 surgical patients, and results were compared with those achieved by total parenteral nutrition (TPN) in a group of 10 patients.

The patients were assigned randomly to receive glucose infusion (GL), lipid infusion (LIP), amino acid infusion (AA), or TPN. The majority of patients in each group had undergone surgery for a malignancy, although sepsis and trauma also were represented. Multiple blood samples were obtained and analyzed for the glucose rate of production (Ra glucose), Ra urea, and net protein catabolism.

The patients assigned to the GL group had a basal net protein catabolism value of 1.53 g/kg/day, decreasing to 1.39 g/kg/day during glucose infusion. Basal net protein catabolism in the LIP group was 2.04 g/kg/day, decreasing to 1.72 g/kg/day during infusion, and for patients in the AA group, it was 1.37

g/kg/day, decreasing to –0.77 g/kg/day during infusion. Net protein catabolism in the patients receiving TPN was 0.79 g/kg/day.

All substrates commonly used in intravenous feeding—glucose, fat, and amino acids—have the capacity to spare protein. Net protein catabolism was reduced more by TPN than by glucose or lipid infusion alone. The effect of amino acids, however, was greater than either of the other substances employed. This effect was not caused solely by insulin secretion. Peripheral vein feeding with amino acid solutions has potential clinical application, especially when TPN is contraindicated or when hospital resources for full TPN are not available.

▶ This is an interesting observation: amino acid infusion into a peripheral vein provides more protein sparing in postsurgical patients than TPN, which must be delivered in a central vein. Fortunately, most patients undergoing elective surgery for cancer can be fed within a few days. It is possible that the peripheral amino acid infusion would be a useful adjunct for those who are malnourished before operation or for those patients who are slow to recover intestinal function.—F.G. Moody, M.D.

Decreased Cholestasis With Enteral Instead of Intravenous Protein in the Very Low–Birth-Weight Infant
Brown MR, Thunberg BJ, Golub L, Maniscalco WM, Cox C, Shapiro DL (Strong Mem Hosp, Rochester, NY)
J Pediatr Gastroenterol Nutr 9:21–27, July 1989   27–7

Cholestasis develops in 30% to 50% of parenterally fed infants with very low birth weights. Whether giving protein enterally instead of giving amino acids parenterally would decrease the incidence of cholestasis was tested in infants with gestational ages of less than 30 weeks. The infants were assigned at random to receive enteral whey feedings and parenteral nutrition without amino acids or to receive standard parenteral nutrition with amino acids. Both groups received premature infant formula enterally.

After 3 weeks' parenteral nutrition, none of the 17 infants in the whey feeding group had a direct serum bilirubin level of more than 3 mg/dL, which was considered to indicate significant cholestasis. The incidence of cholestasis in the 12 control infants who received amino acids, however, was 58%. Infants tolerated the whey protein well. Both groups of infants had equal weight gain and serum albumin level. The major difference between the 2 groups was the significantly earlier first attempt at enteral feeding in the whey group.

The reason for the decrease in cholestasis in the group receiving enteral whey and parenteral amino acid-free nutrition is not clear. The difference may be caused by the early enteral administration of protein or the removal of amino acids from the total parenteral nutrition solution, or both.

▶ I hope that the neonatologists at the Strong Memorial Hospital follow up on their observation that enteral protein supplement in infants of low birth weight decreases the incidence of jaundice, so often observed in these neonates. Because the whey appeared to be well tolerated, its substitution for parenteral amino acids would be cheaper and safer. It is possible they do not need parenteral feedings, even without amino acids. A total enteral approach would reduce greatly the expense and complexity of the cure of these tiny tots.—F.G. Moody, M.D.

Total Parenteral Nutrition and Bowel Rest Modify the Metabolic Response to Endotoxin in Humans
Fong Y, Marano MA, Barber A, He W, Moldawer LL, Bushman ED, Coyle SM, Shires GT, Lowry SF (New York Hosp–Cornell Med Ctr, New York)
Ann Surg 210:449–457, October 1989   27–8

It has been proposed that atrophy of the intestinal mucosa secondary to total parenteral nutrition (TPN) or prolonged bowel rest may enhance the translocation of bowel endotoxin and alter host responses to infection. Twelve healthy persons received either enteral feedings or TPN for 1 week without oral intake. Metabolic studies were carried out during dextrose infusion, starting 12 hours after the last feeding, and continued for 6 hours after an intravenous challenge with 20 units/kg of *Escherichia coli* lipopolysaccharide.

Body weight was maintained with TPN. The pyrogenic response to endotoxin challenge and the heart rate response were greater in the TPN group than in the enteral feeding group. Mean blood pressure did not change significantly in either group. Peak epinephrine and glucagon responses were significantly greater in the TPN group than in the enteral feeding group, and circulating levels of cachectin–tumor necrosis factor were higher than in the enterally fed persons. Peripheral lactate production was significantly increased in the TPN subjects. Hypoaminoacidemia was noted in both groups. Levels of C-reactive protein were higher in the TPN group than in persons fed enterally.

It appears that bowel rest leads to changes in host resistance to injury independent of malnutrition. It seems clear that the route of feeding does affect injury and disease. Total parenteral nutrition can lead to an exaggerated counter-regulatory hormone response and enhanced systemic and splanchnic production of cytokines.

▶ This carefully performed clinical study of normal human volunteers establishes what has been presumed for the past decade: that TPN with bowel rest allows an enhanced splanchnic production of cytokines when the subjects were challenged with parenterally administered endotoxin. But why should TPN be associated with an exaggerated response to endotoxin? Several possibilities exist, the most likely being that endotoxin clearance by the liver is altered when the splanchnic circulation is deprived of the feeding response. It is possible that the gastrointestinal peptides are an important modulator of the immune stress response. I am impressed that only 1 week of bowel rest provides such a marked change in an individual's response to an endotoxin challenge.—F.G. Moody, M.D.

Efficacy of Tube Feeding in Supplying Energy Requirements of Hospitalized Patients

Abernathy GB, Heizer WD, Holcombe BJ, Raasch RH, Schlegel KE, Hak LJ (North Carolina Mem Hosp; Univ of North Carolina, Chapel Hill)
J Parenter Enteral Nutr 13:387–391, July–August 1989   27-9

Patients for whom nutritional support is required may not receive their desirable caloric and protein intake with enteral therapy. The rate of infusion may be low, or complications may reduce feeding time. To test the hypothesis that mechanical and gastrointestinal difficulties often prevent enteral nutrition from meeting patients' energy needs, researchers undertook a prospective 6-week study of all adult patients in a university hospital who were receiving a tube-feeding formula.

Thirty-five patients were identified and calculations of their energy goals were based on general physical parameters and diagnosis. Patients' basal energy expenditures (BEE) were calculated with the Harris-Benedict equation. The amount of enteral formula given was measured daily. A total of 254 patient days were included in the analysis.

The mean daily caloric goal was 1,791 kcal; intakes averaged 61% of this goal, 1,095 kcal/day. On study days 1 through 5, 7, and 8, mean calorie intake was statistically different from mean energy goal. Mean daily calorie intake did not exceed BEE until study day 10. Only 16 patients achieved their energy goal on at least 1 day of the study. In those patients an average of 6 days of therapy was required before the goal was met.

Mechanical complications caused most of the interruptions in therapy. Extubation occurred in 8 patients, and permanent tube obstruction, in 6, resulting in a loss of 415 potential hours of therapy. Gastrointestinal intolerance accounted for a loss of 4.7% of the total study hours. Medical procedures requiring discontinuation of feeding resulted in a loss of 2.8% of potential feeding time. In some cases, physicians had ordered only 75% of calculated energy goals.

Tube feeding under usual hospital conditions does not meet patients' energy requirements. Correct positioning of the tubes and an increase in administration rates, when necessary, can assure that patients actually receive the full measure of prescribed therapy.

▶ The information provided in this study is useful. Enteral feedings must be given in a timely and consistent fashion and to the level of the caloric needs of the patient. Intestinal intolerance accounted for less than 5% of variance from desired intake. The greatest offenders were the physician and his support staff. Insufficient caloric intake was ordered 25% of the time. Obviously, enteral feedings must be monitored with the same care as that given to total parenteral nutrition.—F.G. Moody, M.D.

Utilization of Nasogastric Feeding Tubes in a Group of Chronically Ill, Elderly Patients in a Community Hospital

Quill TE (The Genesee Hosp, Rochester, NY)

The use of nasogastric (NG) feeding tubes in patients with chronic irreversible illness remains controversial. To explore how physicians approach the decision to initiate NG feeding for elderly, chronically ill patients, physician practice, patterns and attitudes about the use of NG tubes among chronically ill, elderly patients in a community hospital were evaluated with a physician questionnaire and chart review.

In responses to the questionnaire, physicians cited predominantly quality-of-life circumstances in considering the placement of an NG tube in an elderly patient with severe, chronic irreversible illness. Overall, 40% of physicians reported that they would recommend NG feeding in an elderly patient with poor prognosis whose wishes are unknown. Given an abstract scenario of a chronically ill, elderly patient, physicians who believed NG feeding was extraordinary treatment (42%) would recommend it less often than those who believed it to be ordinary (21%) or comfort-oriented (37%).

Although 89% of the physicians thought that patients' wishes should guide decisions on using NG feeding tubes, that belief was not translated into practice according to the chart review of 55 patients aged 70 and older who had NG tubes and primary diagnoses of cerebrovascular accident, organic brain syndrome, or metastatic cancer. Patient consent was indirectly documented on the charts of only 2 of 51 patients with NG tubes. Of the 7 charts that indicated a surrogate gave consent, only 1 documented consideration of the patient's actual wishes. Contrary to their replies in the questionnaire, physicians emphasized biomedical concerns, rather than quality of life, in considering the placement of NG tubes. Sixty-four percent of patients died in the hospital, including 90% of those who had comfort-oriented treatment. For only 2 of 55 patients was medical improvement cited as the reason for discontinuing the use of an NG feeding tube. Restraints were used to keep the tube in 53% of patients.

Hospitals must develop policies for the use of NG feeding tubes and other forms of hyperalimentation. These policies should emphasize active patient and family participation in the use of NG feeding tubes, as well as define the potential benefits to, burdens for, and limitations in patients with severe irreversible illnesses.

▶ The aging of our population continues to raise important ethical issues that must be resolved, not by ethicists but by practicing physicians. This study points out that we do not act as we speak. Elderly patients with incurable illnesses are kept alive with a variety of support systems that have no therapeutic benefit, the feeding tube being the most common. Important points in the equation are the wishes of the patient and the patient's family. Often the patient cannot participate in the discussion because of his or her illness. Patients can be kept comfortable without providing them with full nutritional support. The use of restraints to accomplish enteral feedings is likely more disturbing to the patient than the quiet sleep of inanition. A disturbing feature in the article, however, is that 10% of patients provided with enteral feedings for reasons of comfort apparently lived and left the hospital. These patients would have died if they were not provided with tube feedings. This outcome suggests that the supportive care protocols should be flexible for this relatively noninvasive nutritional strategy designed primarily for hydration and metabolic homeostasis.—F.G. Moody, M.D.

Percutaneous Endoscopic Gastrostomy and Jejunostomy

Percutaneous Endoscopic Gastrostomy
Mamel JJ (Univ of South Florida, Tampa)
Am J Gastroenterol 84:703–710, July 1989   27–11

Interest in gastrostomy for nutritional support has been revived since development of endoscopic placement of the gastrostomy feeding tube. Placement is accomplished easily, and the incidence of complications is low.

Either the pull-through technique developed by Ponsky and Gauderer or the push-through technique developed by Sachs and Vine can be used successfully, with little difference in ease of performance and complications. The standard percutaneous endoscopic gastrostomy also may be converted to a feeding jejunostomy.

The complication rate for 1,338 cases reported from 1983 through 1987 was 13.6%. Serious complications included wound infection, pulmonary aspiration, stomal leaks, and dislodgment of the tube. Benign pneumoperitoneum was common. In such cases laparotomy can be avoided if the origin of the pneumoperitoneum is recognized during tube placement. Necrotizing fasciitis has been reported in 3 patients; 1 died. Patients who have achlorhydria as a result of H_2-blocking agents, previous surgery, or atrophic gastritis have an increased risk for such infection.

The endoscopic method has many advantages over surgical placement of a gastrostomy tube, but complications still may occur. Meticulous preoperative assessment of the patient, careful technique during placement, good postoperative care, and early recognition of complications may help to lower morbidity.

▶ The percutaneous endoscopic gastrostomy (PEG) has influenced dramatically the way in which patients who need enteral feedings receive treatment. This report details the complications of the procedure and their management. Only 1 death from the procedure among 1,338 cases attests to the care with which the procedure was performed and attended to at the University of South Florida.—F.G. Moody, M.D.

Gastrointestinal Symptoms Attributed to Jejunostomy Feeding After Major Abdominal Trauma: A Critical Analysis
Jones TN, Moore FA, Moore EE, McCroskey BL (Denver Gen Hosp)
Crit Care Med 17:1146–1150, November 1989   27–12

Enteral feeding via jejunostomy has advantages over parenteral feeding after abdominal trauma, but concern over patient intolerance because of gastrointestinal complaints persists. In an examination of such problems, 123 patients who had emergency laparotomy for major abdominal trauma were randomly assigned to a control group or to a group starting an elemental diet by enteral means 12 hours after surgery.

Gastrointestinal distress affected 50% of the controls and 83% of enterally fed patients. Distress was moderate in 35% of enterally fed patients, but was severe enough to necessitate adjustments in feeding schedule in 15%. Of those with severe complaints, 45% had an abdominal trauma index of more than 40. Of enterally fed patients with symptoms, 13% had to change to total parenteral nutrition. By the fifth postoperative day the average enteral feeding per day included nonprotein, 35 kcal/kg, and nitrogen, 0.24 g/kg; 66% achieved positive nitrogen balance.

In spite of increased gastrointestinal complaints, most patients with major abdominal trauma can tolerate early enteral feeding with close monitoring and management by the nutrition staff. Those whose abdominal trauma indices are more than 40 may do better if enteral nutrition is not initiated for 3 to 5 days postoperatively.

▶ The trauma surgeons at the Denver General Hospital continue to define ways to optimize the use of enteral nutrition in injured patients. In spite of gastrointestinal symptoms, most patients could be fed enterally without adverse effects. Patients with more severe injuries, however, were especially intolerant of early institution of enteral feeding and would have been better served by a 2- to 3-day delay in its use.—F.G. Moody, M.D.

Miscellaneous Considerations

Cholesterol Absorption: Regulation of Cholesterol Synthesis and Elimination and Within-Population Variations of Serum Cholesterol Levels
Miettinen TA, Kesäniemi YA (Univ of Helsinki)
Am J Clin Nutr 49:629–635, April 1989   27–13

Cholesterol absorption is thought to be a regulator of cholesterol synthesis and serum lipoprotein levels. This view was studied in 63 50-year-old men selected at random from a population register.

Obesity and dietary plant sterols had a negative correlation with fractional dietary cholesterol absorption. An increase in dietary cholesterol intake caused a linear increase in absorbed dietary cholesterol. Higher absolute and fractional absorption of dietary cholesterol resulted in a lower rate of biliary secretion, fecal output, and synthesis of cholesterol. The higher the cholesterol absorption, the higher the serum levels of total cholesterol and low-density lipoprotein cholesterol and the lower the cholesterol synthesis. High serum levels of high-density lipoprotein cholesterol were correlated with high cholesterol absorption efficiency and low rates of fecal elimination and cholesterol synthesis.

The efficiency of cholesterol absorption plays an important role in the regulation of cholesterol metabolism. It is also important in serum cholesterol regulation, determining the serum levels of low-density lipoprotein, high-density lipoprotein, and total cholesterol.

➤ The rate of cholesterol absorption was correlated directly with the level of cholesterol intake and, in turn, the concentration of cholesterol in the blood. In addition, the low-density lipoprotein levels also were linked closely to the rate of cholesterol absorption. It is interesting that the role of dietary cholesterol is still so heavily debated. I am sticking to bran, turkey, margarine, and jogging until the green light to a more enjoyable diet and comfortable life-style stays on consistently.—F.G. Moody, M.D.

Reduction of 24-Hour Gastric Acidity by Different Dietary Regimens: A Randomized Controlled Study in Healthy Volunteers
Hopert R, Liehr R-M, Emde C, Riecken E-O (Medizinische Klinik und Poliklinik, Klinikum Steglitz der FU Berlin, Berlin)
J Parenter Enteral Nutr 13:292–295, May–June 1989   27–14

The effect of intraduodenal tube feeding on gastric acidity in clinical situations is not well understood. Results of an orally administered polymer diet and a normal diet, both given 3 times a day, and a liquid hydrolyzed diet applied continuously via portable pump to the duodenum were compared using 10 healthy men and women volunteers.

The 24-hour and prandial gastric pH increased significantly more with the orally given liquid polymer diet than with the normal diet. Continuous intraduodenal administration of the liquid peptide diet caused significantly greater 24-hour, interdigestive, and nocturnal median pH values than the normal diet.

Enteral nutrition may help prevent stress lesions in patients at risk by maintaining high gastric pH values. However, a liquid polymer diet would have to be given more than 3 times a day if gastric acidity were to be reduced continuously. Continuous intraduodenal instillation would not require modification. These conclusions should be substantiated under clinical conditions.

➤ A polymer diet delivered into the duodenum provides a means for the continuous alkalinization of the stomach. This could be a useful way to reduce the risk of stress erosive gastritis in persons for whom intubation is required for support of their nutrition. It is possible that a patient with a head injury would be ideal for this adjuvant to the standard procedures for prophylaxis of stress erosive gastritis.–F.G. Moody, M.D.

The Colon

Chapter 28. Physiology and Pathophysiology
  Studies on Mechanisms of Diarrhea
Chapter 29. Infectious Colitis and Related Disorders
  Hemorrhagic Colitis and *Escherichia coli* 0157:H7
  Shigella
  Associated With Drinking Water
  C. difficile and Antibiotic Associated Diarrhea
  Typhoid Enteritis and Perforation
Chapter 30. Lymphocytic ("Microscopic") Colitis
Chapter 31. Diversion Colitis
Chapter 32. Ileal-Anal Anastomoses
Chapter 33. Rectal Injuries and Colonic Trauma
Chapter 34. Rectal Prolapse and Sigmoid Volvulus
  Rectal Prolapse
  Sigmoid Volvulus
Chapter 35. Colorectal Carcinoma and Other Neoplasms
  Radiologic and Imaging Studies
  Polyps: Cancer Sequence
  Clinical Studies
  Radioimmunolocation and Ablation Studies
Chapter 36. Irritable Bowel Syndrome
  Clinical Studies
Chapter 37. Appendicitis
  Clinical Studies
Chapter 38. Colonic Ischemia
Chapter 39. Miscellaneous Topics
  Total Colectomy for Aganglionosis
  Colon Surgery Without Nasogastric Decompression

28 Physiology and Pathophysiology

Studies on Mechanisms of Diarrhea

Loss of Absorptive Capacity for Sodium Chloride as a Cause of Diarrhea Following Partial Ileal and Right Colon Resection
Arrambide KA, Santa Ana CA, Schiller LR, Little KH, Santangelo WC, Fordtran JS (Baylor Univ, Dallas)
Dig Dis Sci 34:193–201, February 1989   28–1

    Previous studies have emphasized the role of unabsorbed bile acids and fat as the cause of the diarrhea that may follow ileal and right colon resection, via a cathartic effect in the unresected colon. Eight patients with severe postresection diarrhea were studied in a search for a more basic defect in sodium chloride absorption as the cause of postresection diarrhea, such as loss of sodium chloride absorptive capacity as a direct consequence of resection of sites of sodium chloride absorption.

    Diarrhea caused by deficient sodium chloride absorptive capacity may be expected to persist during fasting, whereas diarrhea mediated by bile acid and fat malabsorption should not persist during a fast. During a 48-hour fast diarrhea and large fecal electrolyte losses persisted in all 8 patients with postresection diarrhea (Table 1).

    Sodium chloride and water absorption rates were measured during total gut perfusion with a balanced electrolyte solution to determine whether absorptive capacity during total gut perfusion was reduced by resection or whether adaptive hyperplasia had restored absorptive capacity to normal. Patients with postresection diarrhea had a 23% to 31% reduction in absorptive capacity for water, sodium, and chloride, compared with healthy controls (Table 2).

    Fluid absorptive capacity was studied further in 3 patients under conditions in which there was a concentration gradient between the luminal fluid and plasma for sodium and chloride. The absorptive defect in these patients was markedly accentuated. All patients had severe bile acid malabsorption, but treatment with large doses of cholestyramine resulted in only a modest and insignificant reduction in stool weight, suggesting that bile acid malabsorption did not play a major role in postresection diarrhea.

    These findings suggest that patients with postresection diarrhea may

TABLE 1.—Stool Studies

Pt.	Fat (g/day) reg diet	pH Reg diet	pH 48-hr fast	Wet weight (g/day) Reg diet	Wet weight (g/day) 48-hr fast	Wet weight (g/day) Reg diet + cholestyramine	Fecal electrolyte losses (meq/day) Sodium Reg diet	Sodium 48-hr fast	Potassium Reg diet	Potassium 48-hr fast	Chloride Reg diet	Chloride 48-hr fast	Osmolality (mosm/kg) Reg diet	Osmolality 48-hr fast	Osmotic gap (mosm/kg)† Reg diet	Osmotic gap 48-hr fast
M.G.	7	6.8	6.9	661	203	916	68	21	23	10	37	16	542	458	14	0
D.B.	10	6.0	7.0	738	782	836	60	90	30	24	30	32	423	318	46	2
R.J.	30	5.6	7.0	1007	455		81	35	41	15	27	15	470	349	48	74
T.R.	21	6.3	7.4	1781	1055	1613‡	148	103	62	25	87	70	354	259	54	48
L.G.	12	6.0	7.7	785	525	574	48	46	26	19	27	32	369	316	102	42
S.H.	33	6.1	7.8	1276	962	592	73	77	41	56	51	69	340	300	112	14
B.T.	31	6.8	7.3	1094	667	653	95	52	39	40	64	41	384	325	43	15
J.K.	63	5.4	7.3	1066	398		53	40	26	11	19	20	496	340	143	35
Average	26	6.1	7.3	1051	631	864	79	58	36	25	43	37	385	333	70	29

*Osmolality measured by freezing point depression.
†Osmotic gap calculated using plasma osmolality of 290.
‡Plus belladonna. This patient also studied with double dose (32 g/day) of cholestyramine (stool weight, 1,437 g/day) and with low-fat diet plus 16 g/day of cholestyramine (stool weight 1,441 g/day).
(Courtesy of Arrambide KA, Santa Ana CA, Schiller LR, et al: *Dig Dis Sci* 34:193–201, February 1989.)

TABLE 2.—Water and Electrolyte Absorption Rates During Steady-State Total Gut Perfusion With Balanced Electrolyte Solution

	Water (ml/hr)	Sodium (meq/hr)	Potassium (meq/hr)	Chloride (meq/hr)	Bicarbonate (meq/hr)
Intestinal resection					
M.G.	525	75	0.6	49	28
D.B.	523	74	0.8	42	20
R.J.	610	83	1.3	52	34
T.R.	826	117	1.9	72	44
L.G.	813	117	2.1	80	43
S.H.	538	78	0.3	54	26
B.T.	398	63	0.3	31	31
J.K.	745	106	2.0	71	37
Mean ± SE	622 ± 55	89 ± 7	1.2 ± 0.3	56 ± 6	33 ± 3
Normal subjects					
Mean ± SE	809 ± 26	115 ± 4	4.0 ± 0.8	81 ± 5	37 ± 2.0
Range	552 – 1012	78 – 141	1.2 – 11.7	48 – 126	15 – 47
P value*	<0.005	<0.005	<0.05	<0.02	NS

*Normal subjects vs. intestinal resection patients by group t-test.
(Courtesy of Arrambide KA, Santa Ana CA, Schiller LR, et al: Dig Dis Sci 34:193–201, February 1989.)

have a reduced capacity to absorb sodium chloride, particularly when sodium chloride absorption must take place against a concentration gradient. It appears that loss of ileal and colonic absorptive capacity for sodium chloride, rather than a cathartic effect of unabsorbed bile acids or fat, is the major cause of postresection diarrhea.

▶ The patients described in this report all had diarrhea within a few days of surgical resection of 25–120 cm of terminal ileum and 14% to 50% of colon. The diarrhea was severe and unremitting, did not abate with time, and was poorly responsive to dietary and pharmacologic methods of therapy. The studies by Arrambide and colleagues suggest that a *loss* of ileal and colonic absorptive capacity for sodium chloride rather than a cathartic effect of unabsorbed bile acids or fat is the major cause of diarrhea in these patients. Further, these studies provide an explanation for the fairly frequent failure of cholestyramine, a bile acid sequestering agent, to effect improvement in diarrhea developing after partial ileectomy and right colonic resection.—N. J. Greenberger, M.D.

Studies of Osmotic Diarrhea Induced in Normal Subjects by Ingestion of Polyethylene Glycol and Lactulose
Hammer HF, Santa Ana CA, Schiller LR, Fordtran JS (Baylor Univ Med Ctr, Dallas)
J Clin Invest 84:1056–1062, October 1989   28–2

The pathophysiology of pure osmotic diarrhea and the diarrhea caused by carbohydrate malabsorption was studied. Diarrhea was induced in normal volunteers by ingestion of polyethylene glycol (PEG), a nonabsorbable osmotic solute that is not metabolized by intestinal bacteria and carries no

Stool Weight, Water Content, Frequency, and Fetal Concentration of PEG, Organic Acids, and Carbohydrates in 24-Hour Stool Collections (Mean ±SEM)*

	PEG					Lactulose		
	53 g/d (n = 9)	95 g/d (n = 9)	190 g/d (n = 12)	252 g/d (n = 9)	45 g/d (n = 9)	95 g/d (n = 9)	125 g/d (n = 9)
Stool weight (g/d)	364±41	589±45	1,118±102	1,539±77	254±45	550±115	1,307±111
Stool frequency (times/d)	2±0.2	3±0.3	6±0.3	5±0.7	2±0.2	3±0.3	4±0.6
Average weight of individual bowel movement (g)	226±34	180±19	214±20	398±64†	149±23	175±31	321±36‡
Percent water content	75±0.4	77±0.6	79±0.5	80±0.4	79±1	86±1	90±0.5
Stool water output (g/d)	272±31	451±33	881±58	1,233±64	202±38	483±105	1,184±106
PEG (g/liter)	130±3	158±7	165±2	163±3‡	—	—	—
Organic acids (meq/liter)	81±7‖	60±8	53±8	31±3†	231±23	201±19	114±10‡
Carbohydrate (g/liter)	0.8±0.2‖	1.3±0.2	0.7±0.1	0.9±0.4§	3.6±1.3	17±4	36±3†

*n, 3 consecutive 24-hour samples from each of 3 or 4 subjects. Average weight of individual bowel movements was calculated by dividing daily stool weight by stool frequency. Percent water content was calculated by following formula: $\frac{\text{(original weight)} - \text{(dry weight)}}{\text{original weight}}$. P values, unpaired t-test (252 g/day PEG vs. 53 g/day PEG or 125 g/day lactulose vs. 95 g/day lactulose)

†$P < .01$.
‡$P < .001$.
§Not significant.
‖$n = 7$.

(Courtesy of Hammer HF, Santa Ana CA, Schiller LR, et al: *J Clin Invest* 84:1056–1062, October 1989.)

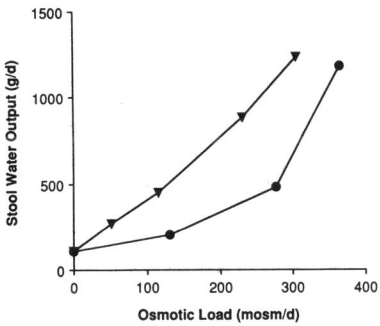

Fig 28–1.—Influence of the osmotic load of PEG *(triangles)* and lactulose *(circles)* on daily stool water output. (Courtesy of Hammer HF, Santa Ana CA, Schiller LR, et al: *J Clin Invest* 84:1056–1062, October 1989.)

electrical charge. Increasing osmotic loads of PEG resulted in a near linear increase in stool weight and stool water output (table). Stool weight or water output was directly correlated with total fecal PEG output. About 40% to 60% of the osmolality of the fecal fluid was caused by PEG, the remainder being contributed by other solutes of either dietary, endogenous, or bacterial origin. The total daily fecal excretions of sodium, potassium, and chloride were very small, despite stool water losses exceeding 1,200 g/day.

Diarrhea also was induced in normal volunteers by ingestion of lactulose, a disaccharide that is not absorbed by the small intestine but is readily metabolized by colonic bacteria. Mean stool weight and water content increased significantly with increasing lactulose dose. A maximum of about 80 g/day of lactulose was metabolized by colonic bacteria to noncarbohydrate moieties (e.g., organic acids). The organic acids were partially absorbed in the colon, whereas the unabsorbed organic acids obligated the accumulation of inorganic cations (e.g., sodium, calcium, potassium, and magnesium), in the diarrheal fluid. Diarrhea associated with low doses of lactulose was mainly a result of unabsorbed organic acids and associated cations, whereas unmetabolized carbohydrates also played a major role in the diarrhea associated with large doses of lactulose. The net effect of bacterial metabolism of lactulose and partial absorption of organic acids on stool water output was dose-dependent.

Comparisons of PEG- and lactulose-induced diarrhea showed that with low or moderate doses of lactulose, stool water losses were reduced by as much as 600 g/day, as compared with equimolar osmotic loads of PEG (Fig 28–1). With larger doses of lactulose, there was an excess of unabsorbed organic acids, which in turn obligated the accumulation of cations. Thus, the increment in osmotically active solutes within the lumen exceeded the increment of the ingested osmotic load, and the severity of diarrhea was augmented after comparable osmotic loads of PEG.

▶ I would like to detail additional points emphasized by the authors in their discussion. First, no correlation between organic acid concentration and the weight of individual bowel movements was found. This is interpreted as an argument against the concept that organic acids may cause rapid colonic emptying because of an effect on colonic motility. Second, the results show that carbohydrate malabsorption can be associated with highly variable stools, that is, formed, mushy, or liquid stools with normal to very high stool weight. One major determinant of stool consistency and weight is the amount of carbohydrate that is malabsorbed, but the substantial variation among subjects when a given amount of lactulose was ingested indicates that other factors also are important. Varying capacities of colonic flora to metabolize carbohydrates and varying colonic absorption rates for organic acids are 2 likely determining influences.—N.J. Greenberger, M.D.

29 Infectious Colitis and Related Disorders

Hemorrhagic Colitis and *Escherichia coli* 0157:H7

Radiologic Findings in Hemorrhagic Colitis Due to *Escherichia coli* 0157:H7
Shortsleeve MJ, Wilson ME, Finklestein M, Gardner RC (Mount Auburn Hosp; Choate Hosp, Cambridge, Mass)
Gastrointest Radiol 14:341–344, Fall 1989   29–1

Patients with hemorrhagic colitis caused by *Escherichia coli* have abdominal cramps, watery diarrhea progressing to bloody diarrhea, and little or no fever. Ischemic colitis and inflammatory bowel disease may be considered more likely than infection because more than 90% of patients are afebrile. The clinical and radiologic findings were reviewed in 3 patients with hemorrhagic colitis caused by *E. coli* 0157:H7.

All 3 patients had a thickened colonic wall, and 2 had areas of submucosal edema with frank thumbprinting (Fig 29–1). The involved colon was spastic on fluoroscopy. The transverse colon was involved in all 3 patients.

In addition to possibly severe abdominal cramps and diarrhea in the absence of significant fever, these patients have moderate leukocytosis and stools negative for pathogens. Typically illness begins about 4 days after exposure to the organism. The young, the elderly, postgastrectomy patients, and those on antibiotic therapy during exposure to the pathogen are at increased risk. Hemolytic uremic syndrome may be seen. The colitis results from production by *E. coli* 0157:H7 of a cytotoxin similar to a Shiga toxin.

▶ *Escherichia coli* 0157:H7 has emerged as an important cause of infectious colitis. The number of patients with bloody infectious diarrhea with this *E. coli* is unknown, but the reported rate of complications is high, with older patients having the hemolytic uremic syndrome. The recognition of *E. coli* 0157:H7 as a cause of hemorrhagic colitis may indicate (1) a phage transfer of a *Shigella*-like toxin to a previously nonpathogenic *E. coli*, or (2) the isolation of an established *E. coli* strain with a specific toxin. A thickened and edematous colonic wall occurs in other hemorrhagic diarrheal states and should be an expected finding in severe cases.—P.B. Miner, Jr., M.D.

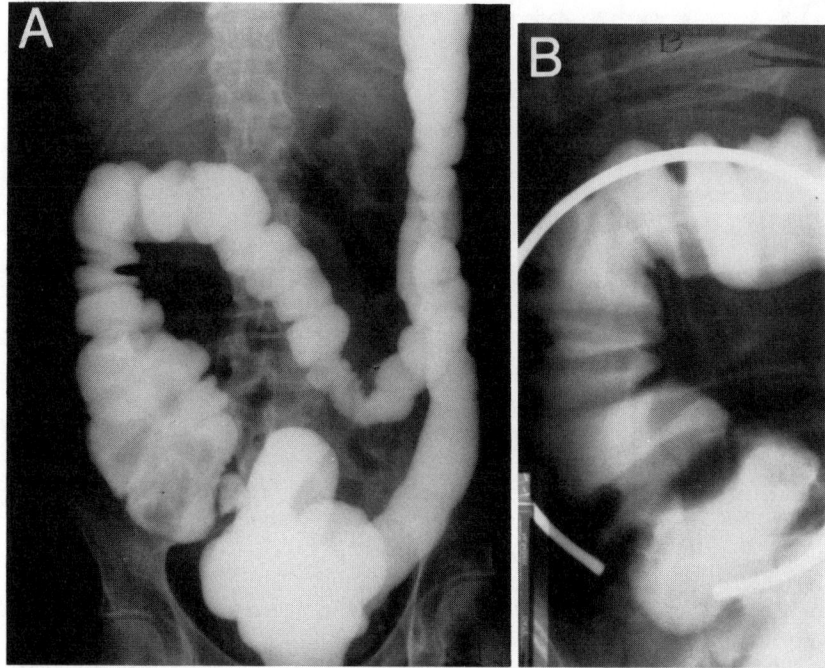

Fig 29-1.—Woman aged 61 years with Escherichia coli O157:H7 hemorrhagic colitis. Note submucosal edema in right and transverse colon (**A**) and thumbprinting in ascending colon (**B**). (Courtesy of Shortsleeve MJ, Wilson ME, Finklestein M, et al: *Gastrointest Radiol* 14:341–344, Fall 1989.)

Shigella

An Outbreak of Shigellosis Associated With the Consumption of Raw Oysters

Reeve G, Martin DL, Pappas J, Thompson RE, Greene KD (Houston Health and Human Services Dept; Texas Dept of Health, Austin; Ctrs for Disease Control, Atlanta)

N Engl J Med 321:224–227, July 27, 1989   29–2

Consumption of raw oysters has been associated with numerous outbreaks of gastroenteritis and hepatitis. *Shigella* infection in persons who have eaten oysters from approved harvesting beds has not been reported previously. An outbreak of *Shigella sonnei* infection occurred in 24 persons who had eaten raw oysters within 5 days before onset of symptoms; all had been served in 8 restaurants in Texas during the summer of 1986.

Inspection of the restaurants involved in the outbreak found them to be in general compliance with regulations pertaining to oyster storage. All 8 restaurants were supplied with fresh oysters by 1 oyster dealer. The oysters had been harvested from approved beds where the waters had been free of fecal contamination just before harvesting. Thus widespread sewage contamination was considered unlikely.

Food-Specific Attack Among the Guests at a Banquet at Restaurant D on July 12, 1986

Food Item	Ate Food Item			Did Not Eat Food Item			Odds Ratio	P Value*
	No. Ill	No. Not Ill	% Ill	No. Ill	No. Not Ill	% Ill		
Oysters	7	10	41	0	24	0	Undefined	<0.001
Crabs	6	16	27	1	18	5	6.8	NS
Mushrooms	6	23	21	1	11	8	2.9	NS
Fruit	2	15	12	5	19	21	0.5	NS
Cheese	5	18	22	2	16	11	2.2	NS
Avocado dip	2	6	25	5	28	15	1.9	NS
Shrimp	7	29	19	0	5	0	Undefined	NS

*The P values were determined with the use of Fisher's exact test. NS, not significant, $P > .05$.

(Courtesy of Reeve G, Martin DL, Pappas J, et al: *N Engl J Med* 321:224–227, July 27, 1989.)

Of 34 stool specimens collected from crew members, 1 yielded *S. sonnei*. The crew member in question was an asymptomatic carrier who reported not having eaten any raw oysters. Isolates from this crew member and from 7 patients with illnesses suggestive of shigellosis had a similar plasmid profile (table). Thus these cases could be linked directly to the *S. sonnei* carrier.

None of the 8 harvesting vessels owned or leased by the oyster dealer were equipped with built-in marine toilets; rather, pails were routinely used as toilets. Several crew members admitted to emptying these pails directly into the waters of the oyster-harvesting sites. This outbreak illustrates the poor sanitary procedures and problems of mishandling human waste on oyster-harvesting vessels. Unfortunately, adherence to public health standards for the handling of human waste on fishing vessels has always been difficult to enforce.

▶ This outbreak of S. *sonnei* resulted from poor sanitary procedures that probably allowed stool from a carrier to contaminate oysters either just before or after they were taken aboard the boat. A convincing argument could be made for not eating raw seafood because consumption of such raw oysters and other shellfish has been associated with numerous outbreaks of disease caused by viruses and several species of bacteria.—N.J. Greenberger, M.D.

Pathogenesis of Shigella Diarrhea: XVI. Selective Targeting of Shiga Toxin to Villus Cells of Rabbit Jejunum Explains the Effect of the Toxin on Intestinal Electrolyte Transport
Kandel G, Donohue-Rolfe A, Donowitz M, Keusch GT (New England Med Ctr/Tufts Univ, Boston; The Johns Hopkins Univ, Baltimore)
J Clin Invest 84:1509–1517, November 1989

Shiga toxin plays a role in the pathogenesis of diarrhea that occurs in *Shigella dysenteriae* infections. To determine the effects of Shiga toxin on intestinal water and electrolyte transport, ligated loops of rabbit jejunum

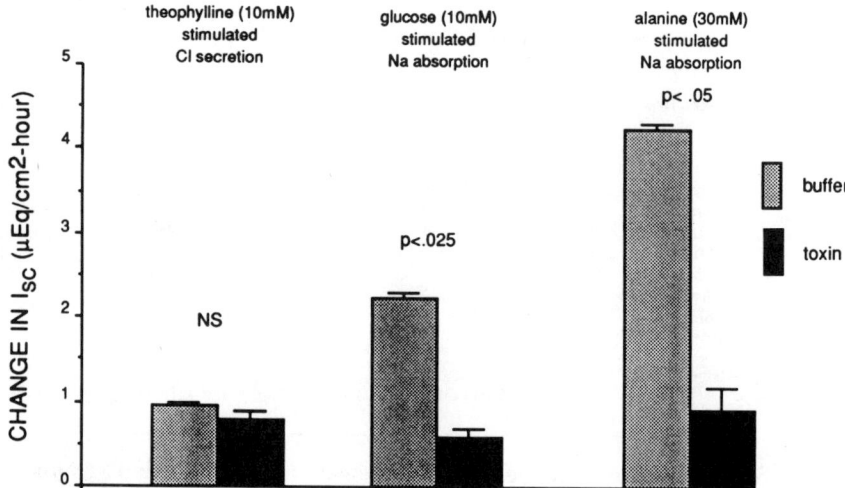

Fig 29-2.—Effect of Shiga toxin on stimulated active electrolyte transport in rabbit jejunum. One hundred twenty minutes after mounting the tissue in Ussing chamber, 10 mM of theophylline was added to the serosal bath, or 10 mM of glucose or 30 mM of alanine were added to the mucosal bath. Results are expressed as the mean ±SE (no. = 9 animals for theophylline and glucose and 3 for alanine). P values are based on the comparison between toxin-incubated and buffer-incubated tissue by paired t-test. (Courtesy of Kandel G, Donohue-Rolfe A, Donowitz M, et al: *J Clin Invest* 84:1509–1517, November 1989.)

were incubated in vivo with purified Shiga toxin and then studied in vivo by single pass perfusion and in vitro by the Ussing chamber voltage-clamp technique.

Toxin-treated loops showed significant accumulation of water in the jejunal lumen, compared with control loops. Net secretion of both sodium and chloride ions occurred as a consequence of diminished mucosa-to-serosa sodium and chloride fluxes. Glucose- and alanine-stimulated sodium absorption also were reduced. In contrast, the Shiga toxin had no effect on either basal short-circuit current (an index of anion secretion) or the secretory response to theophylline (Fig 29-2). Populations of villus and crypt cells from rabbit jejunum were isolated and studied to localize the cellular site of toxin action. There was a 60-fold greater number of binding sites on villus cells than crypt cells. Villus cells were more susceptible to toxin-induced inhibition of protein synthesis than were crypt cells, which was consistent with the presence of a large excess of the neutral glycolipid shiga toxin receptor, G83, on villus cells.

The effect of purified Shiga toxin on intestinal electrolyte transport is demonstrated. Shiga toxin inhibits jejunal fluid absorption without affecting active anion secretion by a preferential effect on the villus cells. This is caused by the differential distribution of toxin receptors on villus cells compared with crypt cells.

▶ As the authors point out in their discussion, all known bacterial enterotoxins, as well as most other protein secretagogues, cause fluid accumulation in the intestinal lumen by inhibiting NaCl absorption while simultaneously stimulating anion secretion. Their results indicate that Shiga toxin is unusual in that, at least in rabbit jejunum, it appears to inhibit Na and Cl absorption without affecting active anion secretion.—N.J. Greenberger, M.D.

Associated With Drinking Water

Chronic Diarrhea Associated With Drinking Untreated Water
Parsonnet J, Trock SC, Bopp CA, Wood CJ, Addiss DG, Alai F, Gorelkin L, Hargrett-Bean N, Gunn RA, Tauxe RV (Ctrs for Disease Control, Atlanta; Illinois Dept of Public Health, Springfield)
Ann Intern Med 110:985–991, June 15, 1989   29–4

No causative agent has been found for "Brainerd diarrhea." An outbreak of a distinct chronic diarrheal illness in Henderson County, Illinois, allowed study of this illness through 72 patients, including truck drivers who ate at the local restaurant suspected as the source (cohorts), local residents, and restaurant patrons who had no diarrhea (controls).

Characteristics of the nonbloody diarrhea included urgency; extreme frequency, with a median of 12 stools per day; fecal incontinence; and a mean weight loss of 4.5 kg. The median incubation period was 10 days. No patient died, but 9 were hospitalized. In 87% of the patients diarrhea persisted after 6 months. No known enteropathogenic agents were detected in stools. Colon biopsy specimens showed normal results or mild inflammation. A local restaurant was implicated as the source, and the untreated well water was the vehicle of transmission. Truck drivers visiting the restaurant increased their risk of illness if they were older, visited more often, and drank more water there.

This is the first outbreak of chronic diarrheal illness linked to untreated water. Physicians should be aware of this syndrome and, recognizing it, should investigate case clusters and possible exposure to untreated water or unpasteurized milk.

▶ This outbreak of chronic diarrhea linked to drinking untreated water is similar to that described in "Brainerd diarrhea" (1). The causative agent and pathophysiologic mechanism of both illnesses remain elusive. The authors suggest a standard case definition for "Brainerd diarrhea" so that responsible vehicles can be identified and transmission interrupted. The criteria would include the following:

1. Acute onset of illness.
2. Nonbloody diarrhea lasting longer than 1 month with negative stool examination for known bacterial and parasitic pathogens.
3. Fecal urgency.
4. Absence of fever.
5. Eight or more stools per day throughout the first week of illness.
6. Normal colonoscopy and normal or mild chronic inflammatory changes on colon biopsy.
7. Normal stool fat or D-xylose test, or both.

The authors assert that this case definition, though untested, would distinguish this chronic diarrheal syndrome from mild diarrheal illness that may be heterogeneous in cause and result from inflammatory bowel or malabsorptive diseases, and collagenous or lymphocytic ("microscopic") colitis.—N.J. Greenberger, M.D.

Reference

1. Osterholin MT, McDonald KL, White KE et al: An outbreak of a newly recognized chronic diarrhea associated with raw milk consumption. JAMA 256:484, 1986.

Large Community Outbreak of Cryptosporidiosis Due to Contamination of a Filtered Public Water Supply

Hayes EB, Matte TD, O'Brien TR, McKinley TW, Logsdon GS, Rose JB, Ungar BLP, Word DM, Pinsky PF, Cummings ML, Wilson MA, Long EG, Hurwitz ES, Juranek DD (Ctrs for Disease Control; Georgia Dept of Human Resources, Atlanta; Environmental Protection Agency, Cincinnati; Univ of Arizona, Tucson; Uniformed Services Univ of the Health Sciences, Bethesda, Md; et al)
N Engl J Med 320:1372–1376, May 25, 1989   29-5

A filtered public water supply was contaminated by *Cryptosporidium*, resulting in the largest outbreak of cryptosporidiosis to date. Between January 12 and February 7, 1987, an outbreak of gastroenteritis affected an estimated 13,000 persons in a county of 64,900 residents in western Georgia. The overall estimated attack rate for the county was 40%. *Cryptosporidium* oocysts were identified in 58 of 147 patients (39%) with gastroenteritis tested during the outbreak. No other enteric pathogens were identified.

Signs and symptoms included diarrhea, stomach pain, nausea, vomiting, fever, and muscle aches. In an random telephone survey, gastrointestinal tract illness was reported by 299 (61%) of 489 household members exposed to the public water supply, compared with 64 (20%) of 322 who were not exposed. The prevalence of Cryptosporidium-specific IgG was significantly higher among exposed respondents to the survey who had been ill than among nonresident controls.

The sudden onset of widespread gastrointestinal tract illness affecting persons of all ages was typical of a waterborne outbreak. *Cryptosporidium* oocysts were identified by a monoclonal antibody test in samples of treated public water. The sand-filtered and chlorinated water met all regulatory agency quality standards, but suboptimal flocculation and filtration probably allowed the parasite to pass into the drinking water supply. Possible contributors to contamination of the surface water supply were low-level *Cryptosporidium* infection in cattle in the watershed and a sewage overflow. Current standards for the treatment of public water supplies may not prevent the contamination of drinking water by *Cryptosporidium*.

▶ As the authors emphasize in their discussion, the results of this investigation demonstrate that *Cryptosporidium* can contaminate filtered public water systems, even when the water quality is within regulatory limits for coliform bacteria, chlorine, and turbidity, causing large epidemics of gastroenteritis in otherwise healthy persons.—N.J. Greenberger, M.D.

C. difficile and Antibiotic-Associated Diarrhea

Nosocomial Acquisition of Clostridium difficile Infection
McFarland LV, Mulligan ME, Kwok RYY, Stamm WE (Univ of Washington; Univ of California, Los Angeles)
N Engl J Med 320:204–210, Jan 26, 1989   29–6

The acquisition and transmission of *Clostridium difficile* were studied by taking rectal swab cultures prospectively from 428 patients admitted within 11 months to a single general medical ward. The hands of health care workers and environmental surfaces also were cultured. Strains of *C. difficile* were distinguished by immunoblot typing.

Thirty of 428 patients (7%) had positive cultures when admitted. Of these 30 patients, 23 had been hospitalized recently, whereas 6 had community-acquired infections. The organism was acquired in the hospital by 21% of patients with negative cultures at admission. Types 1, 2, 4, and 5 were most frequent. Nearly one fourth of incident cases acquired *C. difficile* within a week after admission. Those acquiring it later had more marked underlying disease and had been exposed to more antibiotics. About one third of the patients had diarrhea, but none had colitis.

Time-space clustering of incident cases with the same immunoblot types indicated patient-to-patient transmission. Most of those caring for patients with positive cultures themselves had positive cultures. Hospital rooms occupied by both symptomatic and asymptomatic patients often were contaminated (table). At discharge, 82% of incident cases still had positive cultures, and these patients often went to an extended care facility.

Patient-to-patient transmission of *C. difficile* clearly is important in the hospital environment. In addition to direct spread, hospital personnel and environmental contamination can contribute to transmission. Helpful measures include hand washing, routine body-substance precautions, and frequent environmental disinfection.

	Environmental Isolation of *C. difficile*			
Culture Source	Rooms With Culture-Negative Patients*	Rooms With Asymptomatic Carriers	Rooms With Patients With C. Difficile Diarrhea	Total Positive/ Total Tested (%)
	no. of positive cultures (%)			
Bedrail	0	2	10	12/31 (39)
Commode	1	3	1	5/13 (38)
Floor	5	3	18	26/72 (36)
Call button	1	2	6	9/30 (30)
Windowsill	0	1	2	3/10 (30)
Toilet	0	0	3	3/17 (18)
Other†	0	0	4	4/43 (9)
Total positive cultures	7 (8)	11 (29)	44 (49)	62 (29)
No. of cultures	88	38	90	216

*Rooms in which no patients with positive cultures for *C. difficile* were in residence for more than 48 hours.
†Other sources include the dialysis machine (1), the sink (1), nasogastric alimentation preparation (1), and slipper bottoms (1).
(Courtesy of McFarland LV, Mulligan ME, Kwok RYY, et al: *N Engl J Med* 320:204–210, Jan 26, 1989.)

▶ These findings indicate that nosocomial C. *difficile* infection, which is associated with diarrhea in about one third of cases, is transmitted frequently among hospitalized patients, and that the organism often is present on the hands of hospital personnel caring for such patients. Effective preventive measures clearly are needed to reduce the nosocomial acquisition of C. *difficile*.

That this also is a particularly vexing problem in intensive care is evident from a recent report by Foulk and Silva[1]. Several patients hospitalized in a 12-bed medical intensive care unit were found to have C.-*difficile*-associated colitis. Stool cultures of all patients identified 8 cases (3 culture positive and 5 culture and cytotoxin positive), 7 of which were geographically and temporarily clustered within a 2-week period. At least 1 patient appeared to contract the disease after hospitalization and in the absence of antibiotic therapy or other known major risk factors. The outbreak highlights the problem of C. *difficile* in the intensive care unit. A heightened awareness of the multiple risk factors and preventive measures, along with consideration of possible nosocomial transmission, is necessary to prevent or arrest future clusters of cases in the intensive care unit. The diagnosis of 1 patient with this infection in a unit should prompt a review of all other patients within that unit.—N.J. Greenberger, M.D.

Reference

1. Foulk GE, Silve J Jr: *Clostridium difficile* in the intensive care unit. Management problems and prevention issues. *Crit Care Med* 17:822, 1989.

Prevention of Antibiotic-Associated Diarrhea by *Saccharomyces boulardii*: A Prospective Study
Surawicz CM, Elmer GW, Speelman P, McFarland LV, Chinn J, van Belle G (Univ of Washington)
Gastroenterology 96:981–988, April 1989   29–7

Saccharomyces boulardii, a nonpathogenic yeast, is widely used in Europe to prevent antibiotic-associated diarrhea (AAD). Its effectivity in preventing AAD in an acute care setting was investigated in 180 hospitalized patients in a prospective, double-blind, controlled study. During a 23-month period 116 patients were randomly assigned to receive lyophilized *S. boulardii*, 1 gm, and 64 patients received placebo, within 48 hours of antibiotic therapy and continued for 2 weeks after the last antibiotic dose.

The incidence of diarrhea was significantly decreased in patients receiving *S. boulardii* (9.5%) than in those receiving placebo (21.8%) (Fig 29–3). The efficacy of *S. boulardii* in preventing AAD was 56.7%. Significant risk factors for AAD were multiple antibiotic combinations, particularly those containing clindamycin, cephalosporins, or trimethoprim-sulfamethoxazole, and nasogastric tube feeding. No side effects from *S. boulardii* were noted. The role of *Clostridium difficile* in AAD and the association between *C. difficile* diarrhea and yeast treatment were examined. There was no significant relationship between AAD and the presence of *C. difficile* or cytotoxin in

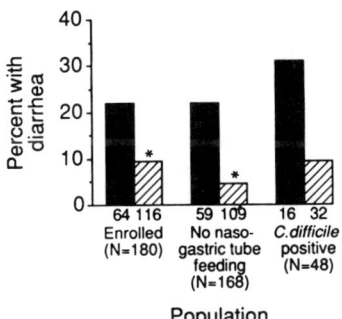

Fig 29-3.—Effectiveness of *S. boulardii* for prevention of antibiotic-associated diarrhea. Solid bars, patients on placebo; hatched bars, patients treated with *S. boulardii*. *Significant difference, P< .05. Numbers at the bottom of the bars denote size of total population at risk. (Courtesy of Surawicz CM, Elmer GW, Speelman P, et al: *Gastroenterology* 96:981–988, April 1989.)

the stools. Of the patients without diarrhea, 35% were culture positive for *C. difficile* and nearly 50% were positive for cytotoxin; similar values were obtained for those with diarrhea. Of the patients at risk of acquiring *C. difficile* (i.e., initial stool sample culture was negative), *S. boulardii* did not prevent such acquisition. Of the *C. difficile*-positive patients, diarrhea occurred in 9.4% of yeast-treated patients compared with 31% of placebo-treated patients.

These data suggest that *S. boulardii* may reduce the risk of AAD in hospitalized patients. Prophylactic *S. boulardii* may be most beneficial in patients for whom the risk of AAD and pseudomembranous colitis is greatest.

Typhoid Enteritis and Perforation

Perforated Typhoid Enteritis: Operative Experience With 108 Cases
Meier DE, Imediegwu OO, Tarpley JL (Baptist Med Ctr, Ogbomoso, Nigeria)
Am J Surg 157:423–427, April 1989   29–8

Typhoid fever remains a serious health problem in developing countries. This chronic systemic illness has a mortality of 15% when untreated. Survivors typically require a prolonged convalescent stage. Perforation, a major cause of death in treated patients, is managed by aggressive surgery at the Nigerian hospital in this study. A retrospective review describes 108 patients with perforated typhoid enteritis confirmed at surgery.

Common presenting symptoms included fever, abdominal pain, vomiting, diarrhea, and constipation. Most patients (73%) had abdominal distention. The average systolic blood pressure was 104 mm Hg, and the average pulse rate was 121 beats per minute. Surgical treatment was undertaken within 24 hours of presentation in most cases (84%).

Moderate or severe intraperitoneal contamination was noted in 80% of the patients. Most perforations were less than 8 mm in size and were in the ileum at an average distance of 22 cm proximal to the ileocecal valve. Débridement and 2-layer bowel closure was the routine treatment method. Surgical complications included intraabdominal abcess in 20 patients, wound dehiscence in 14, and subsequent typhoid perforations in 9. Major laparotomies were repeated in 24 cases.

Of the 35 deaths (32%), 25 (71%) resulted from overwhelming sepsis. A third of the patients died within 24 hours of surgery. Higher mortalities were associated with female sex, systolic blood pressure less than 90 mm Hg on admission, generalized abdominal tenderness, delay in operation, multiple perforations, and subsequent perforations.

In many parts of the developing world, diagnostic and treatment measures are limited. Yet, deaths occur from perforated typhoid enteritis in spite of aggressive surgery, antibiotics, and adequate fluid therapy. Improved survival will come only when safe water supplies and adequate waste disposal are provided throughout the world.

▶ This report is a reminder that a great deal of work remains to be done on the level of public health provided to the Earth's citizens. Typhoid enteritis, a serious complication of typhoid fever, can be eliminated easily by improved environmental conditions in countries where it exists. Surgical treatment of perforations of the gut is the general treatment. The high levels of intra-abdominal abscesses and wound dehiscence probably relate to the poor nutrition and general health of the patients with typhoid. Immunosuppression also must be a prominent feature of the illness because the mode of death usually is sepsis.—F.G. Moody, M.D.

30 Lymphocytic ("Microscopic") Colitis

Lymphocytic ("Microscopic") Colitis: A Comparative Histopathologic Study With Particular Reference To Collagenous Colitis
Lazenby AJ, Yardley JH, Giardiello FM, Jessurun J, Bayless TM (Johns Hopkins Univ; Johns Hopkins Hosp; Hosp de Mexico SS, Mexico City)
Hum Pathol 20:18-28, January 1989

It is proposed that "microscopic colitis" be renamed lymphocytic colitis. This clinicopathologic syndrome is characterized by watery diarrhea, grossly normal colonoscopy, and mucosal inflammatory changes. To delineate the histopathology of lymphocytic colitis, colorectal biopsy specimens obtained from 16 patients with lymphocytic colitis were compared with those of 17 patients with collagenous colitis, 16 with idiopathic inflammatory bowel disease, 1 with acute colitis, and 12 with histologically normal colon. A blinded, semiquantitative analysis of histologic features in the surface epithelium, lamina propria, and crypts was performed.

The most distinctive feature of lymphocytic colitis was a diffuse increase in surface intraepithelial lymphocytes (mean, 24.6 lymphocytes per 100 epithelial cells; Fig 30-1). Other prominent features noted in lymphocytic colitis were surface epithelial flattening, increased crypt lymphocytes, and minimal crypt distortion or active cryptitis. Collagenous colitis had striking similarities with lymphocytic colitis, including increased epithelial lymphocytes, surface epithelial damage, and increased lamina propria mononuclear cells. However, subepithelial collagen thickening was seen only in collagenous colitis. Idiopathic inflammatory bowel disease exhibited prominent crypt distortion, greater active inflammation, and minimal intraepithelial lymphocytes. Acute colitis showed prominent surface epithelial damage but was otherwise dissimilar from lymphocytic colitis.

Because of its characteristic histopathology, including prominent lymphocytic infiltration of the epithelium, "microscopic colitis" should more appropriately be renamed lymphocytic colitis. Clinical and histologic findings between lymphocytic colitis and collagenous colitis are striking, but each entity is distinct on biopsy. Lymphocytic colitis, however, is readily distinguishable from idiopathic inflammatory bowel disease, acute colitis, and normal colorectum.

▶ This carefully done study provides new information on lymphocytic ("micro-

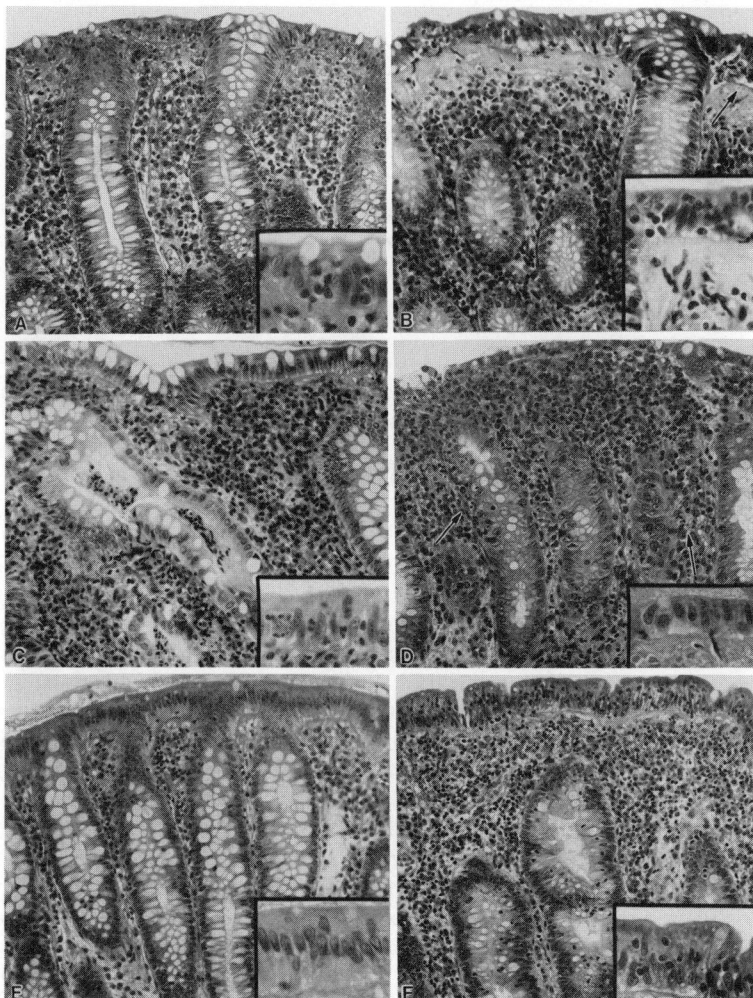

Fig 30–1.—Comparisons of various forms of colitis, histologically normal colon, and small bowel with celiac disease. **A,** lymphocytic colitis. Diffusely increased surface intraepithelial lymphocytes and surface epithelial damage *(inset)* are the major distinguishing features of lymphocytic colitis. Increased lamina propria chronic inflammation, prominent crypt lymphocytes, and mild crypt distortion also can be seen. **B,** collagenous colitis. A distinct subepithelial collagen band is shown, as well as epithelial detachment *(arrow)* and prominent surface intraepithelial lymphocytes *(inset)*. The lamina propria has increased chronic inflammation, and there is mild crypt distortion. **C,** idiopathic inflammatory bowel disease (ulcerative colitis). In idiopathic inflammatory bowel disease, numbers of intraepithelial lymphocytes are minimal, and the surface epithelium is usually tall and columnar (surface epithelial flattening may be present in severe active disease). In active disease, neutrophils are the most numerous intraepithelial inflammatory cells *(inset)*. Prominent crypt distortion, crypt abscesses, and heavy lamina propria chronic inflammation are also present. **D,** acute colitis (*Shigella* sp. infection). In acute colitis, the surface epithelium often is flattened, but intraepithelial lymphocytes are sparse *(inset)*. Chronic inflammatory cells are concentrated in the superficial lamina propria. Neutrophils can be seen in the crypts as well as in the lamina propria *(arrows)*. **E,** "normal colon." This histologically unremarkable colon biopsy has tall columnar epithelial cells and minimal intraepithelial inflammatory cells, and lacks significant crypt distortion and lamina propria chronic inflammation. **F,** celiac disease. The prominent surface damage and increased intraepithelial lymphocytes in this small bowel biopsy of untreated celiac disease are strikingly similar to those changes seen in lymphocytic and collagenous colitis. (All stained with hematoxylin-eosin. All magnifications originally × 200. All inset magnifications originally × 400.) (Courtesy of Lazenby AJ, Yardley JH, Giardiello FM, et al: *Hum Pathol* 20:18-28, January 1989.)

scopic") colitis and collagenous colitis. The striking clinical similarities between the 2 disorders can be summarized briefly as follows: (1) patients are predominantly elderly women; (2) watery diarrhea is secretory in type, with stool volumes of 500–1,000 mL/day frequently noted; (3) colonoscopy and contrast studies of the small and large bowel are normal; and (4) response to treatment with various drugs is often unsatisfactory. Although clinical features and histologic findings obviously are similar, Lazenby et al. believe that each entity is distinct on examination of biopsy specimens.

The same investigators also have reported lymphocytic enterocolitis in patients with "refractory sprue" (1). They describe a patient with refractory sprue who had malabsorption, a flat small bowel biopsy specimen unresponsive to a gluten-free diet, and colonic biopsy specimens consistent with lymphocytic (microscopic) colitis. To investigate further the relationship between celiac disease and lymphocytic or collagenous colitis (a similar and possibly related entity), they examined colorectal and small bowel biopsy specimens in patients indexed histologically as having celiac disease who had been seen at Johns Hopkins Hospital since 1958. Of 135 indexed patients, 21 had colorectal biopsies. Colorectal biopsy specimens were abnormal in 7 of the 21 patients: 4 had biopsy specimens resembling lymphocytic colitis, 2 had acute colitis, and another patient had both lymphocytic and acute colitis. None had collagenous colitis. The 3 patients with lymphocytic colitis and celiac-like changes of the small bowel who never responded to a gluten-free diet may represent a distinctive panintestinal disease for which the term *lymphocytic enterocolitis with malabsorption* is proposed.—N.J. Greenberger, M.D.

Reference

1. Dubois RN, Lazenby AJ, Yardly JH, et al: Lymphocytic enterocolitis in patients with "refractory sprue." *JAMA* 262:935, 1989.

Lymphocytic (Microscopic) Colitis: Clinicopathologic Study of 18 Patients and Comparison to Collagenous Colitis
Giardiello FM, Lazenby AJ, Bayless TM, Levine EJ, Bias WB, Ladenson PW, Hutcheon DF, Derevjanik NL, Yardley JH (Johns Hopkins Univ)
Dig Dis Sci 34:1730–1738, November 1989

Data were reviewed on 18 patients with a mean age of 54 years who had lymphocytic colitis, a form of chronic watery diarrhea with diffuse mucosal inflammatory changes and prominent intraepithelial lymphocytes. These patients had about 25 lymphocytes for each 100 surface epithelial cells. Subepithelial collagen thickening was noted in only 1 patient.

The patients had had an average of 5 bowel movements a day for a mean of nearly 3 years. Twelve had mild diffuse crampy abdominal pain. Only 2 had clinical evidence of malabsorption. Nine of 11 patients had arthritic complaints, and 5 had a nondeforming polyarticular arthritis of unknown cause. Preliminary HLA serotyping in 9 patients showed an increase in

HLA-A1, compared with the control population. Eight of 9 patients had responses to anti-inflammatory agents, but 4 of 5 given nonspecific therapy also improved.

The clinical similarity between lymphocytic colitis and collagenous colitis is considerable, but there also are differences (table), which could reflect etiologic or pathogenic differences. No definite dietary or medication-related cause of lymphocytic colitis has been identified. Two patients did report an onset of symptoms after a Caribbean cruise. The role of immune mechanisms in perpetuating the disorder after an external insult warrants further consideration.

▶ The etiologies of lymphocytic and collagenous colitis remain a mystery. The data provided by this study support the authors' conclusion that lymphocytic and collagenous colitis share many clinical features and may be related, yet distinct, disorders. The paper contains useful information on the natural history and response to treatment of lymphocytic colitis and should be read in its entirety.—N.J. Greenberger, M.D.

Comparison of Lymphocytic and Collagenous Colitis

	Lymphocytic Colitis	Collagenous Colitis
Similarities		
Watery diarrhea	18/18 (100%)	21/21 (100%)
Diarrhea duration (years)	2.8 ± 3.3 (sd) (Range 0.25–10)	5.3 ± 6.0 (0.5–18)
Mean age (years)	53.8 ± 17.2	59.3 ± 16.3
Arthritis	9/11 (82%)	6/7 (86%)
Colonoscopy essentially normal	18/18 (100%)*	9/12 (75%)
Normal Barium Enema	8/10 (80%)	13/14 (93%)
Increased intraepithelial lymphocytes	18/18 (100%)	21/21 (100%)
Differences		
Female-Male ratio	1.3:1	20.0:1
HLA antigens†	(+)A1, (+)DRW53	−DQ2
Autoantibodies	6/12 (50%)	1/11 (09%)
Increased subepithelial collagen	1/18 (6%)‡	20/20 (100%)

*Six patients had nonspecific findings.
†In excess (+); underrepresented (−).
‡Patient later had subepithelial collagen thickening.
(Courtesy of Giardiello FM, Lazenby AJ, Bayless TM, et al: *Dig Dis Sci* 34:1730–1738, November 1989.)

31 Diversion Colitis

Treatment of Diversion Colitis With Short-Chain–Fatty Acid Irrigation
Harig JM, Soergel KH, Komorowski RA, Wood CM (Med College of Wisconsin, Milwaukee)
N Engl J Med 320:23–28, Jan 5, 1989

Diversion colitis often develops in segments of the colorectum after surgical diversion of the fecal stream and persists indefinitely unless the excluded segment is reanastomosed. It is characterized by bleeding from inflamed colonic mucosa, similar to that observed in idiopathic inflammatory bowel disease. Stricture formation may be a sequela. Several mechanisms may account for this condition: bacterial overgrowth of normal colonic flora, invasion by pathogenic organisms, or the absence of short-chain fatty acids (SCFAs), which are the preferred metabolic substrates of colonic epithelium.

Four patients with diversion colitis were studied, none of whom had evidence of Crohn's disease or idiopathic ulcerative or infectious colitis. Breath hydrogen test results suggested that the normal carbohydrate-fermenting anaerobic bacterial flora was absent from the bypassed segment but present in the colon remaining in continuity with the fecal stream. Cultures of the luminal content of the bypassed segments showed no enteropathogenic bacteria. However, the excluded segment of the rectosigmoid contained negligible concentrations of SCFAs. Local instillation of an SCFA solution twice daily for 2–4 weeks resulted in the disappearance of symptoms and inflammatory changes observed at endoscopy. In 1 patient complete remission was achieved for up to 14 months after a maintenance regimen of twice-weekly instillation of the SCFA solution. In contrast, interruption of treatment or administration of enemas containing isotonic saline for 2–7 weeks resulted in definite worsening of the colitis or no improvement at all. Histologic observation revealed a distinctive type of mucosal inflammation that resolved more slowly and less completely than the gross appearance of the inflamed mucosa.

Diversion colitis may represent an inflammatory state resulting from a nutritional deficiency in the lumen of the colonic epithelium, and this condition can be treated effectively with intermittent irrigation with SCFA solution, the missing nutrients.

▶ Short-chain fatty acids are the predominant anions in feces and are produced in the human colon by bacterial fermentation of dietary fiber and other saccharides escaping absorption in the small bowel. Short-chain fatty acids originally were thought to be important in the pathogenesis of diarrhea in carbohydrate malabsorption because of their limited absorption by the colon. However, recent studies indicate that SCFAs are readily absorbed from the colon. It is important that SCFAs have been shown to stimulate active sodium and chloride absorption in the distal colon (1). Binder and Mehta suggest that SCFAs may diminish stool fluid losses that occur as a consequence of altered small intestinal carbohydrate absorption and may be important in the overall regulation of fluid and electrolyte absorption in the large intestine.

Mortensen et al. (2) have demonstrated that colectomized patients with short bowel syndrome have extremely low levels of SCFA in intestinal outputs, whereas patients partially colectomized and patients with small bowel bypass or short bowel syndrome with preserved colon had normal fecal concentrations of SCFA.—N.J. Greenberger, M.D.

References

1. Binder JH, Mehta P: Short chain fatty acids stimulate active sodium and chloride absorption in vitro in the rat distal colon.
2. Mortensen PB, et al: Short chain fatty acids in bowel contents after intestinal surgery. *Gastroenterology* 97:1090; 1989.

32 Ileal-Anal Anastomoses

Ileal Pouch–Anal Anastomosis: Comparison of Results in Familial Adenomatous Polyposis and Chronic Ulcerative Colitis
Dozois RR, Kelly KA, Welling DR, Gordon H, Beart RW Jr, Wolff BG, Pemberton JH, Ilstrup DM (Mayo Clinic and Mayo Found, Rochester, Minn)
Ann Surg 210:268–273, September 1989   32–1

Proctocolectomy with ileal pouch–anal anastomosis (IPAA) maintains anorectal function and avoids the need for permanent abdominal ileostomy in patients with either chronic ulcerative colitis or familial adenomatous polyposis. Although ileorectostomy is still preferred in patients with polyposis, this preference may be based on unsatisfactory results with IPAA in patients with colitis. Results of IPAA in polyposis patients were compared with those in colitis patients.

A series of 758 patients underwent IPAA for chronic ulcerative colitis; in 94 the procedure was used to treat familial adenomatous polyposis. Colitis patients were an average of 4 years older than polyposis patients, but sex, pouch design, and type of diverting ileostomy were similar in both groups.

Two colitis patients died after surgery; no deaths occurred among polyposis patients. Complication rates were similar in both groups as were rates for reoperation for intestinal obstruction. However, sepsis requiring reoperation occurred in 6% of colitis patients but in no polyposis patients. At mean 3-year followup, polyposis patients had fewer daytime stools, less nocturnal fecal spotting, and less pouchitis than colitis patients.

Ileal pouch–anal anastomosis was better tolerated in polyposis patients than in colitis patients, and polyposis patients had less long-term disability. Postoperative sepsis, frequency of daytime stooling, nocturnal incontinence, and pouchitis may be at least in part related to the disease and not the surgeon or the procedure.

▶ Dozois and his associates document that ileal pouch–anal anastomosis after total colectomy is better tolerated by patients with familial polyposis than those operated upon for ulcerative colitis. There are several potential explanations for this outcome, but I favor the one offered by the authors. The debilitating effects of inflammatory bowel disease and the immunosuppressive and metabolic derangements of steroids are likely the adverse factors in the negative outcome. Nevertheless, it is the preferred treatment for the majority of patients with inflammatory bowel disease.—F.G. Moody, M.D.

Alterations in Ileoanal Pouch Technique, 1980 to 1987: Complications and Functional Outcome
Liljeqvist L, Lindquist K, Ljungdahl I (Karolinska Inst, Stockholm)
Dis Colon Rectum 31:929–938, December 1988   32–2

In 1980, the ileoanal pouch technique was relatively new, and unique ways had to be developed to handle complications, to solve evacuation problems with the S-pouch, and to improve operative technique to reduce incontinence and the number of bowel movements. The evolution of experience from 1980 to 1987 was reported.

Thirty-four women and 48 men received an ileoanal pouch. Fifty patients underwent colectomy before pouch surgery; 46 had ileostomy, and 4 had ileorectal anastomosis. Thirty-two patients underwent simultaneous colectomy and pouch surgery. During the first 2 years, S-pouches with long muscle cuffs were used. Later, both J-pouches and S-pouches were used and the muscle cuffs were shortened. In 1985, a more sphincter-preserving technique was adopted, less anal dilatation was introduced, and a strip of transitional epithelium above the dentate line was left intact.

The functional outcome was evaluated in 66 patients followed for a mean 23 months. The mean number of bowel movements in 24 hours was 5; 82% of patients had deferral times of more than 1 hour, and 74% had no leakage or staining. Significantly more men than women had nightly evacuations. Older age was significantly related to leakage and short deferral time.

Ileoanal separations and evacuation problems in early years were significantly reduced by shortening the efferent conduits and muscle cuffs. After reduction of anal dilatation and preservation of the transitional zone, postoperative continence also was significantly improved.

Modifications of the operative technique for construction of the ileoanal pouch has greatly improved the functional outcome. However, perfect continence and low frequency are yet to be achieved in all patients.

▶ The authors share with the reader the trials and tribulations of perfecting the ileal pouch–anal anastomosis. The retrospective provides a clear view of the false paths that were taken in evaluating this important advance in the treatment of ulcerative colitis and familial polyposis. Perfection still eludes even those who have done hundreds of such procedures. Stool frequency and nocturnal soiling require further study.—F.G. Moody, M.D.

Quality of Life After Brooke Ileostomy and Ileal Pouch–Anal Anastomosis: Comparison of Performance Status
Pemberton JH, Phillips SF, Ready RR, Zinsmeister AR, Beahrs OH (Mayo Clinic, Rochester, Minn)
Ann Surg 209:620–628, May 1989   32–3

It has been reported that patients who have undergone proctocolectomy with a Brooke ileostomy in the treatment of chronic ulcerative colitis or familial adenomatous polyposis generally adapt well to the presence of their stomal device. However, other studies found a high incidence of depression and isolation among these patients. To determine whether the newer ileal pouch–anal anastomosis operation improves the quality of life compared with the conventional Brooke ileostomy, 298 patients who had received an ileal pouch and 406 who had a Brooke ileostomy were studied.

The ileostomy patients were sent a questionnaire to determine the impact of the operation and the stomal appliance on their lifestyles. The ileal pouch patients were mostly interviewed by telephone. Questions dealt with the patient's perception of general health, dietary restrictions, social habits, occupation, and daily activities. The median follow-up in Brooke ileostomy patients was 104 months, and in ileal pouch patients, 47 months.

Statistical analysis of the data revealed that 93% of the Brooke ileostomy patients and 95% of the ileal pouch patients were satisfied with the outcome. However, when asked whether they would like a change in the type of ileostomy they had, 39% of the Brooke ileostomy patients desired such a change. Ileal pouch patients had a median of 5 stools per day and 1 at night. During the day, 77% of the patients reported no incontinence, 22% had occasional incontinence, and 1% had frequent incontinence. Brooke ileostomy patients emptied their stomal bag a median of 6 times per day. Sexual limitation was reported by 30% of Brooke ileostomy patients, compared with 13% of ileal pouch–anal anastomosis patients. Examination of quality-of-life results in 7 areas of daily activities revealed that overall, ileal pouch–anal anastomosis was associated with improved performance in each of the 7 categories examined. Patients who undergo ileal pouch-anal anastomosis have significant advantages in performing daily activities compared with patients with Brooke ileostomy, and thus may experience a better quality of life.

▶ Patients with Brooke ileostomies showed remarkable adaptation to their stoma, but their quality of life was inferior to that of patients who had undergone ileal pouch-anal anastomosis. However, the follow-up was 2.5 times less than that for the patients with a Brooke ileostomy; perhaps time will bring the groups closer together with regard to performance criteria, although I doubt it. Anal defecation, even if frequent, would appear to be a more natural way to live.—F.G. Moody, M.D.

33 Rectal Injuries and Colonic Trauma

Colostomy and Drainage for Civilian Rectal Injuries: Is That All?
Burch JM, Feliciano DV, Mattox KL (Baylor College of Medicine, Houston)
Ann Surg 209:600–611, May 1989   33–1

The routine use of colostomy, presacral drainage, antibiotics, and blood transfusions have dramatically decreased the mortality of traumatic rectal injuries. However, the more destructive MK-47 rifle used in the Vietnam War caused severe rectal trauma, which required additional measures (e.g., diverting colostomy, débridement and repair of rectal perforations, and irrigation of the distal rectum). There is no agreement among civilian centers over the utility of some of these additional therapeutic options.

To determine to what extent additional therapeutic options as used in Vietnam are applicable to the treatment of traumatic rectal injuries in civilian urban trauma centers, data were reviewed for a 10-year period in which 88 men and 12 women (average age, 28 years) were treated for extraperitoneal rectal injuries. Mechanisms of injury included firearms in 82 patients, stab wounds in 3, other penetrating injuries in 10, and blunt trauma in 5. Rectal examination was performed in 99 patients; proctoscopy was performed in 67 patients. Treatment of the rectal injury was determined by the operating surgeon's bias, the patient's condition, and the magnitude of the rectal injury.

Diversion of the fecal stream was achieved by proximal loop colostomies in 44 patients, diverting colostomies in 51 patients, Hartmann's procedure in 4 patients (Fig 33–1), and abdominoperineal resection in 1 patient. Extraperitoneal rectal perforations were closed in 21 patients. Forty-six patients underwent rectal irrigation. Transperineal presacral drainage was used in 93 patients (Fig 33–2). Eleven patients had infectious complications directly attributable to rectal wound management. Four patients died of their injuries.

Statistical analysis revealed that only the failure to drain the presacral space increased the likelihood of infectious complications. It could not be determined with certainty that any of the other therapeutic options correlated with outcome. Therefore, a totally diverting colostomy and presacral drainage remain for now the hallmark of treating traumatic rectal injuries.

▶ Civilian rectal injuries, at least in Houston, can be managed effectively by a diverting colostomy and drainage of the presacral space. More extensive procedures such as were required with the destructive lesions seen in Vietnam are not

186 / The Colon

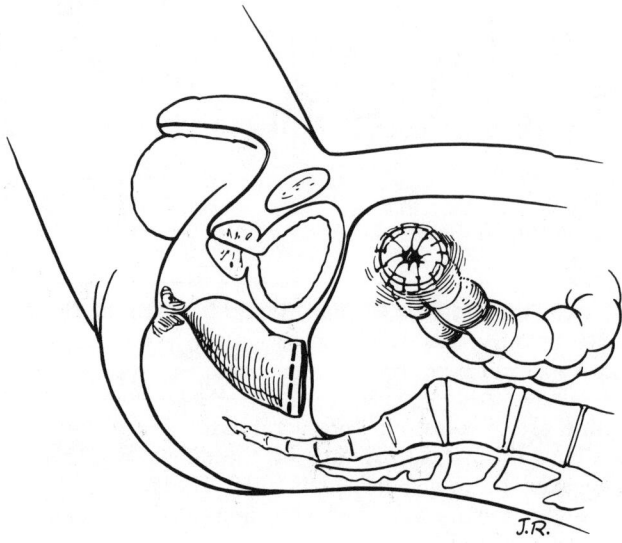

Fig 33–1.—Hartmann's procedure most often is used for large injuries with loss of rectal wall. Resection is performed at level of injury. (Courtesy of Burch JM, Feliciano DV, Mattox KL: *Ann Surg* 209:600–611, May 1989.)

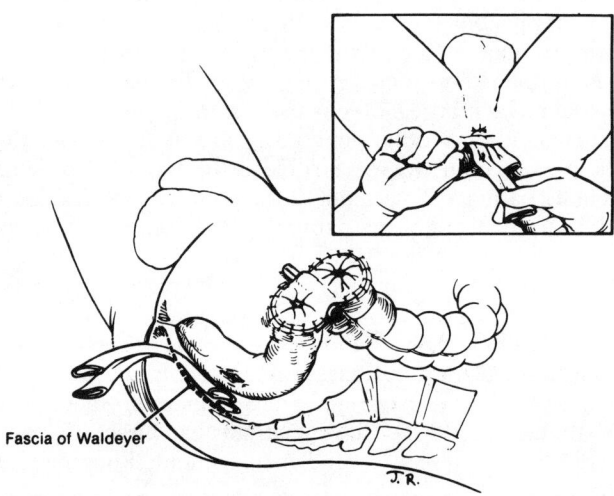

Fig 33–2.—Correct placement of presacral drain via transperineal route. (Courtesy of Burch JM, Feliciano DV, Mattox KL: *Ann Surg* 209:600–611, May 1989.)

indicated except when the injury is from an AK-47-delivered missile or other such high-velocity toys.—F.G. Moody, M.D.

The Influence of Injury Severity on Complication Rates After Primary Closure or Colostomy for Penetrating Colon Trauma

Nelken N, Lewis F (Univ of California, San Francisco; San Francisco Gen Hosp)

Debate on the best way to manage penetrating injury to the colon continues, but there has been little evaluation of primary closure as opposed to diverting colostomy based on the severity of injury. Therefore, 76 patients who survived at least 24 hours after penetrating colon trauma during a 6-year-period were studied retrospectively. Primary repair was used for 37 patients, and 39 had colostomy. Three indices were used to evaluate severity of injury.

One patient in each group died. Major complications, including sepsis, occurred in 49% of the colostomy group and 11% of the primary repair group. The occurrence of such complications was not related to location of injury, age, or stab vs. bullet wound, but with the amount of transfusion and degree of fecal spillage. Morbidity was clearly decreased in patients who had primary repair for mild to moderate injury, that is, when the Penetrating Abdominal Trauma Index was less than 25, the Injury Severity Score was less than 25, and the Flint Colon Injury Score was less than 2. The Penetrating Abdominal Trauma Index was the most useful in identifying patients who would most benefit from primary repair and in predicting complications.

Primary repair should be more widely used in civilian patients with mild or moderate injury to the colon. This approach needs objective comparison with colostomy in a randomized, prospective trial.

▶ The authors propose a randomized controlled trial for the obvious conclusion from their experience and that of centers that treat civilian colon injuries. Most can be repaired primarily, but when associated with severe injuries in a sick patient, the injured segment should be resected and a colostomy performed. The distal end can be brought out of a convenient site for reconstruction or left as a closed end in Hartmann fashion for left colon injuries.—F.G. Moody, M.D.

34 Rectal Prolapse and Sigmoid Volvulus

Rectal Prolapse

Functional Results After Posterior Abdominal Rectopexy for Rectal Prolapse
Yoshioka K, Heyen F, Keighley MRB (Gen Hosp, Birmingham, England)
Dis Colon Rectum 32:835–838, October 1989   34–1

The clinical and physiologic results of posterior abdominal rectopexy in the treatment of rectal prolapse were reviewed. During an 11-year study period, 159 women and 6 men with rectal prolapse, aged 14–90 years (median, 65 years), underwent abdominal rectopexy using polypropylene mesh. Of the 165 patients, 128 had histories of rectal prolapse for less than 5 years; 33, for more than 5 years; and 4 did not know that they had rectal prolapse until it was diagnosed. Thirty-nine patients had undergone operations for rectal prolapse, including 7 who had had unsuccessful rectopexy.

Twenty-two patients died within 2 years of operation, and 8 patients had insufficient follow-up for inclusion, leaving 135 evaluable patients. Before operation, 58% of the patients were incontinent; after operation, 16% were still incontinent. Maximal anal pressure and maximal squeeze pressure were not influenced by rectopexy. Forty patients had constipation before operation, but 60 patients reported constipation after rectopexy. After a median follow-up of 3 years, only 2 patients had a recurrence of full-thickness rectal prolapse and 9 had minor mucosal prolapse. Surgical complications occurred in 32 patients, including wound infection in 15. One patient had intra-abdominal infection around the Marlex mesh, requiring its removal.

Although abdominal posterior rectopexy using Marlex mesh is an effective operation in the treatment of rectal prolapse, approximately one third of the patients in this study had persistent incontinence, and almost half of the patients became constipated after the operation.

► Rectal prolapse appears to occur in epidemic proportions in Birmingham, England. The authors report on the shortcomings of the use of posterior abdominal rectopexy in a large number of patients followed closely over a several-year period. This paper is well worth reading the next time you encounter a patient with this problem.—F.G. Moody, M.D.

Sigmoid Volvulus

Sigmoid Volvulus: A Four-Decade Experience
Mangiante EC, Croce MA, Fabian TC, Moore OF III, Britt LG (Univ of Tennessee, Memphis)
Ann Surg 55:41–44, January 1989   34–2

Morbidity and mortality are high among patients with volvulus of the sigmoid colon. Sigmoid volvulus is the most common cause of strangulated large bowel, accounting for up to 80% of cases. Because about one third of cases recur after sigmoidoscopic detorsion alone, the surgeon must often consider elective colon resection. A review was made of 40 years of management of this disease.

One hundred fifty-nine episodes of sigmoid volvulus were analyzed retrospectively in 140 patients who received treatment at the Regional Medical Center of Memphis from 1945 to 1984. From 1945 to 1964, surgeons performed operative decompression—sigmoid colon detorsion and sigmoidopexy—in 42 of 58 patients. In contrast, operative decompression was used in only 8 of 49 patients from 1964 to 1974 and, in the most recent 10 years, in only 2 of 35 patients. Throughout the entire series, 2 reductions were achieved with barium enema and 2 occurred spontaneously.

In the earliest period, successful nonoperative decompression was achieved in 27% of patients. This percentage rose to 83% in the middle period and 95% in the latest period. Seven deaths occurred among 90 patients with nonoperative decompression; however, the method of reduction was not implicated in the death of any patient. There were 5 deaths among 52 patients when operative reduction was used initially.

Seventeen patients had signs of ischemia at the time of sigmoidoscopy and gangrenous bowel at the time of surgery. Mortality was 39% among patients undergoing resection with colostomy for gangrenous bowel and 53% among those first seen with gangrenous bowel. Subsequent elective sigmoid resection, left hemicolectomy, or both were performed in 92 cases; 5 patients died, for a mortality of 5.4% overall. Combined mortality for all forms of treatment in each period was 13%, 19%, and 8%, respectively. Mortality during the 40-year period was 14%.

In the most recent 10-year period, 71% of cases were associated with neuropsychiatric diseases. One third of patients had had previous episodes of sigmoid volvulus.

Sigmoid volvulus should initially be managed with nonoperative attempts at reduction. Operative reduction should be reserved for refractory cases or those with ischemic bowel. The surgeon can safely perform elective resection during the same hospitalization.

▶ The surgeons from the University of Tennessee in Memphis provide a definitive statement on the management of sigmoid volvulus. Nonoperative decompression is safe and effective in most cases. Only a few will require an emergency or urgent operation. Many, however, will benefit from an elective sigmoid resection during the same hospitalization. The recurrence rate is high; those with recurrence are candidates for resection if the surgical risk is otherwise acceptable.—F.G. Moody, M.D.

35 Colorectal Carcinoma and Other Neoplasms

Radiologic and Imaging Studies

An Evaluation of the Role of Rectal Endosonography in Rectal Cancer
Beynon J (Bristol Royal Infirmary, Bristol, England)
Ann R Coll Surg Engl 71:131–139, March 1989   35–1

The need to improve preoperative staging of rectal cancer has led to the introduction of rectal endosonography. Five layers can be identified in the rectum with ultrasound; these correspond to histologic architecture. An additional layer sometimes appears within the fourth hypoechoic layer, or muscularis propria, which represents an interface of muscle layers of the rectum and another hyperechoic layer, which is an image of the balloon. Extramural extension of cancer requires identification of the fourth hypoechoic layer. If there is a complete hyperechoic third or middle layer, which is the submucosa, tumor has not invaded the muscularis propria.

Clinical study of 100 patients assessed preoperatively for local invasion of rectal adenocarcinoma showed a correlation coefficient of 0.94 when results were compared with those from histologic staging. Invasion beyond the muscularis propria was predicted with a specificity of 91% and a sensitivity of 99%. The positive and negative predictive values were more than 95%. These results were significantly better than those with digital examination, which could not reach several tumors, and CT, which could attest only to the presence or lack of invasions of an adjacent organ or beyond the muscularis propria, and which could not differentiate between T_1 and T_2 stage, unlike ultrasound.

In assessing involvement of mesorectal lymph nodes, a pararectal hypoechoic lesion usually indicated metastasis. Whether it was islands of tumor or involved nodes could not be determined, and false positive results occurred. Endosonography was more accurate and sensitive than CT but less specific.

In 85 patients undergoing endosonography for follow-up after treatment, advanced local recurrences looked the same as the primary tumor and the degree of invasion could be determined. Extrarectal local recurrences could be detected early, but confirmation required transperineal biopsy.

Rectal endosonography shows promise in the preoperative staging of primary tumors and in detecting local recurrences. It is both objective and accurate in assessing local invasion and lymph node involvement.

▶ The use of rectal endosonography for assessment of the extent of involvement of the involved rectal wall and adjacent structures is a unique application of technology. If the high predictive value is confirmed by others, the technique could provide for the first time a precise way to clinically stage rectal cancer before surgery. This capability clearly would enhance the trend toward anal-sparing procedures for low-grade lesions.—F.G. Moody, M.D.

Computed Tomographic Evaluation and Staging of Cecal Carcinoma
Keeney G, Jafri SZH, Mezwa DG (William Beaumont Hosp, Royal Oak, Mich)
Gastrointest Radiol 14:65–69, 1989   35-2

Preoperative CT studies were obtained for 14 patients with biopsy-proved primary cecal adenocarcinoma. Barium enema studies were done for 10 of these patients, and colonoscopy was performed in 4.

Thickening of the cecal wall exceeding 1 cm was the abnormality seen most frequently on CT. All patients but 1 had a distinct cecal mass; the mean size was 5.35 cm. Ten patients had direct tumor extension with hazy margins of the bowel wall or streaked mesenteric fat. Metastatic disease was most frequent in the liver, nodes, and duodenum.

Two of 3 patients with sharply demarcated margins of the bowel wall had histologic tumor extension. In 6 cases tumor stage was upgraded on histologic study because of microscopic nodal metastasis that went undetected with CT. In 2 other cases invasion beyond the bowel wall was not noted on CT study.

Computed tomography tends to underestimate the extent of primary cecal adenocarcinoma. The study is, however, 100% specific for a mass extending beyond the serosa. The differential diagnosis of a cecal mass seen on CT includes right colonic diverticulitis, acute appendicitis, Crohn's disease of the cecum, intestinal tuberculosis, lymphoma, leiomyoma or leiomyosarcoma, carcinoid tumor, and bowel metastasis.

▶ High-quality CT studies have helped in the diagnosis of primary cancers and their metastases. The importance of the study is the emphasis that in cecal carcinoma, CT evaluation underestimates the extent of disease. In more than a third of the patients in this study, the stage of the tumor estimated by CT needed to be upgraded.—P.B. Miner, M.D.

The Value of CT in Rectal Villous Tumors
Hendricks PJ, Keefe B, Wechsler RJ (Thomas Jefferson Univ Hosp, Philadelphia)
J Comp Assist Tomogr 13:269–272, March–April, 1989   35-3

Up to 50% of villous tumors of the rectosigmoid colon may be malignant. Although villous tumors represent 25% of all neoplastic polyps, up to 85% of all colon cancers that arise from adenomas originate in this type of polyp. Computed tomography studies were performed in 7 women and 6 men with

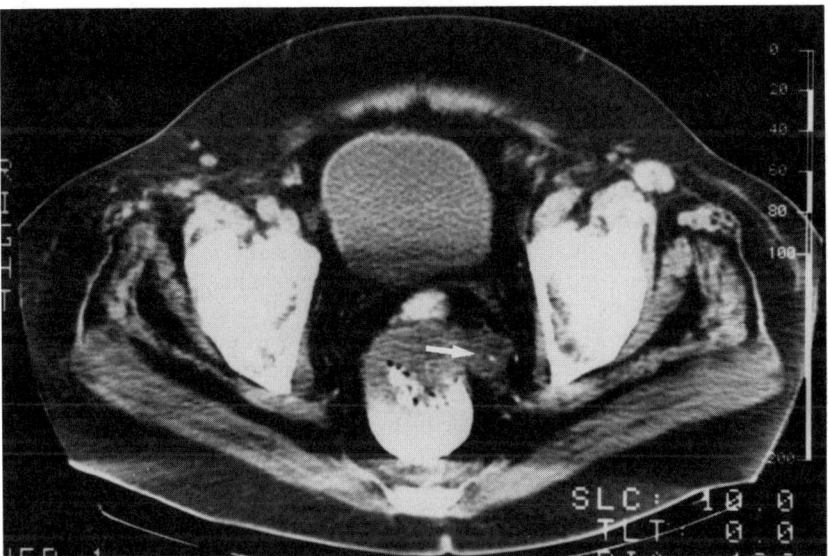

Fig 35–1.—Pelvic CT scan shows large rectal mass with evidence of fronds and perirectal tumor invasion on left (*arrow*). At biopsy malignant villous tumor was found. (Courtesy of Hendricks PJ, Keefe B, Wechsler RJ: *J Comp Assist Tomogr* 13:269–272, March–April 1989.)

villous tumors over a 4-year period. Average age of the 13 was 60.3 years. In all cases CT was carried out within the month preceding pathologic diagnosis. Oral, intravenous and rectal contrast agents were used routinely.

A prospective diagnosis of rectosigmoid tumor had been made in 11 cases; 2 benign lesions were recognized only in retrospect. All 5 benign lesions were manifested as focal colonic wall thickening of less than 2 cm. Seven of the 8 malignant lesions (Fig 35–1) were more than 2 cm in size, with the largest measuring 6 cm. Fronds were seen in 3 of these lesions. At CT examination 2 malignancies were upstaged, 2 were downstaged, and 4 were accurately characterized.

Good correlation was found between the gross pathologic and radiographic appearances of villous adenomas. However, CT is not an accurate means of staging colorectal cancers. When a small tumor is found, biopsy is necessary to rule out a malignancy.

▶ Of the 13 cases of rectal villous tumors reported in this study, 11 were diagnosed prospectively. Computed tomography showed the fronds of the villous adenoma with contrast media between these fingerlike projections. The other abnormalities found with the villous adenoma were indistinguishable from colorectal cancer, though a thickening of the colonic wall was common in all cases, benign or malignant. This study reiterates the difficulty of using CT in staging rectal cancers because of the indistinct evidence of metastatic disease.—P.B. Miner, M.D.

Polyps: Cancer Sequence

Radiological Evidence for the Polyp/Cancer Sequence in the Colon
Rawlinson J, Tate JJT, Brunton FJ, Royle GT (Southampton Gen Hosp, Southampton, England)
Clin Radiol 40:386–388, 1989   35-4

Although the malignant potential of colorectal adenomatous polyps is well recognized, the sequential development of cancer rarely is observed because most polyps are removed when first diagnosed. Frank malignant changes were observed in 3 patients with an untreated polyp. The 2 men and 1 woman were aged 56 to 64 years. The intervals from observation of a polyp to the finding of cancer were 2, 6, and 12 years, respectively. In 1 case the polyp possibly was malignant when first observed.

Because the risk of malignancy is increased with size and with the time a polyp remains in the colon, larger polyps and those in younger patients call for a more aggressive approach. Careful interpretation of radiographs will lessen the risk of overlooking small polyps.

▶ The 3 cases presented confirmed the suspicion that polyps progress to cancer. One of the 3 patients had colonoscopy after the barium enema, and no lesion was found. The failure of colonscopy to identify this polyp is important as endoscopy has become a gold standard for evaluation of polyps and colonic carcinoma. Ott and co-workers (1) indicate they found barium enema was similar to colonoscopy in sensitivity for detecting polyps. They argued that the barium enema should be used as a screening test for polyps because of its lower cost and safety. Another important paper by Glick and associates (2) found 18 patients with important colonic lesions, which were missed by endoscopy. These studies emphasized the importance of careful endoscopic examination as well as reconsidering the role of barium enema in patient evaluation.—P.B. Miner, M.D.

References

1. OH DJ et al: *South Med J* 82:187, 1989.
2. Glick SN et al: *AJR* 152:513, 1989.

Clinical Studies

Sensitivity, Specificity, and Positive Predictivity of the Hemoccult Test in Screening for Colorectal Cancers: The University of Minnesota's Colon Cancer Control Study
Mandel JS, Bond JH, Bradley M, Snover DC, Church TR, Williams S, Watt G, Schuman LM, Ederer F, Gilbertsen V (Univ of Minnesota)
Gastroenterology 97:597–600, September 1989   35-5

Primary prevention of colorectal cancer is not yet possible, as causes have

	Sensitivity, Specificity, and Positive Predictivity		
	Colorectal cancer		
	+	−	Total
Hemoccult test			
+	183	7,047	7,230
−	22 †	89,953	89,975
Total	205	97,000	97,205

Note: Sensitivity, (183/205)100% = 87.3% ± 2.2%. Specificity, (89,953/97,000)100% = 92.7% ± 0.1%. Positive predictivity, (183/7,230)100% = 2.5% ± 0.2%. †Defined as a case diagnosed within 12 months after a negative screening test.
(Courtesy of Mandel JS, Bond JH, Bradley M, et al: *Gastroenterology* 97:597–600, September 1989.)

not been ascertained. Stool testing for occult blood offers some hope for secondary prevention. However, evidence to show its efficacy in reducing mortality from colorectal cancer is not available. The preliminary results of a randomized clinical trial to determine whether the use of the Hemoccult test can decrease death from colorectal cancer were evaluated.

In all, 46,622 persons aged 50–80 years were assigned to 1 of 3 groups: group 1 was screened annually; group 2, biennially; and group 3, not at all. The screening test consisted of 6 guaiac-impregnated slides prepared by placing fecal smears on 2 slides from each of 3 consecutive stools taken while the person was following a meat-free, high-fiber diet.

Rehydrating the slides with a drop of water before processing produced an increase in positivity from 2.4% to 9.8% and an increase in sensitivity from 80.8% to 92.2%. However, it produced a decrease in specificity from 97.7% to 90.4% and a decrease in positive predictivity from 5.6% to 2.2%. The test was more specific for women than for men. Specificity was highest for persons aged less than 60 years and decreased with advancing age. Positive predictivity rose with age from 1.6% for those aged less than 60 years to 3.6% for those aged more than 70 years (table). Because no data are yet available on whether fecal occult blood testing results in decreased colorectal cancer mortality, no specific recommendations on the use of this screening procedure can be given.

▶ Mandel and co-workers point out that definitive data on whether fecal occult blood testing (FOBT) results in a *reduction* in colorectal cancer *mortality* are not yet available and, as such, state that no specific recommendations can be derived from their study. However, FOBT currently is used extensively despite the absence of data on its efficacy, and the University of Minnesota Colon Cancer Control Study does provide some useful information on the sensitivity, specificity, and positive predictive value of the Hemoccult test for colorectal cancer.

For a recent critical review of FOBT for colorectal cancer, see the article by Simon (1).—N.J. Greenberger, M.D.

Reference

1. Simon JB: Occult blood screening for colorectal carcinoma: A critical review. *Gastroenterology* 88:820, 1985.

Clinical Significance of Rectal Cancer in Young Patients
Heimann TM, Oh C, Aufses AH Jr (The Mount Sinai Hosp, New York)
Dis Colon 32:473–476, June 1989

Rectal cancer is fairly rare among patients 40 years or younger. To provide information on differences between them and older patients, data on 39 young patients with rectal cancer seen in a 9-year-period were compared with data on 315 patients aged more than 40 years who underwent resection at the same hospital.

In those aged less than 40 years, the mean duration of symptoms before operation was 6.6 months. None of the 27 undergoing curative resection had early lesions, but 7% in the older group did. Invasion of the muscularis propria but no involvement of lymph nodes was seen in 37% of younger patients and 62% of the older group. Lymph node metastasis was evident in 63% of younger patients undergoing curative resection and 31% of the older population. The differences were significant. More than 1 cancer was evident in 17% of the younger group. However, 30% of younger patients had histories of cancer in first-degree relatives. For younger patients, the overall 5-year survival was 33%; but for those aged less than 30 years, it was only 3%.

Young patients who have rectal cancer compose a high-risk group. They should have preoperative evaluations for synchronous lesions and postoperative follow-up examinations for new lesions. First-degree relatives should be followed up carefully. Awareness of the cancer incidence in younger patients may lead to earlier detection and better survival.

▶ Rectal cancer in young adults is an aggressive disease associated with low rates of survival. The authors emphasize the high incidence of rectal cancer in first-degree relatives of such patients. Translating important information of this type into my clinical practice is always difficult for me. Does this mean that the children of the subject should have colonoscopy at age 20, 30, or 40, or yearly determinations of the carcinoembryonic antigen? They at least should be advised of the risk and the signs that deserve early physician attention. A 55-cm sigmoidoscopic examination at age 30 or so even without symptoms also might be a resolvable approach.—F.G. Moody, M.D.

Endoscopic Laser Treatment for Rectosigmoid Villous Adenoma: Factors Affecting the Results
Brunetaud JM, Maunoury V, Cochelard D, Boniface B, Cortot A, Paris JC (Faculté de Pharmacie, Lille, France)

Endoscopic laser treatment sometimes is used to treat benign rectosigmoid villous adenoma. The long-term results and factors affecting them were assessed in 264 patients. Patients were candidates for the treatment if they were not eligible for surgery, had recurrences after previous nonlaser treatments, or had small, easily treated tumors or tumors that were not surgically resectable by a light surgical procedure. Patients received treatment on an outpatient basis without premedication or anesthesia. Before laser treatment, exophytic villous adenomas were debulked with diathermic snare if possible. Patients were treated twice weekly until the tumor was destroyed. In 67% of the patients, treatment was given with the neodymium:yttrium/aluminum/garnet laser; in 18%, with the argon laser; and in 15%, with both lasers.

Eleven patients were lost to follow-up, 14 died of other causes during treatment, and 13 are still undergoing treatment. Of the 226 remaining patients, treatment was successful in 208 after an average of 6.1 treatments (Fig 35–2). During treatment, invasive carcinoma was detected in 16 patients. At average follow-up of 28 months, 13% of patients had had recurrence. The average time to recurrence was 1 year. In 20 patients, recurrences were easily retreated with an average of 2.9 treatments. Five patients with recurrence are still undergoing treatment, and in 2 patients, cancer was detected.

The circumferential extension of the tumor base was the only factor that affected duration of initial treatment, the rate of cancers occurring during initial treatment, and the occurrence of stenosis requiring dilatation. The cancer rate was 24% in C3 tumors, as compared with 3% in C1 and C2 tumors. The recurrence rate after initial treatment was influenced by the reasons for treatment, initial histology, and the localization, but not by the circumferential extension of the tumor base.

Because treatment is long and difficult and the cancer rate is high, use of endoscopic laser in patients with circumferential villous adenomas should be

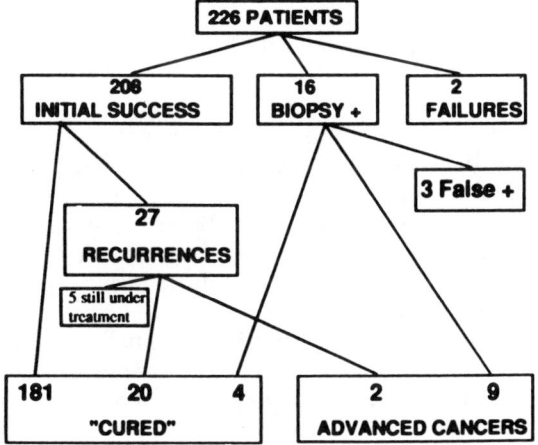

Fig 35–2.—Diagram of laser treatment results in 226 patients with rectosigmoid villous adenoma. (Courtesy of Brunetaud JM, Maunoury V, Cochelard D, et al: *Gastroenterology* 97:272–277, August 1989.)

limited to those in whom surgery is contraindicated. The risk of a fatal complication after surgery should be weighed against the risk of undetected carcinoma in other patients. Indications for endoscopic laser treatment should be evaluated on an individual basis.

▶ This unique report on the treatment of rectosigmoid villous adenomata with laser ablation provides a basis for adopting this relatively tedious but low invasive technique. The incidence of recurrence and the subsequent identification of invasive cancer was high. Therefore, the authors recommend limiting laser ablation to patients with unacceptable surgical risk. Standard surgical procedures should be used for such lesions. The most difficult surgical decision relates to large lesions that lie in the low rectum where an abdominal perineal resection would be required for cure if invasive cancer is present within the depths of the lesion.—F.G. Moody, M.D.

Preoperative Irradiation for Rectal Cancer: Improved Local Control and Long-Term Survival
Kodner IJ, Shemesh EI, Fry RD, Walz BJ, Myerson R, Fleshman JW, Schechtman KB (Washington Univ)
Ann Surg 209:194–199, February 1989   35–8

The role of adjuvant pelvic irradiation in the treatment of rectal cancer is controversial. However, resection alone continues to yield a high local recurrence rate and survival has remained unchanged. Although preoperative irradiation has been shown to reduce local recurrence and allow improved resectability of advanced tumors and pelvic spread, improved survival attributable to preoperative irradiation has not been demonstrated clearly.

Between 1975 and 1986, 68 men and 44 women aged 19–94 years with adenocarcinoma of the rectum received treatment with preoperative irradiation followed by excision surgery. Initial clinical examination suggested that all tumors were transmurally invasive. In 13 patients, tumors were poorly differentiated and in 51 patients tumors were fixed to surrounding tissues.

Between 1975 and 1978, 22 patients received 2,000 cGy external irradiation to the pelvis in 5 fractions over 5 days, followed immediately by excisional surgery for cure. The treatment protocol subsequently was changed to irradiation of 4,500 cGy, delivered in 25 fractions over 5 weeks. Excisional surgery was performed 5–7 weeks after irradiation.

The mean follow-up was 91 months for 16 surviving patients treated with 2,000 cGy and 46 months for 70 surviving patients treated with 4,500 cGY of external radiation. No surgical mortality occurred in either group. The overall surgical complication rate was 12.8%.

Survival at 5 years for 20 patients with potentially curable tumors who received 2,000 cGy of radiation was 81%; there were no local recurrences. Survival at 5 years for 72 patients with potentially curable lesions who received 4,500 cGy of radiation was 86%; there were 2 local recurrences (1.8%). Tumor

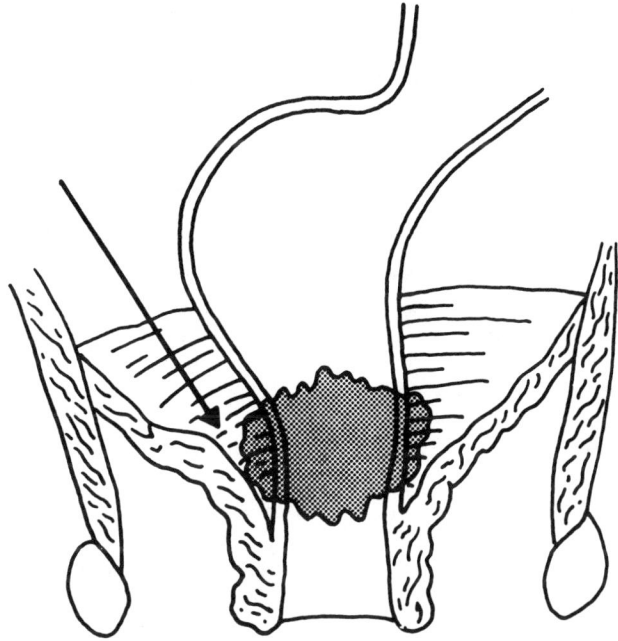

Fig 35–3.—A rectal cancer below the peritoneal reflection. The *arrow* indicates the tangential margin. (Courtesy of Kodner IJ, Shemesh EI, Fry RD, et al: Ann Surg 209:194–199, February 1989.)

fixation and histologic dedifferentiation were the only factors influencing survival.

Preoperative external beam irradiation to the pelvic area improves survival, local control, and resectability in patients with rectal cancer. The beneficial effect of pelvic irradiation may be caused by the treatment of tangential margins and local lymph node metastases (Fig 35–3). Because of comparable survival rates and low recurrence rates with either irradiation dose, it is suggested that small lesions without fixation and a favorable histology be treated with the 5-day 2,000-cGy protocol, and large, fixed lesions, with the 5-week, 4,500-cGy protocol.

▶ This is not a randomized controlled trial, but Kodner and his associates present convincing evidence that preoperative irradiation coupled with well-performed extirpative surgery offers long-term survival with low morbidity and low recurrence rates. A 5-day, 2,000 cGy preoperative course of irradiation appeared to be as effective as 5 weeks of 4,500 cGy. The latter should be reserved for patients with large fixed lesions. I imagine that this will not be the last word on the subject, but it is most welcome and encouraging for those who will be afflicted with this relatively common cancer.—F.G. Moody, M.D.

Radioimmunolocation and Ablation Studies

Radioimmunolocation of Hepatic and Pulmonary Metastasis of Human Colon Adenocarcinoma
Takahashi H, Carlson R, Ozturk M, Sun S, Motte P, Strauss W, Isselbacher KJ, Wands JR, Shouval D (Massachusetts Gen Hosp, Boston; Harvard Med School)
Gastroenterology 96:1317–1329, May 1989   35-9

A monoclonal antibody reactive with a 125-kilodalton cell surface protein, MAb SF-25, reacts with colonic adenocarcinomas obtained surgically but not with adjacent normal mucosa. The antibody was produced against an antigen expressed on a human hepatoma cell line, FOCUS. Because both the liver and colon are of endodermal origin, the possibility of antigen expression in colonic tumors was studied with a view toward radioimmunodetection of metastatic tumor.

Antigen was found in all 23 surgical specimens of colonic adenocarcinoma examined and was absent from adjacent normal mucosa. When athymic mice were immunosuppressed by intravenous injection of anti-NK cell antibodies and then injected with LS 180 cells from a human metastatic colon adenocarcinoma cell line, gross pulmonary and lymphatic metastases developed within 2–3 weeks and liver metastases, in 3–4 weeks. Hepatic, pulmonary, and lymphatic tumor spread was localized by imaging with ^{125}I-labeled SF-25. Hepatic micrometastases were detected autoradiographically 5–10 days after nuclide injection.

Monoclonal antibody SF-25 may prove useful, both for localizing colon adenocarcinoma and for treatment either alone or in conjunction with other monoclonal antibodies conjugated to radionucleotides or chemotherapeutic agents.

▶ This and the following article highlight important developments in the immunolocation of metastatic colonic adenocarcinoma and the selective destruction of established human colon carcinoma transplants by ^{131}-I-labeled monoclonal carcinoembryonic antigen antibody F(ab')$_2$ fragments. These studies may well prove useful as reference points for the planning of radioimmunotherapy in colorectal carcinoma patients.—N.J. Greenberger, M.D.

Ablation of Human Colon Carcinoma in Nude Mice by ^{131}I-Labeled Monoclonal Anti-Carcinoembryonic Antigen Antibody F(ab')$_2$ Fragments
Buchegger F, Pfister C, Fournier K, Prevel F, Schreyer M, Carrel S, Mach J-P (Ludwig Inst for Cancer Research; Univ of Lausanne, Switzerland)
J Clin Invest 83:1449–1456, May 1989   35-10

Limited regression of colon carcinoma has been achieved in nude mice using a mixture of intact monoclonal antibodies and their F(ab')$_2$ fragments labeled with ^{131}I. Greater success now has been achieved by using exclusively F(ab')$_2$ fragments of the same anti-carcinoembryonic antigen (CEA) mono-

Chapter 35–Colorectal Carcinoma and Other Neoplasms / 201

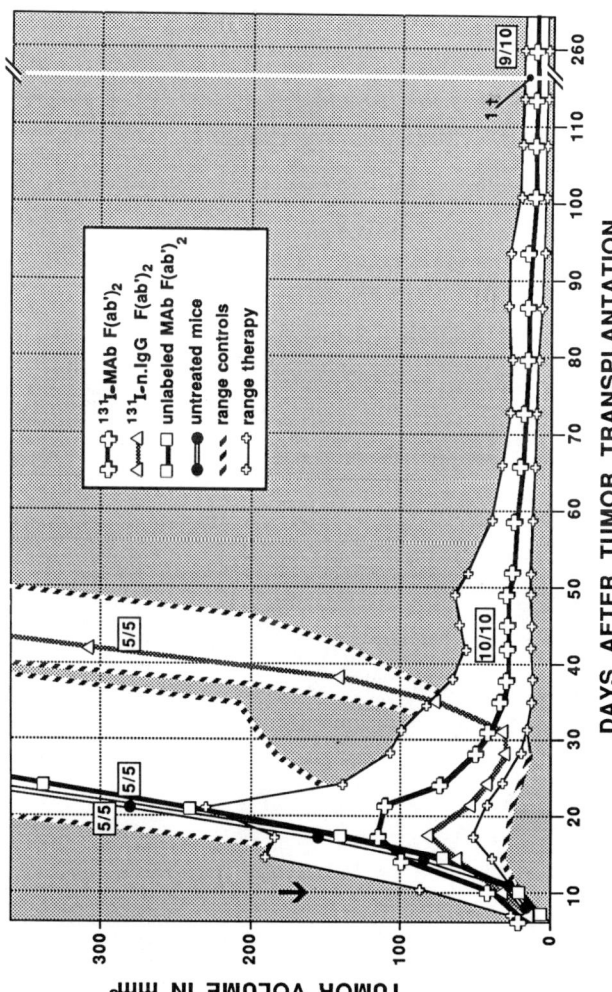

Fig 35-4.—Tumor size in mice injected with a single dose of 2,200 µCi MAb F(ab')$_2$. Three groups were injected 10 days after tumor transplantation, either with a single dose of 2,200 µCi ^{131}I-anti-CEA MAb F(ab')$_2$, the same amount of ^{131}I coupled to control IgG F(ab')$_2$, or the corresponding amount of unlabeled anti-CEA MAb F(ab')$_2$ (275 µg). A fourth group of mice was untreated. The mean tumor size for each group is represented by *thick lines*. The range in tumor size in the control groups is represented by *dashed lines*, whereas the range in tumor size of ^{131}I-anti-CEA MAb F(ab')$_2$-treated animals is shown by 2 *thin lines*. A mouse in the antibody-treated group killed at 4 months because of ulcerative skin disease is indicated by †. (Courtesy of Buchegger F, Pfister C, Fournier K, et al: *J Clin Invest* 83:1449–1456, May 1989.)

clonal antibodies labeled with greater amounts of ^{131}I. Antibody was given intravenously to 36 mice starting 9–10 days after tumor transplantation.

Mice given a single dose of 2,200 µCi had complete tumor remission (Fig 35–4) and were free of tumor when killed after a year of good health. Mice given 4 fractionated doses of 400 µCi had no relapse on follow-up for longer than 9 months. Tumor growth was retarded only transiently when control ^{131}IgG F(ab')$_2$ was administered. When given unlabeled anti-CEA F(ab')$_2$, mice had ongoing tumor progression. Treatment was well tolerated; only 4 animals with complete remission needed marrow transplantation.

Established human colon cancer transplants may be destroyed selectively by either single or fractionated doses of ^{131}I-labeled monoclonal antibody F(ab')$_2$ fragments. These findings may help in planning radioimmunotherapy for patients with colorectal carcinoma.

36 Irritable Bowel Syndrome

Clinical Studies

Effect of Dietary Fiber on Symptoms and Rectosigmoid Motility in Patients With Irritable Bowel Syndrome: A Controlled, Crossover Study
Cook IJ, Irvine EJ, Campbell D, Shannon S, Reddy SN, Collins SM (McMaster Univ, Hamilton, Ont; Royal Adelaide Hosp, Adelaide, Australia)
Gastroenterology 98:66–72, January 1990   36–1

The symptoms of irritable bowel syndrome (IBS) appear to be related to disordered intestinal motility and hyperresponsiveness to endogenous and exogenous stimuli. Epidemiologic evidence suggests that deficiency in dietary fiber may predispose to colonic motor disorders, including IBS.

The effects of fiber supplementation were examined with 14 patients in a double-blind crossover study which lasted 7 months. Nine completed the study. All patients received 4 cookies each day which contained 20 g of corn fiber or placebo.

Improvement in symptom scores over time was not significantly greater in patients given fiber than in those given placebo (Fig 36–1). Scores declined substantially for all patients within the first 4 weeks. Meal-stimulated increases in rectosigmoid motility were unrelated to fiber intake, and declining motility over time also was unrelated to fiber intake. Fasting proximal motility was not correlated with symptoms, but distal motility was correlated moderately with the severity of abdominal pain.

The authors conclude that both corn fiber and placebo relieved symptoms of IBS. Fasting and postprandial rectosigmoid pressures tended to decrease after fiber intake.

▶ Though the pathophysiology of IBS commonly is attributed to dysfunction of the large intestine, evidence exists to incriminate the small bowel. To further explore the role of the small bowel in IBS, Kellow and colleagues (1) applied several stimuli in an attempt to unmask the dysmotility of the jejunum and ileum. These included infusions of cholecystokinin-octapeptide (CCK-OP), a high-fat meal, neostigmine, and balloon distention of the ileum. Three groups (no. = 8) each of age- and sex-matched healthy volunteers were studied; patients with IBS reported predominant constipation (no. = 8) or diarrhea (no. = 8). Patients with IBS responded excessively to stimulation by CCK-OP, fatty meal, and ileal distention. In general, patients with diarrhea were more sensitive to stimuli than those with constipation were. The ileum responded more to stimulation than the jejunum. As in the large bowel, stimuli

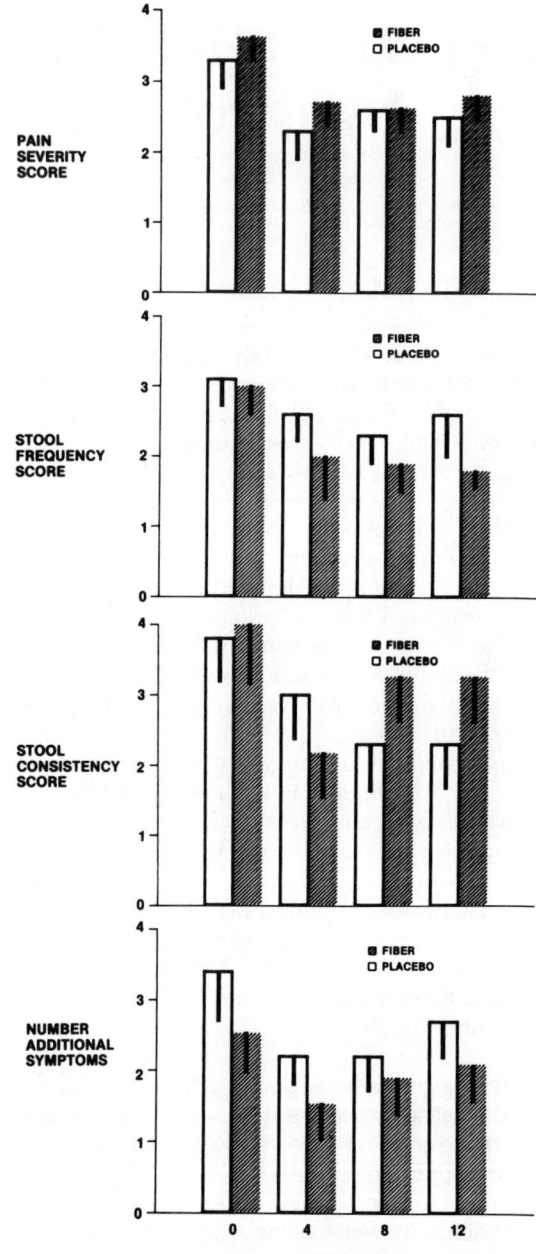

Fig 36-1.—Symptom scores in response to fiber and placebo. Represented are individual scores for symptoms evaluated by standardized questionnaire. Significant improvement in scores for pain severity ($P = .001$), stool frequency ($P = .001$), stool consistency ($P = .001$), and number of additional symptoms ($P = .02$) was observed during both placebo and fiber interventions. (Courtesy of Cook IJ, Irvine EJ, Campbell D, et al: *Gastroenterology* 98:66–72, January 1990.)

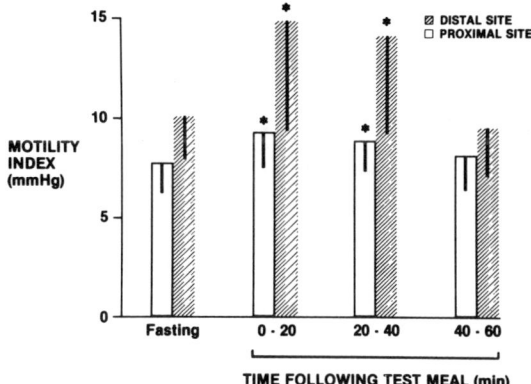

Fig 36–1. (Continued).

appear to unmask intestinal dysmotility in patients with IBS. Motor abnormalities often were accompanied by abdominal symptoms, raising the possibility that dysfunction of the small bowel contributes to the symptoms of IBS.—N.J. Greenberger, M.D.

Reference

1. Kellow JE, Phillips SF, et al: Dysmotility of the small intestine in irritable bowel syndrome. *Gut* 29:1236–1243, 1988.

Food Intolerance and the Irritable Bowel Syndrome
Nanda R, James R, Smith H, Dudley CRK, Jewell DP (Radcliffe Infirmary, Oxford, England)
Gut 30:1099–1104, 1989   36–2

The irritable bowel syndrome (IBS) accounts for about 50% of referrals to many gastroenterology clinics, but treatment is notoriously unsatisfactory. To determine the proportion of patients with IBS who would have good responses to exclusion diets, and to document the long-term effects of dietary manipulation, 200 patients received treatment for 3 weeks with dietary exclusion. Of these, 189 completed the study.

About half (91) of the patients had symptomatic improvement (Fig 36–2). When these patients had subsequent challenges with individual foods, 73 of them could identify 1 or more food intolerances, usually dairy products and grains. All but 1 of these remained well with a modified diet during a mean follow-up period of 14.7 months. Of the 98 patients without improvement after the 3-week diet, only 3 were symptomatically well at follow-up. Response and symptom complex were not significantly correlated.

Dietary manipulation is effective in about half of the patients with IBS. A

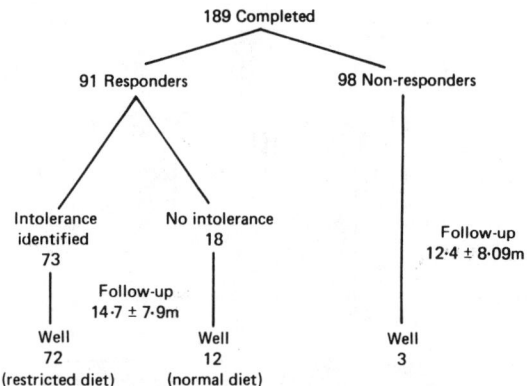

Fig 36–2.—Response to dietary therapy in patients completing the study. (Courtesy of Nanda R, James R, Smith H, et al: *Gut* 30:1099–1104, 1989.)

high probability of prolonged symptomatic benefit is possible in patients who respond to this treatment, but compliance is the main problem with this approach.

▶ I have emphasized repeatedly the importance of carefully recording a dietary history for patients with IBS. Not infrequently, just the exclusion of specific putative foods results in symptomatic improvement. The food intolerances most frequently identified by patients in the study of Nanda and associates were milk and milk products, wheat products, chocolate, and coffee. I frequently find that patients have been advised at proprietary nutrition centers or health food stores to sharply increase their intake of fiber and bran products, and not surprising, they have had crampy abdominal pain, loose bowel motions, and excessive flatus. Approximately one third of patients with lactose intolerance still have irritable bowel symptoms after deleting milk and milk products from their diets, in part because they may be sensitive to other carbohydrates.—N.J. Greenberger, M.D.

37 Appendicitis

Clinical Studies

Localized Ileus of the Proximal Jejunum: A New Sign for Acute Appendicitis
Mowji PJ, Jones MD, Cohen AJ (Univ of California, Irvine)
Gastrointest Radiol 14:173–175, 1989   37–1

Both a small distended loop of proximal jejunum in the left upper quadrant and a paucity of gas and fecal material in the right lower quadrant may be present early in the course of appendicitis. Supine and upright radiographs and chest films were reviewed for 100 consecutively seen patients with pathologically confirmed acute appendicitis. Data on 30 patients with Crohn's disease of the terminal ileum, 25 with pancreatitis, and 25 with pelvic inflammatory disease also were reviewed.

Focal ileus was present in 51 patients with appendicitis, including 35 of 59 patients with simple appendicitis. Focal ileus also was present in 2 patients with Crohn's disease and 1 with pelvic inflammatory disease (table).

In addition to an inverted "C loop" at the level of the proximal jejunum, a paucity of gas and fecal material in the cecal region is evidence of acute appendicitis. The localized ileus may represent bowel irritation by the upper ileocolic nodes. A sympathetic response is not a likely cause of focal bowel dilatation. Focal ileus occasionally is associated with other disorders, including Crohn's ileitis and ureteral stone disease.

▶ The presence of a localized ileus in the proximal jejunum as a sign of acute appendicitis is an interesting, though an etiologically perplexing, finding. Although this study is retrospective, the review of 30 cases of Crohn's disease, 25 cases of pancreatitis, and 25 cases of pelvic inflammatory disease as controls indicate high specificity, with few false positives. The authors suggest the localized ileus is from an upper group of ileocolic nodes that correlate with early symptoms of appendicitis.—P.B. Miner, Jr., M.D.

Ultrasonography in the Diagnosis of Acute Appendicitis: A Prospective Study
Schwerk WB, Wichtrup B, Rothmund M, Rüschoff J (Philipps-Univ of Marburg, West Germany)
Gastroenterology 97:630–639, September 1989   37–2

The overall accuracy of the preoperative clinical diagnosis of acute appen-

Pathological Findings Associated With Localized Ileus (Inverted C Sign) of Proximal Jejunum

Pathologic diagnosis	No. of cases	No. of cases with C sign
Appendicitis		
Simple	59	35
Gangrenous	18	7
Perforative	10	4
Appendiceal abscess	13	5
Total cases	100	51
Control	100	1
Crohn's ileitis	30	2
Pancreatitis	25	0
Pelvic inflammation	25	1

(Courtesy of Mowji PJ, Jones MD, Cohen AJ: *Gastrointest Radiol* 14:173–175, 1989.)

dicitis ranges from 70% to 78% because the typical clinical signs and symptoms are nonspecific and, before high-resolution sonography, no noninvasive imaging technique was available to enable direct visualization of the inflamed vermiform appendix. A prospective study was made of the routine use of high-resolution sonography in 523 patients with suspected acute appendicitis.

Criteria for ultrasound diagnosis included visualization of a noncompressible aperistaltic appendix with a target-like appearance in transverse view and a diameter of at least 7 mm. In 115 of 130 patients with proved appendicitis, or appendiceal abscess the inflamed appendix was visualized, yielding a sensitivity of 88.5%. Ultrasonically visible appendices had a mean diameter of 11.4 mm. The overall accuracy of sonography was 95.7%, and specificity was 98%. The predictive value of a positive test was 94.5%, and that of a negative test, 96.3%. In 24 (89%) of the 27 patients with appendiceal rupture the correct diagnosis was made with ultrasound. In the other 3 (11%) the diagnosis was missed.

High-resolution, real-time sonography is a sensitive, specific imaging technique for diagnosing acute appendicitis and its complications. Routine use of ultrasonography significantly improved the diagnostic accuracy in patients with suspected appendicitis and reduced the negative laparotomy rate from 22.9% to 13.2%.

▶ Several recent studies attest to the validity and utility of sonography in the diagnosis of acute appendicitis (1,2). Larson and co-workers (1) examined 206 patients with suspected appendicitis with sonography over a 6-month period in 3 community teaching hospitals. Of 41 patients for whom the surgeons judged the clinical findings severe enough to warrant immediate surgery (group A), 34 (83%) had appendicitis. Sonography had a sensitivity of 0.76, a specificity of 0.71, and an accuracy of 0.76. Of 165 patients for whom the surgeons judged the clinical findings severe enough to warrant hospitalization for observation but not immediate surgery (group B), 51 (32%) had appendicitis at subsequent surgery. Sonography had a sensitivity of 0.96, a specificity of 0.94, and an accuracy of 0.95. Of 49 surgeons surveyed, the mean testing threshold (i.e., the probability of appendicitis below which they would send the patient home without further tests or observation) was 0.11, and the mean treatment threshold (i.e., the probability of appendicitis above which they would operate immediately) 0.82. The posttest probability of appendicitis with findings indicating appendicitis present on sonography was 0.93 in group A and 0.88 in group B, and with findings absent on sonography it was 0.62 in group A and 0.02 in group B. Larson and co-workers conclude that in group A patients the use of sonography remains controversial in the diagnosis of appendicitis, but in group B patients it is both valid and useful.

Fa and Cronan (2) reassessed 70 ultrasonographic examinations and retrospectively reanalyzed these studies using the most recently published criterion, which requires a maximal appendiceal diameter of more than 6 mm. Ultrasonography was shown to be 80.0% sensitive, 95.0% specific, and 92.9% accurate in diagnosing appendicitis, with a positive predictive value of 72.7% and a negative predictive value of 96.6%. Ultrasonographic examination provided additional findings, predominantly gynecologic or obstetric, in 52% of the women, leading to an alternative diagnosis in a third of these patients who complained of abdominal pain. Ultrasonographic study provided additional findings in 12% of the men, leading to alternative diagnoses in 12%. Ultrasonographic results directly influenced clinical management in 18% of the patients.

Appendiceal ultrasonographic examination is a reliable ancillary technique in diagnosing or excluding appendicitis. It is indicated for patients with atypical or equivocal presentation; those with sound clinical grounds for the diagnosis do not require ancillary diagnostic aids and should proceed immediately to surgical intervention. Fa and Cronan conclude that the predominant role of ultrasonography in evaluating appendicitis is not as an independent diagnostic determinant. Rather, it is most useful as a means of improving decision making when considered in combination with a thorough history and physical examination for those patients who represent diagnostic dilemmas.—N.J. Greenberger, M.D.

References

1. Larson JM et al: The validity and utility of sonography in the diagnosis of appendicitis in the community setting. *AJR* 153:687, 1989.
2. Fa EM, Cronan JJ: Compression ultrasonography as an aid in the differential diagnosis of appendicitis. *Surg Gynecol Obstet* 169:290, 1989.

The Consequences of Current Constraints on Surgical Treatment of Appendicitis
Cacioppo JC, Diettrich NA, Kaplan G, Nora PF (Columbus Hosp, Chicago)
Am J Surg 157:276–281, March 1989   37–3

During the past decade, policies aimed at cost containment have altered many aspects of health care. Patients with cholelithiasis and inguinal hernias have suffered as a result of constraints on elective surgical referral. A condition that does not offer options for medical or elective operative treatment—acute appendicitis—was selected for study to determine whether similar trends affect these patients.

Records of patients undergoing appendectomy were studied for the years 1980 (76 patients), 1986 (61 patients), and 1987 (73 patients). Information was obtained on the stage of the disease, delay in referral, morbidity and mortality, and length of hospitalization. Three stages of acute appendicitis were identified: uncomplicated (group A), complicated (group B), and advanced (group C).

The rate of negative appendectomy remained unchanged over the years. Most (82%) patients underwent surgery within 6 hours of evaluation by the surgeon. No patient appeared to have had perforation between referral and surgery, and no deaths occurred, but compared with 1980, significantly more patients progressed to advanced appendicitis with abscess (group C) in 1986 and 1987. A prolonged delay in hospitalization or surgical referral occurred in 37% of patients in 1986 and in 29% in 1987. As a result, over the course of the 1980s, morbidity more than quadrupled. This increase in morbidity resulted in an extended length of stay.

For patients whose condition requires urgent operative treatment, current policies result in deterioration in patient care and failure in cost containment. When acute appendicitis is suspected, immediate referral, hospitalization, and surgery—even though results may be negative—will actually lower financial expenditures.

▶ This is a timely indictment of the extreme measures currently being pursued to contain medical costs. The authors provide evidence that restraint on hospital referral for the treatment of acute appendicitis is contributing to delay in therapy and therefore increased costs associated with treatment of a more advanced stage of the disease. Attempts at cost containment have been effective in reducing lengths of hospital stays and bed utilization at community hospitals, but at the expense of health care in rural areas and a marked increase in the costs devoted to the bureaucracy of health care. There must be a more rational way to deploy $600 billion for a more uniform and effective delivery of the highly refined medical technology and services we have developed in this country.—F.G. Moody, M.D.

Antibiotic Prophylaxis in Acute Nonperforated Appendicitis: The Danish Multicenter Study Group III
Bauer T, Vennits B, Holm B, Hahn-Pedersen J, Lysen D, Galatius H, Kristensen ES, Graversen P, Wilhelmsen F, Skjoldborg H, Malmfred S, Villadsen J, Bendix J, Danish Multicenter Study Group III (Bauer T, Herlev Hosp, Herlev, Denmark)
Ann Surg 209:307–311, March 1989   37–4

Cefoxitin is at least as effective as a combination of ampicillin and metronidazole in the prevention of wound infection and formation of intraabdominal abscess after operation for perforated appendicitis. Whether a single preoperative cefoxitin dose given to patients undergoing appendectomy for acute nonperforated appendicitis would lower postoperative wound infection and intra-abdominal abscess rates was determined.

During a 2-year study period, 2,387 patients undergoing appendectomy were randomly assigned to receive cefoxitin, 2g, intravenously for 20–30 minutes before operation or no prophylaxis. Patients found to have a perforated or ruptured appendix during operation were subsequently excluded because antibiotic treatment could not be withheld. The study criteria were met by 1,735 patients (median age, 23 years); 845 received cefoxitin preoperative and 890 served as controls.

Wound infection after appendectomy occurred in 95 of the 1,735 patients. Infection developed in 21 of the 845 treated patients and in 74 of the 890 untreated controls. Both wound infection and an intra-abdominal abscess developed in 7 patients. Twenty-one patients (1.2%) had intra-abdominal abscess formation after appendectomy; of these, 8 were treated patients (38%) and 14 were controls (62%). The difference statistically was not significant. Only 41 of the 95 wound infections occurred during hospitalization; the other 54 developed between the time of hospital discharge and the follow-up examination 4 weeks after operation. None of the patients given cefoxitin had side effects, and the drug was well tolerated.

A single preoperative cefoxitin dose can reduce the overall postappendectomy wound infection rate from 8.3% to 2.5% in patients with nonperforated appendicitis. However, the cefoxitin prophylaxis does not affect the postoperative intra-abdominal abscess rate.

▶ The Danes have an advantage over Americans when they conduct multicenter trials; they have a relatively homogeneous population and health care system. A single preoperative dose of cefoxitin reduces the postoperative wound infection rate threefold but does not influence the occurrence of intra-abdominal infections in patients who undergo appendectomy for acute nonperforated appendicitis. This approach is safe, effective, cheap, and substantiated by a well-conducted trial.— F.G. Moody, M.D.

38 Colonic Ischemia

A Prospective Study of Clinically and Endoscopically Documented Colonic Ischemia in 100 Patients Undergoing Aortic Reconstructive Surgery With Aggressive Colonic and Direct Pelvic Revascularization, Compared With Historic Controls
Zelenock GB, Strodel WE, Knol JA, Messina LM, Wakefield TW, Lindenauer SM, Eckhauser FE, Greenfield LJ, Stanley JC (Univ of Michigan; VA Med Ctr, Ann Arbor, Mich)
Surgery 106:771–780, October 1989   38–1

Although intestinal ischemia after abdominal aortic reconstruction is uncommon but not rare, its clinical recognition often is delayed. Unrecognized colonic ischemia may cause transmural infarction of the colon, which is associated with a mortality of 60% to 100%. To identify and treat factors contributing to colonic ischemia in patients undergoing reconstruction of the abdominal aorta, 100 men with a mean age of 62.4 years who underwent elective or urgent reconstruction of the abdominal aorta over a 3-year period were prospectively studied.

Fifty patients were treated for aneurysmal disease, and 42 were treated for chronic aortoiliac occlusive disease; 88 patients had conventional aortic reconstructions with an aortofemoral bypass graft, and 12 had 14 adjunctive procedures to preserve or enhance pelvic and colonic blood flow. Colonic blood flow was assessed intraoperatively with Doppler ultrasonography. Intraoperative assessment included gross inspection of the colon. Colonoscopy was performed within 24–48 hours of aortic reconstruction. Three patients had endoscopic evidence of colonic ischemia. None of the patients had transmural infarction, and bowel resections or diverting colostomies proved unnecessary. Three patients died, but none had evidence of colonic ischemia. Preoperative clinical information was not sufficiently sensitive to enable identification of patients in whom colonic ischemia would develop. Intraoperative assessments were helpful only when distinct abnormalities were observed.

No specific factors contributing to colonic ischemia as a complication of abdominal aortic reconstruction could be identified. Any preoperative or intraoperative findings suggestive of potential colonic ischemia should be treated with adjunctive vascular procedures to enhance pelvic perfusion, as such procedures may decrease the incidence of this complication of aortic reconstructive surgery.

▶ The vascular surgeons at the University of Michigan have carried out an important clinical study. Only 3 of 100 patients having colonoscopy within 3 days of a major aortic reconstructive procedure had evidence of ischemia. None had transmural infarction, and none required surgical intervention. These patients could not be distinguished from those with normal colonoscopies. Apparently, their use of intraoperative colonic blood flow by Doppler ultrasonography led to the relatively low incidence of even mucosal ischemic lesions in their patient population.—F.G. Moody, M.D.

Computed Tomographic Findings in Bowel Ischemia
Pérez C, Lllanger J, Puig J, Palmer J (Univ Autonoma de Barcelona, Barcelona, Spain)
Gastrointest Radiol 14:241–245, 1989

Computed tomography was used to assess 11 patients with ischemic bowel lesions before confirmation by surgery or autopsy. The patients had abdominal pain of unknown origin. Nine patients had involvement of the small bowel, 1 had colonic ischemia alone, and 1 had diffuse involvement of the small bowel and colon. Five patients had adhesive bands causing volvulus or intestinal obstruction, 5 had occlusive vascular lesions, and 1 had low cardiac output. Four patients with massive mesenteric vascular occlusion died before attempting bowel resection.

Bowel wall thickening was the most frequent finding (table). Postcontrast enhancement was the rule. Nine patients had fluid-filled bowel loops (Fig 38–1), and 5 had intramural zones of low attenuation. Focal or diffuse intraperitoneal fluid was present in 5 cases. The "whirl sign" of volvulus was seen in 3 patients (Fig 38–2).

The CT findings in bowel ischemia are a combination of those seen with plain radiography, barium study, and angiography. Intramural zones of low attenuation probably represent edema. Intramural or intravascular gas is a more specific CT finding of bowel infarction. Portal or mesenteric venous gas or both are characteristic of advanced bowel ischemia. Angiography is a more sensitive means of determining the site and nature of arterial occlusive disease. Computed tomography is helpful in diagnosing bowel ischemia resulting from occlusive volvulus.

▶ Mucosal edema (thumbprinting) is a classic finding on traditional barium examinations used to diagnose ischemia. The CT findings observed in this study confirm this finding and provide additional signs of ischemia. Unfortunately, some of the signs the authors use to document ischemia suggest the presence of gangrene, which is accompanied by a poor prognosis. Recognition of edematous bowel is useful, as many patients will have a CT scan as one of the early tests for abdominal pain. Early clinical awareness of a thickened bowel wall will allow clinicians to focus on infectious, inflammatory, or ischemic causes of the patients' symptoms.—P.B. Miner, M.D.

Computed Tomographic Findings in 11 Patients With Proven Bowel Ischemia

CT finding	No. cases
Thickened bowel wall	10
Postcontrast enhancement of thickening of bowel wall	9
Fluid-filled loops	9
Intramural low attenuation zones ("target" image)	5
Free intraperitoneal fluid	5
Diffuse	4
Localized	1
Intramural gas	8
Mesenteric vein gas	1
Mesenteric twisting	3
Other findings	
Aortic aneurysm	2
Emphysematous pyelonephritis	1
Chronic pancreatitis	1
Neoplasm of the bladder	1

(Courtesy of Pérez C, Llanger J, Puig J, et al: *Gastrointest Radiol* 14:241–245, 1989.)

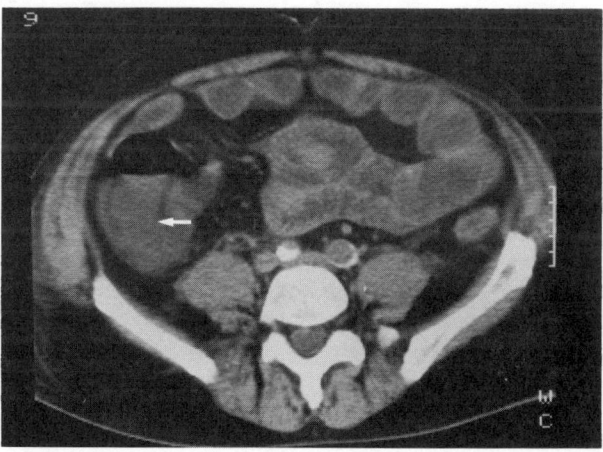

Fig 38–1.—Mesenteric ischemia: distended fluid-filled intestinal loops with thickened bowel wall. Double wall image in the cecal area (*arrow*). (Courtesy of Pérez C, Llanger J, Puig J, et al: *Gastrointest Radiol* 14:241–245, 1989.)

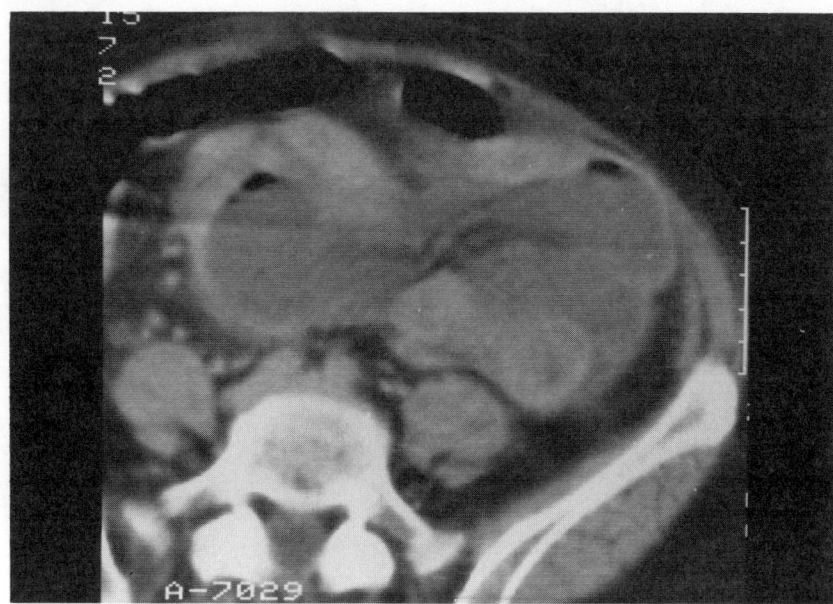

Fig 38–2.—Volvulus of the small bowel: signs of ischemia (intramural gas) and twisted mesentery (whirl sign). (Courtesy of Pérez C, Llanger J, Puig J, et al: *Gastrointest Radiol* 14:241–245, 1989.)

39 Miscellaneous Topics

Total Colectomy for Aganglionosis

Total Colectomy and Ileorectal Anastomosis in the Treatment of Total Colonic Aganglionosis: A Long-Term Follow-up Study of Six Patients
Bergmeijer J-H, Tibboel D, Molenaar JC (Sophia Children's Hosp, Rotterdam, The Netherlands)
J Pediatr Surg 24:282–285, March 1989   39–1

The treatment of total colonic aganglionosis is controversial. Recent reports have advocated Martin's modified Duhamel technique, but it may have serious complications. Experience with low anterior resection and ileorectal anastomosis by the method of Rehbein and Von Zimmermann is evaluated. After total colectomy and ileorectal anastomosis, the patients received total parenteral nutrition, then gradual introduction of an elementary low-residue, low-osmolar diet, followed by a soybean diet, and then normal feeding. Supplementary salt was given to stimulate salt and water absorption. Loperamide was administered to reduce bowel motility, and bowel deflation was accomplished regularly with cannulas to prevent excessive fecal stasis.

For the 6 patients receiving treatment with this method, delays in diagnosis, which delayed surgery, ranged from 4 weeks to 9 months. The extent of the aganglionic bowel was 30 cm in 1 patient, 20 cm in 2 patients, and 10 cm in 3 patients.

No deaths were encountered during the 1- to 7-year follow-up. A short period of frequent, loose stools was followed by 2 to 3 semisolid stools a day by the end of the first year after surgery. Most patients achieved normal growth.

The Rehbein procedure is preferred to Martin's modification of the Duhamel procedure for treatment of total colonic aganglionosis. The method is relatively simple, the final results are satisfactory, and the complications are manageable.

▶ Ileorectal anastomosis after total colectomy is surprisingly effective in patients with total colonic aganglionosis.—F.G. Moody, M.D.

Colon Surgery Without Nasogastric Decompression

Elective Colon and Rectal Surgery Without Nasogastric Decompression: A Prospective, Randomized Trial
Wolff BG, Pemberton JH, van Heerden JA, Beart RW Jr, Nivatvongs S, Devine RM, Dozois RR, Ilstrup DM (Mayo Clinic, Rochester, Minn)
Ann Surg 209:670–674, June 1989

Postoperative nasogastric decompression is standard in surgery, but questions raised about its value remain unresolved. To study the benefits of this practice, 535 patients were assigned randomly to nasogastric decompression or no decompression. Excluded were patients who had chronic obstruction, peritonitis, pelvic irradiation, abscess, intra-abdominal infection, extensive fibrous adhesions, difficult endotracheal intubation, or prolonged operating time.

No major complications occurred in either group. Significantly more nausea, vomiting, and abdominal distention occurred in the group without decompression. Patients with decompression had a 5% tube replacement rate in contrast to a 13% placement rate for those without decompression. The rates for nasopharyngeal or gastric bleeding, respiratory or wound infection, inability to cough effectively, return of bowel function, and hospital stay were similar in both groups.

Nasogastric decompression is not required for most patients after colon and rectal surgery, and it is expensive and uncomfortable. The routine use of nasogastric decompression in colon and rectal surgery is unwarranted.

▶ I agree with the authors' conclusions and strongly encourage surgeons to only use nasogastric suction when it is needed. Only 1 of 10 patients undergoing colonic surgery will need a nasogastric tube; such patients can be identified easily by lack of bowel sounds, emesis, or abdominal distention in the early postoperative period. Adopting the approach used by the Mayo surgeons, the incidence of postoperative pulmonary complications should decrease to a very low level.—F.G. Moody, M.D.

The Liver

- **Chapter 40. Jaundice and Disorder of Bilirubin Metabolism**
- **Chapter 41. Fulminant Hepatitis and Liver Failure**
- **Chapter 42. Viral Hepatitis Type B**
  - Clinical Studies
  - Chronic Hepatitis B
- **Chapter 43. Non-A, Non-B Hepatitis (Hepatitis C)**
  - Development of Specific Tests for Hepatitis C
  - Clinical Studies
  - Treatment with Interferon
  - Hepatitis C and Hepatocellular Carcinoma
- **Chapter 44. Alcoholic Hepatitis**
- **Chapter 45. Cirrhosis and Related Problems**
  - Ascites
  - Portal Hypertension, Bleeding Varices, Sclerotherapy, and Shunts
  - Portal Systemic Encephalopathy
- **Chapter 46. Drug-Associated Hepatic Injury**
- **Chapter 47. Liver Neoplasms**
  - Primary Liver Cancer
  - Metastatic Liver Disease
  - Imaging Studies
- **Chapter 48. Liver Transplantation**
- **Chapter 49. Primary Biliary Cirrhosis**
- **Chapter 50. Miscellaneous Topics**
  - Major Hepatic Resection
  - Wilson's Disease
  - Hepatic Hemangiomas
  - Hydatid Cysts
  - Blunt Trauma

40 Jaundice and Disorder of Bilirubin Metabolism

Less Is Better: The Diagnostic Workup of the Patient With Obstructive Jaundice
Olen R, Pickleman J, Freeark RJ (Loyola Univ, Maywood, Ill)
Arch Surg 124:791–795, July 1989   40–1

Patients with suspected obstructive jaundice typically undergo an extensive preoperative work-up to obtain information that will aid the surgeon at exploration. Data were reviewed on 50 men and 33 women aged 30 to 94 years who were seen in a 15-year period with jaundice caused by common periampullary carcinomas. Sixty of the 83 patients had pancreatic cancer.

Seven of 53 patients had normal or nondiagnostic findings on abdominal ultrasound studies. Findings on computed tomography scans were normal for 3 of these patients. Nine of 43 patients had normal findings on liver-spleen scans. Only 6 of 30 patients with no preoperative vomiting had abnormal findings on upper gastrointestinal roentgenograms. Percutaneous transhepatic cholangiography produced major complications in 8 of 31 patients. Attempted endoscopic retrograde cholangiopancreatography failed in 7 of 37 patients, and 3 patients had major complications.

Abdominal sonography is indicated for patients with histories and liver function tests that suggest obstructive jaundice. If distal bile duct obstruction is found, no further tests generally are required before surgery. Preoperative biliary drainage is not recommended and preoperative percutaneous aspiration or biopsy is not favored. Positive findings on surgical biopsy specimens are not necessary before pancreatic resection in a nonalcoholic patient with an obstructing pancreatic mass.

▶ The diagnostic work-up of a jaundiced patient has been greatly modified by the ability to more clearly define the reason for its occurrence. Pickleman and Freeark are satisfied with demonstrating a dilated biliary tree with ultrasonography and whatever other indirect evidence this technology might provide about the nature of the obstructing lesion. Their negative experience with other, more specific tests have led to the impression that the nature of the problem can be worked out easily at operation. My experience over the past 30 years had led me to the opposite conclusion. Computed tomography scan is a useful staging procedure to assess the presence of node or vascular involvement or metastatic spread to the liver. An endoscopic retrograde cholangiogram may provide a tissue diagnosis and offers a means for biliary drainage in advanced cases. In the situation of an obstruction from a mass in the head of the pancreas, I prefer a thin-needle aspiration for purposes of diagnosis. I am convinced that the surgeon can perform the appropriate surgical procedure if fully informed about the nature and extent of the lesion before operation.—F.G. Moody, M.D.

Abnormalities in Bilirubin and Liver Enzyme Levels in Adult Patients With Bacteremia: A Prospective Study

Sikuler E, Guetta V, Keynan A, Neumann L, Schlaeffer F (Ben Gurion Univ of the Negev, Beer-Sheva, Israel)
Arch Intern Med 149:2246–2248, October 1989   40–2

Hyperbilirubinemia as a complication of bacteremia has been well documented, but the incidence and extent of liver enzyme abnormalities in septic patients have received less attention. Liver enzyme and bilirubin levels were assessed prospectively in 84 adult patients with bacteremia, none of whom had a preexisting malignant neoplasm or hepatobiliary disease.

The 42 males and 42 females, aged 17–89 years, all had positive blood cultures. Laboratory testing included assessment of aspartate aminotransferase (AST), alanine aminotransferase (ALT), alkaline phosphatase, and bilirubin. Blood samples were obtained on hospital admission or as soon as bacteremia was suspected and again a mean of 5.4 days after onset of illness.

Fifty-five patients had an elevation of at least 1 liver enzyme or bilirubin level on the first determination after onset of illness. The AST level was elevated in 44 patients, ALT in 39, alkaline phosphatase in 45, and bilirubin in 5. However, total bilirubin elevation was mild in 4 of these 5 patients; only 1 had severe jaundice. The elevation in liver enzyme levels rarely exceeded 3 times the upper limit of normal. At the second determination of liver enzyme and bilirubin levels, AST was elevated in 11 patients, ALT in 17, alkaline phosphatase in 26, and bilirubin in only 1. Thus all measures indicated significant improvement. There was no statistically significant difference between septic patients with or without biochemical liver abnormalities with respect to

TABLE 1.—Clinical Diagnosis and Frequency of Liver Biochemical Abnormality in 84 Bacteremic Patients

Diagnosis	No. (%) of Patients	No. (%) of Patients With LBA
Urinary tract infection	42 (50.0)	27 (64.3)
Cellulitis	10 (11.9)	7 (70.0)
Bacteremia without obvious cause	10 (11.9)	6 (60.0)
Pneumonia	8 (9.5)	6 (75.0)
Bacterial endocarditis	3 (3.6)	1 (33.3)
Other.	11 (13.1)	8 (72.7)

*Includes meningitis, diverticulitis, gastroenteritis, septic abortion, trauma, and line sepsis.
(Courtesy of Sikuler E, Guetta V, Keynan A, et al: Arch Intern Med 149:2246–2248, October 1989.)

TABLE 2.—Organisms Isolated and Frequency of Liver Biochemical Abnormality in 84 Bacteremic Patients

Organism	No. (%) of Cases	No. (%) of Patients With LBA
Escherichia coli	33 (39.3)	24 (72.7)
Pneumococcus	7 (8.3)	4 (57.1)
Proteus mirabilis	7 (7.1)	4 (66.7)
Klebsiella	6 (7.1)	3 (50.0)
Streptococcus group A	6 (7.1)	6 (100.0)
Pseudomonas aeruginosa	5 (6.0)	1 (20.0)
Staphylococcus aureus	5 (6.0)	4 (80.0)
Streptococcus group D	4 (4.8)	3 (75.0)
Other*	12 (14.3)	6 (50.0)
All gram-negative	54 (64.3)	34 (63.0)
All gram-positive	30 (35.7)	21 (70.0)

*Undefined gram-negative organisms, Staphylococcus epidermidis, Streptococcus viridans, and Streptococcus group G.
(Courtesy of Sikuler E, Guetta V, Keynan A, et al: Arch Intern Med 149:2246–2248, October 1989.)

infection site, type of bacteria isolated, or clinical outcome (Tables 1 and 2). These findings indicate that elevation of liver enzymes and serum bilirubin in adult patients with bacteremia is common, usually mild, of short duration, and of no prognostic significance.

▶ Several factors have been postulated to account for liver test abnormalities and jaundice in patients with bacteremia; these include (1) bacterial endotoxins that can cause intrahepatic cholestasis, (2) hemolysis, (3) metabolic abnormalities secondary to hypermetabolism during sepsis, (4) decreased hepatic blood flow, (5) hepatic hypoxia, (6) malnutrition, and (7) fever. Note that Sikuler and associates found liver biochemical abnormalities to be as common in bacteremia caused by gram-negative organisms as in that caused by gram-positive organisms, suggesting that such abnormalities are not related to a single bacterial toxin and may well be multifactorial in origin.

Hyperbilirubinemia, however, may be more significant than liver enzyme abnormalities in septic patients. Quale and associates (1) have provided data suggesting that the presence of hyperbilirubinemia in patients with S. aureus sepsis may identify persons at high risk of dying from overwhelming sepsis. Further, these investigators suggest that lipoteichoic acid may play an important role in causing defective hepatic excretory function, which is responsible for hyperbilirubinemia.

Eleven of 47 consecutively seen patients with S. aureus endocarditis had hyperbilirubinemia without clinical or laboratory evidence of hepatic bacterial infection. Compared with the remaining 36 patients, these 11 patients had a significantly lower mean platelet count and a higher serum creatinine level and white blood cell count. Although none of the 47 patients was hypotensive on admission, 4 of the 11 hyperbilirubinemic patients died of overwhelming sepsis, compared with 2 of the 36 remaining patients. When 1 of the clinical isolates of S. *aureus* or lipoteichoic acid was infused into conscious rabbits, the hepatic transport maximum was markedly decreased and the relative hepatic storage capacity of sulfobromophthalein was increased. Similar changes were noted after the administration of lipopolysaccharide.—N.J. Greenberger, M.D.

Reference

1. Quale JM, Mandel LJ, Bergasa NV: Clinical significance and pathogenesis of hyperbilirubinemia associated with staphylococcus aureus septicemia. *Am J Med* 85:615–618, 1990.

Benign Recurrent Intrahepatic Cholestasis: Altered Bile Acid Metabolism
Bijleveld CMA, Vonk RJ, Kuipers F, Havinga R, Boverhof R, Koopman BJ, Wolthers BG, Fernandes J (Univ Hosp, Groningen, The Netherlands)
Gastroenterology 97:427–432, August 1989   40–3

Benign recurrent intrahepatic cholestasis (BRIC) is characterized by multiple episodes of cholestatic jaundice in the absence of extrahepatic bile duct obstruction. The etiology of BRIC is unknown, but altered bile acid metabolism is thought to play a role in its pathophysiology. Bile acid metabolism was investigated in 3 children and 10 adults aged 2–65 years with BRIC.

None of the patients had overt cholestasis at the beginning of the trial. To measure the bile acid pool size, each patient was given 1% bicarbonate solution containing 50 mg of deuterated cholic acid and 50 mg of deuterated chenodeoxycholic acid (CDCA), after which blood and stools were sampled for 4 days. A test meal of cream was given on day 5. Serum bile acids were measured at 0, 1, 2, and 3 hours after test meal ingestion. The Entero-Test was swallowed so that duodenal juice could be sampled for determination of bile acid pool composition. Because an increase in the postprandial hydroxy-bile acid concentration is an early sign of liver dysfunction in BRIC patients, this response was measured in all patients. Three patients subsequently were excluded from the final analysis on the basis of their abnormal postprandial responses (Fig 40–1).

The pool sizes of cholic acid and CDCA in BRIC patients were contracted significantly and the fractional turnover rates for these 2 primary bile acids were increased significantly when compared with control values (table). The BRIC patients also had increased fecal bile acid loss and increased serum 7a-hydroxycholesterol levels when compared with controls. An increased serum 7a-hydroxycholesterol level is considered an indication of accelerated bile acid synthesis in response to increased activity of cholesterol 7a-hydroxylase. Because this enzyme catalyzes the first step in the major pathway of bile acid synthesis, a contracted bile acid pool in BRIC patients probably increases the liver's susceptibility to cholestatic agents.

▶ The authors interpret their data as indicating that intestinal malabsorption of 3a-hydroxy-bile acids occurs in BRIC patients. They have developed the following strategy for treatment, which is currently being evaluated in their department.

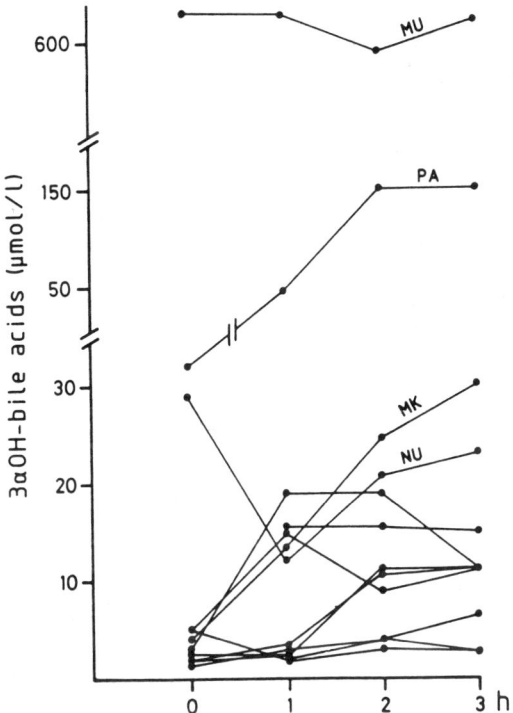

Fig 40–1.—Postprandial response of 3α-hydroxy-bile acids in patients with benign recurrent intrahepatic cholestasis. Patient MU, age 2.5 years, had an unexpected cholestatic episode; patient PA had a patent portocaval shunt; patient NU mentioned mild itching some days before the test; patient MK at 0 time was in the normal range and the postprandial response suggested prodromal stage. (Courtesy of Bijleveld CMA, Vonk RJ, Kuipers F, et al: *Gastroenterology* 97:427–432, August 1989.)

	Pool Size and Fractional Turnover Rate of Primary Bile Acids			
	Cholic acid		Chenodeoxycholic acid	
Patient	Pool size (μmol/kg)	FTR (day^{-1})	Pool size (μmol/kg)	FTR (day^{-1})
D.D.E.	4.9	0.62	10.9	0.30
J.H.	12.8	1.13	7.5	0.94
H.H.K.	—	—	13.9	0.53
A.K.	7.1	1.06	13.1	1.00
L.K.	14.1	0.36	19.4	0.24
L.K.B.	2.0	0.52	6.2	0.47
R.B.	7.8	0.72	15.5	0.63
M.K.	7.3	0.52	6.8	0.49
Mean	8.0 ± 4.2^a	0.70 ± 0.29^a	11.7 ± 4.7^a	0.58 ± 0.27^a
Seven healthy young adult volunteers				
Mean	24.1 ± 11.7	0.29 ± 0.12	22.9 ± 7.8	0.23 ± 0.10

Abbreviation: FTR, fractional turnover rate.
*Significantly different from control value ($P < .05$).
(Courtesy of Bijleveld CMA, Vonk RJ, Kuipers F, et al: *Gastroenterology* 97:427–432, August 1989.)

1. Enlarge the bile acid pool with unconjugated cholic acid or ursodeoxycholic acid during a cholestasis-free period.

2. During a prodromal phase with elevated serum 3a-hydroxy-bile acids, patients should be treated with bile acid binding resins such as cholestyramine. However, irregular treatment with cholestyramine may provoke a period of cholestasis induced by an iatrogenic small bile acid pool.

3. During an episode of cholestasis with a reduction or absence of bile flow, synthesis of bile acid may be blocked with ketoconazole or cholesterol synthesis inhibitors; it would be useful to bind residual intestinal bile acids with cholestyramine.—N.J. Greenberger, M.D.

41 Fulminant Hepatitis and Liver Failure

Early Indicators of Prognosis in Fulminant Hepatic Failure
O'Grady JG, Alexander GJM, Hayllar KM, Williams R (King's College, London)
Gastroenterology 97:439–445, August 1989   41–1

Orthotopic liver transplantation is a successful treatment for patients with fulminant hepatic failure. Thus early prognostic indicators are needed to select those patients most likely to benefit. A definition of prognosis was attempted by deliberately using standard and easily obtainable parameters, including static variables definable on admission and dynamic laboratory variables that could be followed sequentially.

Data on 588 patients with acute liver failure managed medically between 1973 and 1985 were analyzed by univariate and multivariate methods. In acetaminophen-induced fulminant hepatic failure, survival was correlated with arterial blood pH, peak prothrombin time, and serum creatinine level. A pH of less than 7.3, a prothrombin time of more than 100 seconds, and creatinine of more than 300 µmol/L indicated a poor prognosis. In patients with viral hepatitis and drug reactions, etiology, age less than 11 years and more than 40 years, duration of jaundice before onset of encephalopathy, a serum bilirubin level of more than 300 µmol/L, and prothrombin time longer than 50 seconds indicated poor prognosis.

Guidelines are needed for selecting patients with fulminant hepatic failure to undergo orthotopic liver transplantation.

▶ Based on the findings in this study, the Kings College Liver Unit now has adopted the above criteria for referring patients with fulminant hepatic failure for liver transplantation and anticipates that these will improve the speed and accuracy of selecting appropriate candidates for liver transplantation.

Akriviadis and Redeker (1) have reported fulminant hepatitis A in intravenous drug users with chronic parenchymal liver disease. All 4 patients had chronic parenchymal liver disease, which may have contributed to the development of hepatic failure. During the last 2 years, 16 of 113 patients with hepatitis A seen at the liver unit of the University of Southern California required hospitalization. Among the 16 hospitalized patients, fulminant hepatitis developed in 6 and 4 patients died (the patients reported here). The 2 patients who survived were not intravenous drug users nor did they have evidence of chronic liver disease. In all 4 fatal hepatitis A cases, heroin was self-injected, creating a distinct identifiable risk factor. Recent reports show a striking increase in hepatitis A infection among intravenous drug users, and injection or ingestion of contaminated drugs has been suggested as the cause of common-source spread of the virus.

This report by Akriviadis and Redeker suggests that intravenous drug users are at high risk for chronic liver disease, which superimposed on hepatitis A infection may cause unusually severe hepatic injury.—N.J. Greenberger, M.D.

Reference

1. Akriviadis EA, Redeker AG: Fulminant hepatitis A in intravenous drug users with chronic liver disease. *Ann Intern Med* 110:838–839, 1989.

Biochemical and Clinical Response of Fulminant Viral Hepatitis to Administration of Prostaglandin E: A Preliminary Report
Sinclair SB, Greig PD, Blendis LM, Abecassis M, Roberts EA, Phillips MJ, Cameron R, Levy GA (Univ of Toronto)
J Clin Invest 84:1063–1069, October 1989

Prostaglandin (PG) is a promising, efficacious agent in the treatment of fulminant hepatic failure (FHF). The effect of prostaglandin E_1 (PGE_1) on patients with fulminant and subfulminant viral hepatitis were studied in 17 patients with FHF secondary to hepatitis A (no. = 3), hepatitis B (no. = 6), and non-A, non-B hepatitis (no. = 8). Fourteen patients had stage III or IV hepatic encephalopathy.

Initially, all patients had elevated aspartate transaminase (AST) and bilirubin levels, prolonged prothrombin time and partial thromboplastin time, and decreased synthesis of coagulation factors V and VII. Intravenous PGE_1 infusion was started 24–48 hours later after a steady rise in AST, bilirubin, prothrombin time, and partial thromboplastin time. Twelve of 17 patients responded to PGE_1. There was a prompt and marked decrease in serum AST activity (Table 1), improvement in coagulopathy (Table 2), and resolution of hepatic encephalopathy. Five responders with non-A, non-B hepatitis had relapses after initial cessation of therapy; improvement was observed upon retreatment. Two of these patients recovered completely and remained in remission 6 and 12 months after cessation of therapy. Another 2 patients continued in remission after 2 and 6 months of PGE_2. In contrast, none of the patients with hepatitis A and hepatitis B virus infection who survived had a relapse on cessation of PGE_1 therapy. Liver biopsy specimens in all 12 survivors returned to normal. Five patients did not have responses to PGE_1 therapy. They had a more aggressive disease with a short prodrome and development of stage IV hepatic coma within 12–18 hours of onset of FHF. Three died of cerebral edema, and 2 underwent liver transplantation. Overall survival was 71%. None of the patients discontinued PG therapy because of side effects.

Prostaglandin E_1 may prove beneficial in patients with fulminant and subfulminant hepatitis.

▶ These exciting studies are an extension of earlier work by the same investigators (1). Their studies in mice injected with murine hepatitis virus 3 demonstrated that

TABLE 1.—The Effect of PGE$_1$ Infusion on Hepatic Function in Patients with FHF

	Pre-PGE$_1$ infusion			At start of treatment			Post-PGE$_1$ infusion	
	At presentation							
Patient No.	AST	Bilirubin	HE	AST	Bilirubin	HE	AST	Bilirubin	HE
	U/liter	μmol/liter	stage	U/liter	μmol/liter	stage	U/liter	μmol/liter	stage
1	1,460	164	I	1,530	225	III	48	136	0
2	2,160	280	I	1,840	410	III	31	210	0
3	1,810	310	I	2,960	365	III	24	286	0
4	680	140	II	456	370	IV	84	160	0
5	1,550	180	II	1,420	214	III	65	110	0
6	1,420	210	II	2,295	345	IV	55	85	0
7	1,445	75	I	1,280	410	III	42	210	0
8	2,850	110	III	4,100	175	IV	978	320	IV
9	4,800	145	III	6,365	192	IV	3,950	184	IV
10	3,140	140	I	2,810	460	I	565	70	0
11	460	220	I	345	150	IV	45	20	0
12	1,740	458	II	1,585	680	IV	1,100	55	0
13	820	340	IV	810	355	IV	640	410	IV
14	663	536	III	1,367	522	IV	401	576	IV
15	1,200	184	I	846	410	II	41	38	0
16	916	384	I	1,116	410	I	156	11	0
17	4,240	60	III	6,195	110	IV	4,740	165	IV
Mean	1,844	232		2,195	341		763	179	
SD	1,246	135		1,810	148		1,398	150	

Note: Normal range: AST, less than 35 units/L; bilirubin, less than 18 μmol/L.
(Courtesy of Sinclair SB, Greig PD, Blendis LM, et al: *J Clin Invest* 84:1063–1069, October 1989.)

TABLE 2.—Effect of PGE$_1$ Infusion on Coagulation

Patient No.	At presentation				At start of treatment Pre-PGE$_1$ infusion				Post-PGE$_1$ infusion			
	PT* s	PTT† s	Factor V‡ %	Factor VII‡ %	PT s	PTT s	Factor V %	Factor VII %	PT s	PTT s	Factor V %	Factor VII %
1	22	58	8	12	26	61	7	9	12	31	45	36
2	36	64	4	18	38	72	4	12	11	29	85	75
3	21	57	6	8	29	58	7	9	12	31	57	82
4	28	67	7	22	31	90	5	11	13	32	74	65
5	38	68	5	11	40	54	7	9	13	29	100	90
6	36	72	12	6	32	81	4	8	12	30	65	74
7	28	68	11	3	29	71	7	6	11	29	45	69
8	26	90	7	6	28	110	5	8	24	85	43	71
9	62	90	2	3	58	84	3	4	27	60	38	81
10	16	40	9	14	22	51	7	11	11	31	82	65
11	24	60	5	7	28	72	6	9	14	32	55	42
12	26	54	11	6	32	61	7	6	14	34	58	65
13	84	150	2	6	78	110	3	5	65	>150	4	11
14	28	75	8	11	34	81	7	9	20	49	18	22
15	31	72	11	9	36	81	6	8	11	29	89	110
16	16	48	17	11	21	52	12	9	11	29	69	84
17	59	110	7	6	54	91	8	7	28	41	22	28
Mean	34	73	8	9	36	75	6	8	18	44	56	63
SD	18	26	4	5	15	18	2	2	13	31	26	26

*Normal range, less than 11 s.
†Normal range, less than 35 s.
‡Normal range, 70% to 110%.
(Courtesy of Sinclair SB, Greig PD, Blendis LM, et al: J Clin Invest 84:1063–1069, October 1989.)

treatment with dimethyl PGE_2 prevented biochemical toxicity and confluent liver necrosis.

As the authors point out, the mechanism of the beneficial effects of prostaglandins in patients with fulminant hepatic failure remains to be clarified. The observation of a marked and sustained decrease in AST levels after initiation of therapy suggests that prostaglandins may be antiviral. Alternatively, the ameliorative effects of prostaglandins may be through their immunosuppressive properties. In this regard, prostaglandins have been shown to decrease expression of HAV class I and II antigens and to inhibit T-cell-mediated cytotoxicity against isolated mouse liver cells.

The striking results of this study suggest efficacy of prostaglandins in fulminant hepatic failure; further investigations, possibly including controlled trials, are warranted.—N.G. Greenberger, M.D.

Reference

1. Abecassis M, Fack JA, Makowka L, et al: 16,16 Dimethyl prostaglandin E_2 prevents the development of fulminant hepatitis and blocks the induction of monocyte/macrophage procoagulant activity after murine hepatitis virus strain 3 infection. *J Clin Invest* 80:881–889, 1987.

Liver Transplantation in the Management of Fulminant Hepatic Failure
Emond JC, Aran PP, Whitington PF, Broelsch CE, Baker AL (Univ of Chicago)
Gastroenterology 96:1583–1588, June 1989   41–3

Orthotopic liver transplantation now is performed in patients with fulminant hepatic failure because other approaches have proved unrewarding. In the cases reviewed, patient selection for transplantation was based on worsening hepatic encephalopathy, clinical evidence of brain edema, and a prolonged prothrombin time despite up to 48 hours of intensive medical care. Twenty-seven of 37 patients admitted with fulminant hepatic failure deteriorated despite medical treatment and 19 of them underwent liver transplantation. All those who deteriorated but who were not operated on died.

The 1-year actuarial survival rate after liver transplantation was 58%. Primary graft failure caused 3 deaths. Five of 6 patients with cerebral edema preoperatively survived. Three patients who were discharged after liver transplantation later died, one of them after retransplantation for chronic rejection.

More than half of the critically ill patients with fulminant hepatic failure can be expected to survive after orthotopic liver transplantation. The liver biopsy findings may help identify those patients who are unlikely to survive with supportive care alone. When feasible, transplantation is presently the best approach to such patients.

▶ Liver transplantation sounds like a heroic approach to fulminant hepatic failure, but it is life-saving in more than half of appropriately selected patients. It is always a problem to know which patients will live and which will die from this catastrophic illness, but now that liver transplantation is a common and relatively nonmorbid operation, it should be offered more frequently to this easily identified group of patients. Transplantation early in the course of this illness likely would lead to an even higher survival rate.—F.G. Moody, M.D.

42 Viral Hepatitis Type B

Clinical Studies

Half-Life of HBs Antibody After Hepatitis B Vaccination: An Aid to Timing of Booster Vaccination
Nommensen FE, Go ST, MacLaren DM (Free Univ, Amsterdam)
Lancet 2:847–849, Oct 7, 1989   42–1

Vaccination against hepatitis B virus (HBV) generally is administered to persons at increased occupational risk for HBV infection. Because the protection provided by vaccination against HBV is of limited duration, booster vaccination is indicated. It has been assumed that the duration of antibody persistence is directly related to the peak antibody level achieved after vaccination, and that antibody levels fall at about the same rate in most persons. It therefore has been proposed that the booster vaccination against HBV should be scheduled based on an individual's postvaccination peak antibody level. However, some evidence suggests that antibody levels decrease rapidly in some persons. Accordingly, the rate of decline of anti-HBV antibody was assessed in 54 healthy hospital employees vaccinated against HBV.

All employees were vaccinated with HBV vaccine at 0, 1, and 6 months. Postvaccination serum samples were obtained at month 7 to assess the vaccination response and again at 21–869 days thereafter to assess antibody decline.

The anti-HBV antibody half-life in 10 of the 48 evaluable persons was less than 90 days, whereas another 12 persons had anti-HBV antibody half-lives of more than 190 days. The rate of antibody decline seemed unrelated to the height of the postvaccination antibody level (Fig 42–1). To maintain protection against HBV, the date for revaccination should be scheduled on the basis of postvaccination anti-HBV antibody levels, as well as antibody half-lives, as measured in each person.

▶ This study indicates that the protection afforded by vaccination against hepatitis B virus is highly variable. Approximately 30% of the persons had a serum antibody level of only 1:4 at the end of 1 year and more judged to be susceptible to infection with the hepatitis B virus. The authors, therefore, suggest that half-life determinations on completion of vaccination provide a rational basis for estimating when booster vaccination is needed. Whether this proves cost-effective (by avoiding unnecessary vaccination) remains to be determined.—N.J. Greenberger, M.D.

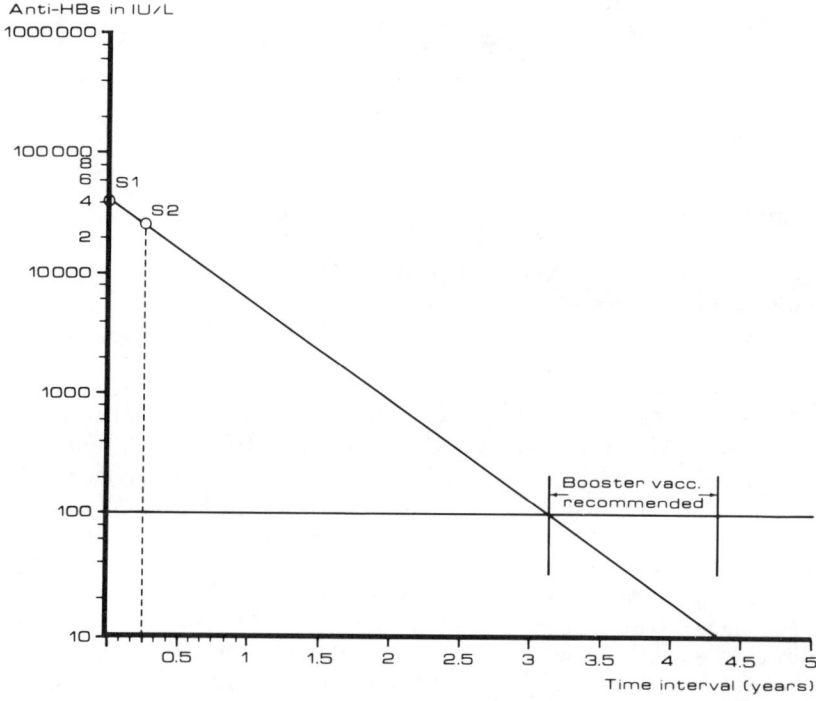

Fig 42–1.—Estimated duration of vaccine-induced protection. *S1*, antibody level of the first serum sample plotted at time 0 on a logarithmic scale; *S2*, level of the second sample plotted at the time intervening between sampling dates; *vacc*, vaccine. The time to expiration of protection (at 100 IU/L) is estimated by extension of S1 - S2. (Courtesy of Nommensen FE, Go ST, MacLaren DM: *Lancet* 2:847–849, Oct 7, 1989.)

Hepatitis B Virus Infection Among Children Born in the United States to Southeast Asian Refugees
Franks AL, Berg CJ, Kane MA, Browne BB, Sikes RK, Elsea WR, Burton AH (Ctrs for Disease Control; Georgia Dept of Human Resources; Fulton County Health Dept, Atlanta)
N Engl J Med 321:1301–1305, Nov 9, 1989   42–2

Infection with hepatitis B virus (HBV) is hyperendemic in Southeast Asia. In a cross-sectional seroprevalence study, the frequency and patterns of transmission of HBV infection among the children of refugees from Southeast Asia were studied in 196 refugee families with 257 children born in the United States.

Of the 31 children born in the United States to mothers with infectious disease, 17 (54.8%) had been infected with HBV. Of the 226 children born to mothers who did not have infectious disease, 15 had HBV infection, for a prevalence of 6.6% (95% confidence interval, 4.1–10.7). This is 10 times more than the prevalence among age-matched white children in the general population. The risk of infection was highest among children living in households with children with infectious disease (table), and the risk was greater for those who lived with children aged 1 to 5 years with infectious disease than for those who lived with older children with infectious disease. Having fathers or adults with infectious disease in the household was not significantly associated with risk of infection. Of the 128 children from households with no members with infectious disease, 3.9% were infected (95% confidence interval, 1.7–8.8). Perinatal transmission from mothers with infectious disease was not a factor in 46% of the cases of HBV infection among children born in the United States.

These findings suggest that child-to-child transmission remains an important route of infection among Southeast Asian refugees living in the United States. Current recommendations to immunize the newborns of mothers with infectious disease are not sufficient to protect all children of Southeast Asian refugees from HBV infection in early life, when the risk of chronic sequelae and premature death is greatest. The authors recommend that hepatitis B vaccination policy should expand to include all newborn children of Southeast Asian immigrants.

▶ The diagnosis of HBV infection is based on sensitive standardized radioimmunoassays and the enzyme-linked immunosorbent assay for the detection of viral hepatitis B surface antigen (HBsAg) and antibodies to the core antigen (anti-HBcAg) and surface antigen (anti-HBsAg). Negative results with these tests have implicated a group of viruses defined as non-A, non-B viruses. However, DNA sequences hybridizing under highly stringent conditions with an HBV DNA probe have been shown in the liver, serum, and mononuclear blood cells of persons without serum HBV markers by conventional tests.

In an important study, Thiers and co-workers (1) used the polymerase chain reaction (PCR) to identify and characterize serum HBV DNA sequences in 3 patients without HBV serologic markers. By use of sets of primers on the S and pre-S parts of the HBV genome, the presence of HBV DNA was demonstrated in the serum of

Risk of HBV Infection Among U.S.-Born Children of Mothers Without Infectious Disease, According to the Presence of Other Persons With Infectious Disease in the Household

Status	U.S.-Born Children			Relative Risk*
	TOTAL NUMBER	NUMBER INFECTED	PERCENT INFECTED	
Father†				
Uninfectious	177	9	5.1	1.0
Infectious	32	3	9.4	1.8 (0.5–6.4)
Other adult‡				
Uninfectious	147	8	5.4	1.0
Infectious	50	3	6.0	1.1 (0.3–4.0)
Child§				
Uninfectious	191	9	4.7	1.0
Infectious	23	6	26.1	5.5 (2.3–13.4)

*Values in parentheses are 95% confidence intervals.
†Category excludes 16 children whose fathers' HBV status was not known.
‡Category excludes 28 children for whom the HBV status of all household adults other than their parents was not known.
§Category excludes 11 children for whom the HBV status of all other children in the household was not known.

(Courtesy of Franks AL, Berg CJ, Kane MA, et al: *N Engl J Med* 321:1301–1305, Nov 9, 1989.)

all 3 patients. Inoculation of 2 chimpanzees with human sera induced acute hepatitis in both animals; 1 became positive for HBsAg and anti-HBcAg, and the other, only for anti-HBsAg. Thiers and colleagues conclude that PCR with HBV primers may identify unambiguously HBV infectious particles among non-A, non-B viruses and is a potentially useful diagnostic test for detection of HBV DNA sequences in serum.—N.J. Greenberger, M.D.

Reference

1. Thiers V, Kremsdorf D, Schellekens H, et al: Transmission of hepatitis B from hepatitis B seronegative subjects. Lancet 2:1273–1276, 1988.

Chronic Hepatitis B

Mutation Preventing Formation of Hepatitis B e Antigen in Patients With Chronic Hepatitis B Infection
Carman WF, Jacyna MR, Hadziyannis S, Karayiannis P, McGarvey MJ, Makris A, Thomas HC (St Mary's Hosp Med School, London; Hippocration Hosp, Athens, Greece)
Lancet 2:588–591, Sept 9, 1989   42-3

Patients with chronic hepatitis B virus infection include those with HB e antigen (HBeAg), viremia, and chronic liver disease; those with HBeAg negative results and anti-HBe positive results, yet have viremia and often have especially severe chronic hepatitis; and those with anti-HBe but without viremia or liver disease. Hepatitis B e antigen is derived from the viral precore/core open reading frame, and its expression might modify the course of the disease. Whether the absence of HBeAg in some patients might be caused by mutations in the precore region of the viral genome was investigated. Using the polymerase chain reaction (Fig 42–2) viral DNA from sera of 18 Greek and 3 non-Greek patients, comprising all 3 categories described above, was amplified and sequenced.

All 8 anti-HBe-positive patients with viremia were found to have a mutation from guanosine to adenosine at position 1896 at the end of the precore region. This mutation results in a new translation stop codon, which is predicted to prevent HBeAg protein synthesis. Seven of these patients also had a mutation at position 1899 that may enhance ribosomal binding and translation. Four of 5 patients positive for HBeAg had sequences in this region identical to known HBV sequences. Patients positive for anti-HBeAg without viremia had heterogeneous viral genomes detectable by enzymatic amplification, although they were HBV negative by dot-blot hybridization.

These findings provide evidence consistent with the hypothesis that some patients with chronic hepatitis B but negative for HBeAg are infected with viral genomes that contain 1 or 2 particular mutations in the precore region. The rest of the precore region in these patients was similar to those of known viruses and to those of HBeAg-positive sequences. The small amount of HBV-DNA detected in patients without viremia or liver disease may have been either intact virions or free viral DNA released from cells.

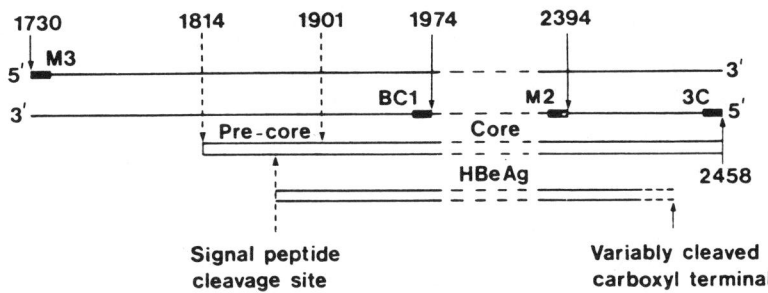

Fig 42-2.—Target sequence for DNA amplification. Upper strand has positive polarity. In vivo derivation of translated peptides is shown. Precore ATG begins at position 1814, and that of core at 1901. Positions of DNA amplification primers ME (5'CTGGGAGGAGTTGGGGGAGGAGATT) and M2 (5'GGCGAGGGAGTTC-TTCTTCTAGGGG) and sequencing primer BCl (5'GGAAAGAAGTCAGAAGGCAA) are shown. (Courtesy of Carman WF, Jacyna MR, Hadziyannis S, et al: *Lancet* 2:588–591, Sept 9, 1989.)

▶ Only 1 type of hepatitis B virus is known; it has a nucleocapsid bearing the HBc specificity and an envelope containing S, pre S_1, and pre S_2 proteins. Subtypes have a common specificity "a" on the envelope, but different subtype specificities: d, r, y, or w.

Coursaget and colleagues have reported HBsAg positive reactivity in human beings that is not caused by hepatitis B virus (1). These investigators observed a new type of HBsAg-positive infection in Senegal. Infection was characterized by the presence of HBsAg without anti-HBc, and after the loss of HBsAg neither anti-HBc nor anti-HBs became detectable. Moreover, HBeAg was not detected in infected patients. Viral particles 45–60 nm in diameter and some 22–30-nm spherical forms were observed in such HBsAg-positive sera. HBsAg-DNA complementary sequences were detected, weakly, in only 1 of 15 serum samples from persons with HBsAg-positive, anti-HBc-negative infection. This observation may result from the low concentration of the virus in the serum and the partial nucleic acid homology with HBV. The virus responsible for the infection is probably a hepadnavirus because it shares with other members of this family a common ultrastructure and shows some cross-reactive antigenic determinants. They have named this new virus HBV_2.—N.J. Greenberger, M.D.

Reference

1. Coursaget P, Bourdel C, Adomowicz P, et al: HBsAg positive reactivity in man not due to hepatitis B virus. *Lancet* 1:1354–1357, 1987.

Which Patients With Chronic Hepatitis B Virus Infection Will Respond to α-Interferon Therapy? A Statistical Analysis of Predictive Factors

Brook MG, Karayiannis P, Thomas HC (St Mary's Hosp Med school, London)
Hepatology 10:761–763, 1989

The success rates of α-interferon therapy in chronic hepatitis B virus (HBV) infection vary from 25% to 50%, indicating the heterogeneous nature of

Pretreatment Variables Significantly Predicting Response

Variable	Responders	Nonresponders	Significance
Acute hepatitis			
Yes	22	16	
No	21	55	$p < 0.005$
Histology *			
CAH	37	37	
CPH	6	34	$p < 0.005$
Anti-HIV status			
Positive	1	22	
Negative	42	49	$p < 0.001$
Mean $\log_{10}$ AST ± S.D.	2.00 ± 0.25	1.77 ± 0.22	$p < 0.001$
Mean DNA (pg/ml) ± S.D.	1,446 ± 1,086	2,204 ± 905	$p < 0.001$

*Abbreviations: CAH, chronic active hepatitis; CPH, chronic persistent hepatitis.
(Courtesy of Brook MG, Karayiannis P, Thomas HC: Hepatology 10:761–763, 1989.)

patients. To assess factors predictive of response, 114 patients given α-interferon for chronic HBV infection were studied. Treatment response was defined as the loss of HBeAg and HBV DNA maintained for 12 months after therapy.

Of the 114 patients who received α-interferon, 90 million units/m² over 12 weeks, 43 responded to therapy. Univariate analysis showed that a history of acute icteric hepatitis, chronic active hepatitis on liver biopsy, high levels of aspartate aminotransferase (AST), low hepatitis B virus DNA level, and a negative anti-HIV antibody status were associated significantly with response (table). Treatment response was significantly more likely to occur in patients with chronic infection of less than 2 years' duration. Stepwise logistic regression analysis showed that HBV DNA, AST, and a history of acute hepatitis were independent predictive variables. The most reliable combination of predictive factors was a negative anti-HIV antibody status and either a history of acute icteric hepatitis and AST greater than 45 IU/L or no history of acute icteric hepatitis and AST greater than 85 IU/L. This combination had a sensitivity of 77% and a specificity of 79%.

This predictive model, which includes anti-HIV antibody status, a history of acute icteric hepatitis, and AST levels, may be useful in predicting response to a-interferon therapy of patients with chronic HBV infection.

► Recombinant human a-interferon is now under intensive investigation as therapy for chronic type B hepatitis. Recent reports have suggested that prolonged a-interferon therapy may induce autoimmune reactions. Werner and associates (1) have evaluated the problem of autoimmunity related to a-interferon therapy by testing for 15 different antibodies in the sera of 31 patients given α-interferon. No patient had autoantibodies before treatment; in 27 (87%) of 31 patients at least 1 autoantibody developed. Eleven patients had antinuclear antibodies, and 21 had smooth muscle antibodies, both types of which usually developed during α-interferon therapy. In contrast, antibodies to endocrine organs such as thyroid microsomal, thyroglobulin, and parietal cell antibodies arose in 12 patients, but usually several months after treatment with α-interferon. The appearance of these autoantibodies were not correlated with disease activity or response to α-interferon. No patient had autoantibodies specifically associated with autoimmune liver diseases such as liver kidney microsomal antibodies, autoantibodies to soluble liver antigen, and the primary biliary cirrhosis-specific subtypes of antimitochondrial antibodies.

Werner and colleagues suggest that prolonged α-interferon therapy can induce autoantibody production, which in susceptible patients might lead to autoimmune disorders.—N.J. Greenberger, M.D.

Reference

1. Werner J, Mayet Hess G, Rossal S, et al: Treatment of chronic type B hepatitis with recombinant a-interferon induces autoantibodies not specific for autoimmune chronic hepatitis. *Hepatology* 10:24–28, 1989.

Detection of Hepatitis B Virus X Gene Protein and Antibody in Type B Chronic Liver Disease
Katayama K, Hayashi N, Sasaki Y, Kasahara A, Ueda K, Fusamoto H, Sato N, Chisaka O, Matsubara K, Kamada T (Osaka Univ, Osaka, Japan)
Gastroenterology 97:990–998, October 1989   42–5

The genome of hepatitis B virus (HBV) contains a sequence, the X gene, whose role is uncertain. The region of this gene was expressed in *Escherichia coli* by constructing a recombinant plasmid pOCTX, containing the Bam HI-Bgl II fragment of the HBV genome (Fig 42–3). The resultant protein had a molecular weight of about 17 kilodaltons. Sera from 139 persons were analyzed for anti-X with the Western blot method. Most of the persons tested had positive results for hepatitis B surface antigen.

Anti-X was present in 41% of patients with chronic hepatitis, 46% of those with hepatocellular carcinoma, and 63% of those with cirrhosis (table), but was not found in patients with acute hepatitis. In chronic hepatitis, anti-X was most frequent in patients positive for antibody to hepatitis B e antigen. The X protein was identified in the livers of 87.5% of 26 patients with chronic hepatitis and in 4 of 6 patients with cirrhosis. Hepatitis B core antigen often was expressed along with X protein in the liver.

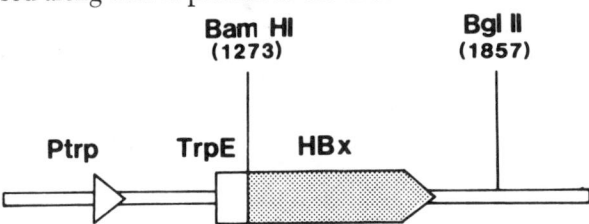

Fig 42–3.—Structure of pOCTX. A 584 base pairs fragment (from Bam HI to Bgl II) was excised from pBRadr4 and inserted after the seventh codon of pOCT2-5. This fragment included 145 amino acids (from the 10th to the 154th) of the X gene. The nucleotide number marked along the HBV genome starts from the Xho I site. *Ptrp*, tryptophan operon promoter; *TrpE*, TrpE gene. (Courtesy of Katayama K, Hayashi N, Sasaki Y, et al: *Gastroenterology* 97:990–998, October 1989.)

Occurrence of Antibody to Hepatitis B Virus X Antigen in Sera From Patients With Hepatitis B Virus Infection

Diagnosis	HBeAg/anti-HBe			Total
	+/−	−/−	−/+	
HBsAg-positive				
Acute hepatitis	0/4		0/2 *	0/6 (0%)
Healthy carrier	0/7		0/5	0/12 (0%)
Chronic hepatitis	10/32 (31%)		11/19 (58%)	21/51 (41%)
Liver cirrhosis	7/10 (70%)	1/1 (100%)	7/13 (54%)	15/24 (63%)
Hepatocellular carcinoma	3/7 (43%)	1/2 (50%)	8/17 (47%)	12/26 (46%)
HBsAg-negative				
Chronic liver disease †				3/14 (21%)
HBV markers negative ‡				0/8 (0%)

Abbreviations: anti-HBe, antibody to hepatitis B e antigen; *HBeAg*, hepatitis B e antigen; *HBsAg*, hepatitis B surface antigen.
*Of 4 patients with acute hepatitis, the serial sera of 2 patients were studied.
†These patients with chronic liver disease had antibody to hepatitis B surface antigen.
‡These patients did not have hepatitis B surface antigen, antibody to hepatitis B surface antigen, or antibody to hepatitis B core antigen.
(Courtesy of Katayama K, Hayashi N, Sasaki Y, et al: *Gastroenterology* 97:990–998, October 1989.)

Expression of X protein in the liver and of anti-X in the serum in type B liver disease indicate that the X gene may be associated with HBV replication. Anti-X is found more often as the duration of infection increases. Anti-X may suppress the expression of X protein in the liver.

▶ Hepatitis B virus is a causative agent for type B viral hepatitis, which has been linked to hepatocellular carcinoma in human beings. Molecular cloning and nucleotide sequencing have indicated that the genome of HBV contains at least 4 open reading frames: S, C, P, and X. The roles of the S, C, and P regions have been reported, but the function of the X region is still unclear. This paper provides tentative evidence suggesting that X protein may be related to viral replication.—N.J. Greenberger, M.D.

43 Non-A, Non-B Hepatitis (Hepatitis C)

Development of Specific Tests for Hepatitis C

An Assay for Circulating Antibodies to a Major Etiologic Virus of Human Non-A, Non-B Hepatitis
Kuo G, Choo Q-L, Alter HJ, Gitnick GL, Redeker AG, Purcell RH, Miyamura T, Dienstag JL, Alter MJ, Stevens CE, Tegtmeier GE, Bonino F, Colombo M, Lee W-S, Kuo C, Berger K, Shuster JR, Overby LR, Bradley DW, Houghton M (Chiron Corp, Emeryville, Calif; Clinical Ctr, Bethesda, Md; Univ of California, Los Angeles; Univ of Southern California, Downey; Natl Inst of Allergy and Infectious Diseases, Bethesda, Md; et al)
Science 244:362–364, Apr 24, 1989   43-1

Non-A, non-B (NANB) hepatitis represents more than 90% of transfusion-associated hepatitis, and up to 10% of transfusions have resulted in NANB hepatitis. At least half of these infections result in chronic hepatitis, of which 20% have led to cirrhosis. The genome of the NANB agent, cloned recently, is designated as hepatitis C virus (HCV). Data on the development and use of a recombinant-based assay for HCV antibodies were reviewed.

A polypeptide synthesized in recombinant yeast clones of the HCV was used to capture circulating viral antibodies. Detection of bound antibodies was achieved with a radioactive second antibody. A high sensitivity and specificity of this antibody assay for bloodborne NANB hepatitis was demonstrated in 7 NANB hepatitis human serum samples shown previously to transmit NANB hepatitis in chimpanzees. Assays of 10 blood transfusions in the United States that resulted in chronic NANB hepatitis demonstrated that there was at least 1 positive blood donor for 9 of these patients and that all 10 recipients seroconverted during their illnesses. More than 50% of NANB hepatitis patients from the United States with no identifiable source of parenteral exposure to the virus were positive for HCV antibody. In addition, about 80% of chronic, posttransfusion patients with NANB hepatitis from Japan and Italy had circulating HCV antibody; a much lower frequency (15%) was observed in acute, resolving infections.

Hepatitis C virus is a major cause of chronic NANB hepatitis throughout the world. The advent of this recombinant-based assay for HCV antibody should improve the safety of the blood supply and provide an important clinical diagnostic tool. In addition, this assay and the availability of HCV hybridization probes may help to identify the existence of other parenteral NANB hepatitis agents.

▶ This landmark study details the characterization of a virus associated with blood-borne NANB hepatitis and provisionally names this virus hepatitis C. Recent surveys of blood donor populations have indicated that the incidence of antibodies to hepatitis C (anti-HCV) ranges from 0.4% of 3,123 patients (1) to 0.68% of 25,137 patients (2) to 0.87% of 11,117 patients (3).

Alter and associates (4) studied patients with acute NANB hepatitis from 4 geographic areas in the U.S. (no. = 131), followed for 6–48 months after onset of illness to determine risk factors, frequency, and severity of chronic hepatitis. These patients were tested for antibody to hepatitis C virus (anti-HCV) using a newly developed radioimmunoassay. Anti-HCV was found in 54% of acute-phase sera drawn within 30–60 days of onset of illness and in 67% of chronic-phase sera drawn within 6–36 months after onset. Chronic phase sera were positive for anti-HCV in 60% of patients with a history of transfusions, 89% of intravenous drug users, 80% of health care workers, 63% of those with household or sexual exposure, and 57% of those with no known source of infection. Liver enzyme abnormalities persisted in 51% of patients and were more likely to persist in patients positive for anti-HCV (58%) than in those negative for anti-HCV (36%).

Emerging evidence suggests that approximately 85% of patients with post-transfusion hepatitis will have anti-HCV, but the seroconversion may be delayed as long as 6 months. As noted above anti-HCV is more likely to persist in patients with chronic hepatitis and to regress in patients in whom hepatitis C resolves. As noted in a recent editorial (5) many questions have yet to be settled. How many other agents are involved? Is there a short-incubation agent? What is the cause of the negative cases of sporadic NANB hepatitis in the community? Are any of these related to the enterically transmitted NANB virus so common on the Indian subcontinent? Will the assay help to select patients for interferon treatment?—N.J. Greenberger, M.D.

References

1. Kühnl P, et al: Antibodies to hepatitis C virus in German blood donors. *Lancet* 2:324, 1989.
2. Janst C, et al: Antibodies to hepatitis C in French blood donors. *Lancet* 2:796–797, 1989.
3. Sirchia G, et al: Antibodies to hepatitis C virus in Idahoan blood donors. *Lancet* 2:797, 1989.
4. Alter MJ, Margolis AS, Krawczyaski K, et al: Clinical outcome and risk factors associated with hepatitis C in the United States. *Hepatology* 10:581, 1989.
5. Will the real hepatitis C stand up? *Lancet* 2:307–308, 1989 (editorial).

Clinical Studies

Detection of Antibody to Hepatitis C Virus in Prospectively Followed Transfusion Recipients With Acute and Chronic Non-A, Non-B Hepatitis
Alter HJ, Purcell RH, Shih JW, Melpolder JC, Houghton M, Choo Q-L, Kuo G (Natl Inst of Allergy and Infectious Diseases, Bethesda, Md; Chiron Corp, Emeryville, Calif)

Non-A, non-B hepatitis remains a serious consequence of blood transfusions, and the virus may be associated causally with hepatocellular carcinoma. Detection has been difficult, although recent advances have followed cloning of the hepatitis C virus (HCV). The antibody to HCV (anti-HCV), which causes non-A, non-B hepatitis, was measured by immunoassay in transfusion recipients and their donors.

Adult patients with no preexisting liver disease who underwent open-heart surgery were tested during the year after transfusion for development of non-A, non-B hepatitis. The diagnosis was determined when clinical and laboratory studies excluded other hepatotropic viruses and nonviral causes of hepatocellular injury. Fifteen of 70 cases were thought to be unequivocal for chronic non-A, non-B hepatitis; 5 patients with acute, resolving non-A, non-B hepatitis were also included in the study. Each patient with chronic disease was negative for anti-HCV before transfusion; all became positive at some later time (table).

The 5 patients with resolving disease were compared with the 15 chronic cases. Seroconversion to anti-HCV occurred in only 3 of the 5 self-limited cases. Those who did not seroconvert differed from the other 3 cases only in a short period (less than 6 weeks) of abnormal alanine aminotransferase. At a mean follow-up of 6.9 years, antibody persisted in 14 of 15 patients with

Anti-HCV Seroconversion in Prospectively Followed Patients in Whom Chronic Transfusion-Associated Non-A, Non-B Hepatitis Developed*

PATIENT NO.	AGE/SEX	ACUTE PHASE			CHRONIC PHASE		ANTI HCV SEROCONVERSION
		ONSET (WEEKS AFTER TRANSFUSION)	PEAK ALT (IU/liter)	PEAK BILIRUBIN (μmol/liter)	DURATION (yr)	LIVER HISTOLOGIC FEATURES	
1	61/M	10	978	5.1	$\geq$13	CAH	Yes
2	46/M	5	610	15.4	$\geq$11	CAH	Yes
3	57/F	6	468	13.7	10½	CPH	Yes
4	54/F	9	768	10.3	8	CPH	Yes
5	71/M	9	421	17.1	>10†	CAH/cirrhosis	Yes
6	29/M	6	678	13.7	$\geq$9	CAH	Yes
7	55/F	7	434	13.7	$\geq$12	CAH	Yes
8	53/M	9	450	100.9	>6‡	CAH/cirrhosis	Yes
9	63/F	7	1200	153.9	4‡	CAH/cirrhosis	Yes
10	62/M	5	525	12.0	$\geq$7	CAH/cirrhosis	Yes
11	25/M	8	505	17.1	7	CPH	Yes
12	60/M	6	2112	106.0	$\geq$12	CAH	Yes
13	35/F	8	555	27.4	$\geq$1	No biopsy	Yes
14	63/M	8	1600	143.6	6	CAH	Yes
15	55/M	7	785	20.5	4	CAH	Yes

*Abbreviations: ALT, alanine aminotransferase; CAH, chronic active hepatitis; CPH, chronic persistent hepatitis; CAH/cirrhosis, CAH on initial biopsy and cirrhosis on later biopsy.
†Patient died of causes unrelated to liver disease.
‡Patient died of causes directly or indirectly related to liver disease.
(Courtesy of Alter HJ, Purcell RH, Shih JW, et al: N Engl J Med 321:1494–1500, Nov 30, 1989.)

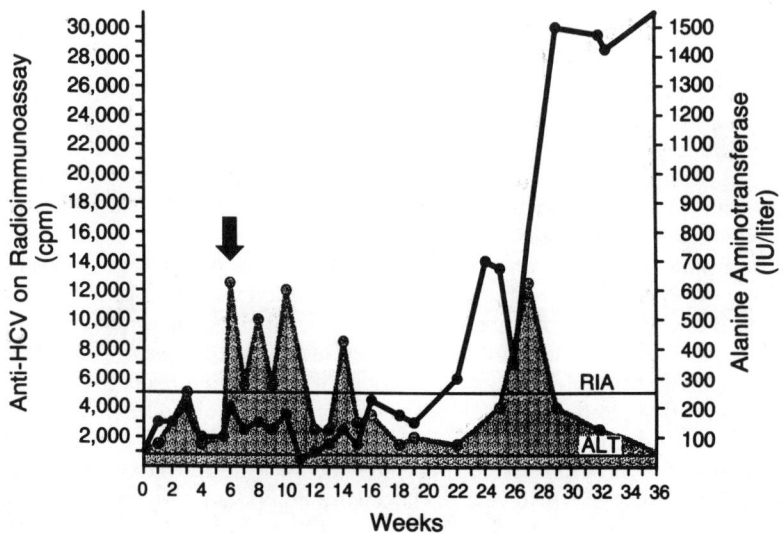

Fig 43-1.—Serial alanine aminotransferase and anti-HCV levels in patient, demonstrating the characteristic long interval between transfusion and the first appearance of detectable antibody. The *shaded area* shows the level of alanine aminotransferase, and the *heavy line* shows anti-HCV. The *horizontal lines* show the upper limits of normal for alanine aminotransferase *(ALT)*, and anti-HCV on radioimmunoassay *(RIA)*. The *arrow* represents the onset of hepatitis. The interval between exposure and the appearance of detectable antibody was 20 to 22 weeks. There was a correspondingly long interval (14 to 16 weeks) between the onset of hepatitis and the first appearance of the antibody. Note the fluctuating alanine aminotransferase pattern characteristic of non-A, non-B hepatitis. Antibody has persisted for more than 10 years. (Courtesy of Alter HJ, Purcell RH, Shih JW, et al: *N Engl J Med* 321:1494–1500, Nov 30, 1989.)

chronic disease. In contrast, only 2 of 5 patients with acute resolving disease have evidence of antibody at 4.1 years.

A typical delayed response was seen in a patient with chronic hepatitis. The antibody was detected at 20 to 22 weeks after exposure, 14 to 16 weeks after the onset of hepatitis. Anti-HCV rose to a plateau and persisted for more than 10 years, whereas alanine aminotransferase levels showed a characteristic fluctuating pattern (Fig 43–1). The status of both donors and recipients could be analyzed in 16 cases; in 14 (88%), an anti-HCV-positive donor was detected. Use of the surrogate assays, primarily that for anti-HBC, would have excluded 53% of the positive donors.

The primary cause of chronic, transfusion-associated non-A, non-B hepatitis appears to be HCV. Seroconversion may not take place for more than 1 year and may not be detected if sampling is inadequate. The antibody may disappear in patients with the acute, resolving form of the disease. Routine use of the assay might detect 85% of donors capable of transmitting non-A, non-B hepatitis.

Hepatitis C Virus Antibodies Among Risk Groups in Spain
Esteban JI, Esteban R, Viladomiu L, López-Talavera JC, González A, Hernández JM, Roget M, Vargas V, Genescà J, Buti M, Guardia J, Houghton M, Choo Q-L, Kuo G (Hosp Vall d'Hebron; Universitat Autonoma, Barcelona, Spain; Chiron Corp, Emeryville, Calif)

Non-A, non-B (NANB) hepatitis accounts for more than 90% of transfusion-associated hepatitis, including a substantial proportion of infections among patients with frequent parenteral exposure to blood and more than 25% of patients with sporadic hepatitis without obvious percutaneous exposure. Recently, a blood-borne NANB hepatitis agent was isolated: hepatitis C virus (HCV). A recombinant-based immunoassay for detecting specific anti-HCV antibodies was developed, and the frequency of HCV infection in Spain was determined using this assay on 836 serum samples from 676 patients. The patients were selected on the basis of their risk for blood-borne viral infections and the presence of liver disease.

Among patients at high risk of infection, anti-HCV antibodies were detected in 85% of prospectively followed patients with posttransfusion NANB hepatitis, 62% of patients with chronic hepatitis or cirrhosis and a history of blood transfusion, 70% of hemophiliac persons receiving replacement therapy, 70% of intravenous drug abusers, and 20% of patients undergoing hemodialysis. Only 8% of homosexual men with HIV infection and 6% of female contacts of drug abusers tested positive. Among those with liver disease and no history of parenteral exposure to blood, anti-HCV antibodies were found in 38% of patients with cryptogenic, alcoholic, or primary biliary cirrhosis and in 44% with chronic active hepatitis. The overall prevalence of anti-HCV in healthy persons without risk factors for hepatitis was 1.2%.

Hepatitis C virus accounts for most posttransfusion hepatitis in Spain. Although seroconversion may occur in the acute phase of infection, anti-HCV antibodies were first detected 4–6 months after transfusion in more than half of these patients, and in some the antibody response occurred considerably later. Because the finding of anti-HCV appears to be associated with chronic infection, HCV may be an important pathogen in nearly half of the patients whose liver disease is currently attributed to nonviral causes.

▶ At the 1989 meeting of the American Association for the Study of Liver Diseases there were 25 presentations on hepatitis C. It seems clear that this agent can be implicated in the vast majority of patients with chronic non-A, non-B hepatitis as well as in patients with various chronic liver diseases. The report by Di Bisceglie and colleagues (1) is a representative study.

To characterize the diseases associated with chronic HCV infection, these investigators have tested serum from 206 patients with chronic liver disease for antibody to HCV (anti-HCV). They studied all patients with chronic NANB hepatitis and autoimmune hepatitis seen at NIH between 1979 and 1988. Diagnoses were made using standard criteria before anti-HCV testing was available. In addition, patients with chronic type B and type D (delta) hepatitis, primary biliary cirrhosis, and sclerosing cholangitis were studied. Samples were tested by radioimmunoassay (Chiron Corporation) or by enzyme-linked immunoassay (Ortho Diagnostic Systems) (table).

Infection with HCV in 73 patients with chronic NANB hepatitis was associated with blood transfusion (55%), intravenous drug abuse (27%), and occupational exposure to blood (10%); 7 patients had no known parenteral exposure to blood. Of 7 patients with chronic hepatitis B, delta infection, and primary biliary cirrhosis

Results of Testing for Hepatitis C Virus Antibody in 206 Patients

Disease	No.	Anti-HCV positive	(%)
Chronic NANB Hepatitis	92	73	(79)
Autoimmune Hepatitis	14	6	(43)
Chronic Hepatitis B	36	3	(8)
Chronic Delta Hepatitis	22	1	(5)
Primary Biliary Cirrhosis	35	3	(9)
Sclerosing Cholangitis	7	0	(0)

(Courtesy of DiBisceglie AM, Alta H, Kao G, et al: *Hepatology* 10:581, 1989.)

who had anti-HCV detectable, 5 had had transfusions, 1 had used intravenous drugs and only 1 had no apparent source of infection. Six patients with autoimmune hepatitis were seropositive for anti-HCV; 1 had been transfused, 2 had medical occupations, whereas 3 others had no obvious source of infection. Thus the large majority of patients with chronic blood-borne NANB hepatitis have detectable anti-HCV in serum. A substantial proportion with autoimmune hepatitis also appears to have HCV infection, suggesting that the original diagnoses were incorrect. Most other patients with anti-HCV had histories of parenteral exposure to blood.—N.J. Greenberger, M.D.

Reference

1. Di Bisceglie AM, Alta H, Kao G, et al: Detection of antibody to hepatitis C virus in patients with various chronic liver diseases. *Hepatology* 10:581, 1989 (abstract).

Importance of Heterosexual Activity in the Transmission of Hepatitis B and Non-A, Non-B Hepatitis

Alter MJ, Coleman PJ, Alexander WJ, Kramer E, Miller JK, Mandel E, Hadler SC, Margolis HS (Ctrs for Disease Control, Atlanta; Jefferson County Dept of Health, Birmingham, Ala; Tacoma–Pierce County Health Dept, Tacoma, Wash)
JAMA 262:1201–1205, Sept 1, 1989

Non-A, non-B (NANB) hepatitis in the United States has been associated with parenteral exposures, primarily blood transfusions and intravenous drug use. Personal contact with persons who had hepatitis in the past and contact with infected persons within households have occasionally been identified as risk factors for NANB hepatitis. However, the role of person-to-person contact in disease transmission has not been well defined. Sexual activity has apparently not played an important role in the transmission of this type of hepatitis. An attempt was made to identify previously unrecognized sources of acute hepatitis B and NANB hepatitis.

Comparison of NANB Hepatitis Patients With Matched Controls by Selected Risk Factors Associated With Acquiring NANB Hepatitis

No. (%) Positive

Risk Factor	Non-A, Non-B Hepatitis Patients (n = 52)	Control Subjects (n = 104)	Crude Odds Ratio	P	Adjusted Odds Ratio	P
≤12 y of education	35 (67)	45 (43)	2.25	.01	2.91	<.01
Multiple sexual partners (>2)	6 (12)	1 (1)	12.00	.01	10.70	<.05
History of hepatitis in household/sexual contact*	6 (12)	1 (1)	6.00	.03	5.58	.06

*Includes household or sexual contact with a person who had an episode of hepatitis that occurred in the preceding 6 months or at some other time in the past.
(Courtesy of Alter MJ, Coleman PJ, Alexander WJ, et al: JAMA 262: 1201–1205, Sept 1, 1989.)

Patients with these types of hepatitis in 2 county health departments and matched controls were interviewed. Of 218 patients with hepatitis B and 140 patients with NANB hepatitis, no commonly recognized source was evident for 46% and 53%, respectively. Compared with matched controls, significantly more patients with hepatitis B had multiple heterosexual partners, accounting for 14% of all hepatitis B infections. More patients with NANB hepatitis had either sexual or household contact with a person who had hepatitis in the past or had multiple heterosexual partners, accounting for 11% of all NANB infections (table). Heterosexual transmission may play an important role in the spread of NANB hepatitis.

▶ Sexual transmission of hepatitis B virus (HBV), primarily between homosexual men, has been well documented. In recent years, heterosexual activity as a risk factor for acquiring HBV has been reported with increasing frequency. The study by Alter and colleagues is the first to suggest that heterosexual transmission may play an important role in the spread of NANB hepatitis.—N.J. Greenberger, M.D.

Treatment With Interferon

Treatment of Chronic Hepatitis C With Recombinant Interferon Alfa: A Multicenter Randomized, Controlled Trial

Davis GL, Balart LA, Schiff ER, Lindsay K, Bodenheimer HC Jr, Perrillo RP, Carey W, Jacobson IM, Payne J, Dienstag JL, VanThiel DH, Tamburro C, Lefkowitch J, Albrecht J, Meschievitz C, Ortego TJ, Gibas A, Hepatitis Interventional Therapy Group (Univ of Florida; Ochsner Clinic, New Orleans; Univ of Miami; Univ of California, Los Angeles; Brown Univ; et al)
N Engl J Med 321:1501–1506, Nov 30, 1989

Approximately 5% to 10% of patients who receive transfusions will be infected with hepatitis C (non-A, non-B hepatitis). In about half of these patients, chronic hepatitis C will develop. No effective treatment currently exists for chronic hepatitis C. The results of recombinant interferon-α in the treatment of this viral liver disease were evaluated in 166 adults who were randomly assigned to 1 of 3 groups. Of the 126 patients tested, 86% had antibody to the hepatitis C virus. Fifty-one patients received no treatment; 57 were treated 3 times a week with 1 million units of interferon per dose; and 58 were assigned to a 3-times-weekly dose of 3 million units of interferon. After completion of the 24-week treatment period, patients were followed at 4-week intervals.

A complete response (normal serum alanine aminotransferase levels) occurred in 38% of those given 3 million units, in 16% treated with 1 million units, and in 4% of untreated patients. Near-complete remissions in the 3 groups ranged from 4% to 12%, not a significant difference. In both treatment groups, maximal responses to interferon occurred within the first 12 weeks of therapy. The probability of response after 6 months of treatment was 46% for the larger dose of interferon, 28% for the smaller dose, and 8% with no treatment (Fig 43–2). The probability of relapse at 6 months was similar (about 50%) for the 2 treatment groups (Fig 43–3).

Liver biopsy specimens showed significant improvement with respect to the degree of lobular inflammation in patients in the higher-dose group. This histologic improvement was noted even in 13 of 25 patients who received 3 million units of interferon but showed no biochemical response. Side effects of interferon caused 16 patients (14%) temporarily to reduce their dosage. None of the 5 deaths in the follow-up period were attributed to therapy.

A 6-month course of recombinant interferon-α, 3 million units injected 3 times a week, was tolerated generally well and brought about both biochemical and histologic improvement in some patients with chronic hepatitis C. About

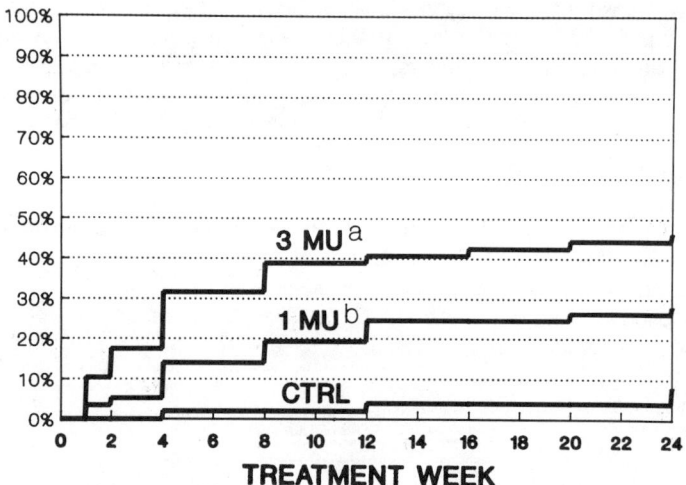

Fig 43–2.—Probability of complete or near-complete response during treatment with recombinant interferon-α in patients with chronic hepatitis C. [a]$3\ MU$, a dose of 3 million units of interferon thrice weekly; [b]$1\ MU$, a dose of 1 million units thrice weekly; $CTRL$, untreated. $P < .0001$ for the difference between the 3-million-unit group and the untreated group; $P < .05$ for the difference between the 2 treatment groups; and $P < .02$ for the difference between the 1-million-unit group and the untreated group. (Courtesy of Davis GL, Balart LA, Schiff ER, et al: *N Engl J Med* 321: 1501–1506, Nov 30, 1989.)

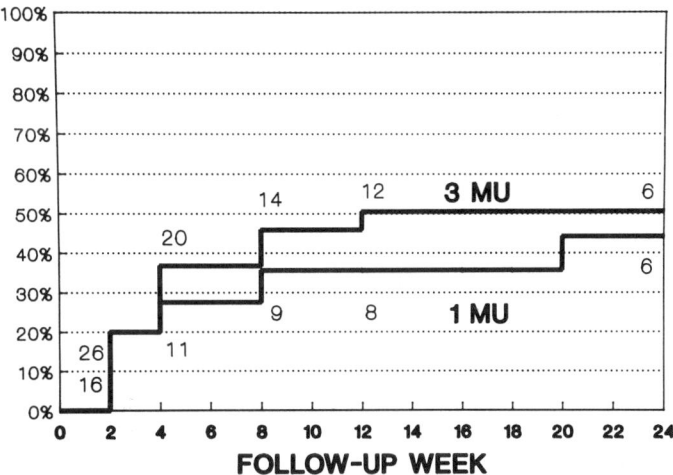

Fig 43-3.—Probability of relapse after discontinuation of treatment with recombinant interferon-α in patients with chronic hepatitis C. The numbers of patients studied at each time are shown for each group. The probability of relapse in each group was similar. *3 MU*, a dose of 3 million units of interferon thrice weekly; *1 MU*, a dose of 1 million units thrice weekly; *CTRL*, untreated. (Courtesy of Davis GL, Balart LA, Schiff ER, et al: *N Engl J Med* 321:1501–1506, Nov 30, 1989.)

half of these patients, however, had relapses; longer follow-up may reveal additional recurrences of disease activity.

▶ Di Bisceglie (1) and his colleagues also have studied the effects of recombinant human interferon-α in a prospective, randomized, double-blind, placebo-controlled trial in patients with well-documented chronic hepatitis C. Forty-one patients were enrolled in the trial, 37 of whom later were found to have antibody to hepatitis C virus. Twenty-one patients received interferon-α (2 million units) subcutaneously 3 times weekly for 6 months, and 20 received placebo. The mean serum aminotransferase levels and the histologic features of the liver improved significantly in the patients treated with interferon but not in the patients given placebo. Ten patients treated with interferon (48%) had a complete response, defined as a decline in mean serum aminotransferase levels to the normal range during therapy; 3 others had a decrease in mean aminotransferase levels of more than 50%. After treatment ended, however, serum aminotransferases usually returned to pretreatment levels; 6 to 12 months after the discontinuation of interferon therapy, only 2 patients (10%) still had normal values.

Di Bisceglie and colleagues conclude that interferon-α therapy is beneficial in reducing disease activity in chronic hepatitis C; however, the beneficial responses are often transient.—N.J. Greenberger, M.D.

Reference

1. Di Bisceglie AM, Martin P, Kassianides C, et al: Recombinant interferon alfa therapy for chronic hepatitis C: A randomized, double-blind, placebo-controlled trial. *N Engl J Med* 321:1506–1510, 1989.

Hepatitis C and Hepatocellular Carcinoma

Prevalence of Antibodies to Hepatitis C Virus in Italian Patients With Hepatocellular Carcinoma
Colombo M, Kuo G, Choo QL, Donato MF, Del Ninno E, Tommasini MA, Dioguardi N, Houghton M (Univ of Milan, Italy; Chiron Corp, Emeryville, Calif)
Lancet 2:1006–1008, Oct 28, 1989   43-6

The incidence of hepatocellular carcinoma is increasing in Italy, and factors other than hepatitis B virus and alcohol may be involved in its pathogenesis. A sensitive radioimmunoassay was used to detect antibodies to hepatitis C virus (HCV) in 132 patients with histologically proven hepatocellular carcinoma and 139 patients with non-A, non-B chronic hepatitis and cirrhosis.

Antibodies to HCV (anti-HCV) were detected in 86 (65%) patients with hepatocellular carcinoma and in 103 (74%) patients with chronic hepatitis (table). The prevalence of anti-HCV in patients with hepatocellular carcinoma had no relation to the presence or absence of hepatitis B surface antigen (HBsAg). The prevalence of anti-HCV was lower in HBsAg-negative patients with hepatocellular carcinoma than in patients with non-A, non-B chronic hepatitis (16% vs. 55%), and the prevalence of serum antibodies to hepatitis B core antigen (anti-HBc) was higher in the former (70% vs. 28%, respectively). Anti-HCV and anti-HBc occurred together nearly 3 times more often in HBsAg-negative patients with hepatocellular carcinoma as in patients with chronic hepatitis.

The data indicate that in Italy, HCV is an important factor in the pathogenesis of hepatocellular carcinoma and non-A, non-B chronic hepatitis.

▶ Similar results have been reported by Bruix and associates for Spanish patients with hepatocellular carcinoma and cirrhosis. The prevalence of antibodies against HCV was investigated in 96 patients with hepatocellular carcinoma, 106 patients with liver cirrhosis without evidence of cancer, and 177 controls without liver disease. Seventy-five percent of patients with hepatocellular carcinoma had HCV

Prevalence of Anti-HCV and Anti-HBc in Patients With Hepatocellular Carcinoma and Chronic Hepatitis

	No	Anti-HCV-positive *	Anti-HBc-positive *
Hepatocellular carcinoma			
HBsAg-positive	41	22 (54)	41 (100)
HBsAg-negative	91	64 (70)	64 (70)
Total	132	86 (65)	105 (80)
Chronic hepatitis			
Post-transfusion	19	16 (84)	2 (11)
History of transfusion	82	60 (73)	28 (34)
Community-acquired	38	27 (71)	9 (24)
Total	139	103 (74)	39 (28)

*Shown as number (%).
(Courtesy of Colombo M, Kuo G, Choo QL, et al: Lancet 2:1006–1008, Oct 28, 1989.)

antibodies (anti-HCV), a significantly higher proportion than that observed in patients with cirrhosis (55.6%) or controls (7.3%). The prevalence of anti-HCV was significantly higher in patients with alcoholic cirrhosis and hepatocellular carcinoma (76%) than in patients with alcoholic cirrhosis alone (38.7%), whereas in patients with cryptogenic cirrhosis there was no significant difference between those with and those without primary liver cell cancer (81.4% and 77.5%, respectively). Bruix and co-workers interpret these results to indicate that HCV infection may have a role in the pathogenesis of hepatocellular carcinoma, even in patients with chronic liver disease apparently related to other agents such as alcohol, and that this recently identified hepatitis virus may be found in a large proportion of patients with cryptogenic cirrhosis.—N.J. Greenberger, M.D.

Reference

1. Bruix J, Colvet X, Costa J, et al: Prevalence of antibodies to hepatitis C virus in Spanish patients with hepatocellular carcinoma and hepatic cirrhosis. *Lancet* 2:1004–1006, 1989.

44 Alcoholic Hepatitis

Methylprednisolone Therapy in Patients With Severe Alcoholic Hepatitis: A Randomized Multicenter Trial
Carithers RL Jr, Herlong HF, Diehl AM, Shaw EW, Combes B, Fallon HJ, Maddrey WC (Med College of Virginia, Richmond; Johns Hopkins Univ; Thomas Jefferson Univ; Southwestern Med Ctr, Dallas)
Ann Intern Med 110:685–690, May 1, 1989

Several studies have shown that a subgroup of patients with alcoholic hepatitis may benefit from corticosteroid therapy. A randomized, double-blind, placebo-controlled, multicenter trial was undertaken to determine the efficacy of corticosteroids in reducing the short-term mortality of patients with severe, life-threatening alcoholic hepatitis. The series included 66 patients with alcoholic hepatitis and either spontaneous hepatic encephalopathy or a discriminant function value greater than 32; the latter was calculated using the formula: 4.6 (prothrombin time − control time) + serum bilirubin (in micromoles per liter)/17.1. The patients were randomly assigned to receive either methylprednisolone, 32 mg, or placebo within 7 days of admission. Therapy was continued for 28 days, and the doses were tapered over 2 weeks and discontinued. The end point of the study was death.

The cumulative 28-day mortality was significantly higher in placebo recipients (11 of 31, 35%) than in those receiving methylprednisolone (2 of 35, 6%) (Fig 44–1). The 95% confidence interval for the difference in mortality was

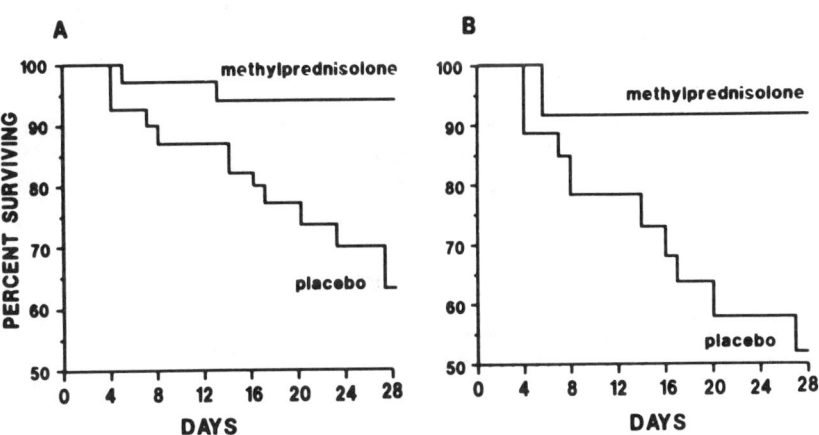

Fig 44–1.—**A,** cumulative survival in methylprednisolone and placebo recipients ($P = .0049$). **B,** cumulative survival in methylprednisolone and placebo recipients with hepatic encephalopathy at study entry ($P = .025$). (Courtesy of Carithers RL Jr, Herlong HF, Diel AM, et al: Ann Intern Med 110:685–690, May 1, 1989.)

12% to 70%. Similarly, in a subgroup of patients with spontaneous hepatic encephalopathy at entry, the cumulative 28-day mortality was significantly higher in placebo recipients, (9 of 19, 47%) than in patients who received methylprednisolone (1 of 14, 7%). The 95% confidence interval for the difference in mortality was 14% to 66%. After adjustment for other potentially important prognostic variables, the Cox proportional hazards regression model showed the advantage of methylprednisolone over placebo with regard to survival.

Methylprednisolone therapy increases short-term survival in patients with severe alcoholic hepatitis, as manifested by spontaneous hepatic encephalopathy or a markedly elevated discriminant function value.

▶ Alcoholic hepatitis (AH), a serious form of acute liver injury with a hospital mortality as high as 65%, has no widely accepted treatment. The efficacy of corticosteroids in treating AH remains controversial despite 11 randomized clinical trials; 4 report that corticosteroids significantly reduce mortality compared with placebo, whereas 7 report no difference. To determine whether corticosteroids affect short-term mortality from alcoholic hepatitis, Imperiale and McCullough (1) performed a meta-analysis of the 11 randomized clinical trials. Two independent critical appraisers evaluated and abstracted quantitative data from the trials. The appraisers assigned a quality score to each trial to assess compliance with selected methodologic standards for randomized clinical trials: clear inclusion and exclusion criteria, baseline equivalence of groups, and equal performance of therapies.

Interobserver agreement was excellent. Overall, the protective efficacy of corticosteroids was 37% and was greater in the higher quality score trials and in trials that excluded subjects with active gastrointestinal bleeding. Protective efficacy was less in the lower quality score trials and was absent in trials without the gastrointestinal bleeding exclusion. It is important that in patients with hepatic encephalopathy the protective efficacy was 55% overall; it was greater in the higher quality score trials and in trials with the gastrointestinal bleeding exclusion, but was not observed in the lower quality score trials or in the trials without the gastrointestinal bleeding exclusion. These results are in accord with the study by Carithers and colleagues and suggest (l) that corticosteroids reduce short-term mortality in patients with alcoholic hepatitis who have hepatic encephalopathy; (2) that this effect depends on a high-quality score and excluding patients with active gastrointestinal bleeding; and (3) that corticosteroids have a smaller and less consistent benefit among alcoholic hepatitis patients without hepatic encephalopathy.—N.J. Greenberger, M.D.

Reference

1. Imperiale TF, McCullough AJ: Corticosteroids reduce mortality from alcoholic hepatitis: A meta-analysis. *Hepatology* 10:580, 1989.

45 Cirrhosis and Related Problems

Ascites

Total Paracentesis Associated With Intravenous Albumin Management of Patients With Cirrhosis and Ascites
Titó L, Ginès P, Arroyo V, Planas R, Panés J, Rimola A, Llach J, Humbert P, Badalamenti S, Jiménez W, Rodés J (Hosp Clínic i Provincial of Barcelona, Spain; Germans Trias i Pujol of Badalona; Hosp Mútua of Terrassa, Catalunya, Spain)
Gastroenterology 98:146–151, January 1990   45–1

Repeated large-volume paracentesis plus intravenous injections of albumin is an effective approach to cirrhotic patients with ascites. To determine whether tense ascites can be safely mobilized in a single paracentesis session "total paracentesis" without adversely affecting systemic hemodynamics and renal function, 38 cirrhotic patients with tense ascites underwent total paracentesis and were given albumin intravenously, 6–8 g/L of ascites removed. Three fourths of the patients had had previous episodes of ascites.

Ascites were eliminated by paracentesis in all patients but 1; the mean volume of fluid removed was 10.7 L. During the first hospital admission 2 patients had hepatic encephalopathy, 2 had gastrointestinal bleeding, and 1 had culture-negative bacterial peritonitis. Renal impairment developed in no patient.

Twenty-three patients required a total of 43 readmissions during a mean follow-up of 32 weeks. More than half the readmissions were for new episodes of ascites.

Tense ascites in cirrhotic patients may be totally mobilized within 1–2 hours without adverse effect so long as albumin is given to expand the intravascular volume. Later administration of diuretics prevents reaccumulation of ascites in patients with responses. Tense ascites now can be treated effectively in a single hospital day.

▶ These results provide additional evidence indicating that total paracentesis associated with intravenous albumin can be performed safely in cirrhotic patients with tense ascites and suggest that these patients can receive treatment in a single-day hospitalization regimen.

Runyon and colleagues have assessed the effect of diuresis vs. therapeutic paracentesis on ascitic fluid opsonic activity and serum complement. This study was done because patients with adequate ascitic fluid opsonic activity have been reported to be protected from spontaneous bacterial peritonitis. In a randomized controlled trial, 19 patients with cirrhotic ascites had diuresis or daily therapeutic paracenteses during 20 hospitalizations. Serum and ascitic fluid complement concentrations and ascitic fluid opsonic activity were measured at the beginning and end of treatment. Although opsonic activity increased significantly in patients having diuresis, this parameter was stable in the paracentesis group. The stability of the ascitic fluid opsonic activity and complement concentration in the paracentesis group were maintained at the expense of a decrease in serum complement, whereas serum and ascitic fluid complement increased in the diuresis group. The authors conclude that diuresis may have the advantage over therapeutic paracentesis of providing better protection from spontaneous bacterial peritonitis. However, study of larger numbers of patients will be necessary to determine whether these changes in complement concentrations and opsonic activity translate into an increased risk of spontaneous bacterial peritonitis in vivo.—N.J. Greenberger, M.D.

Reference

1. Runyon BA, Antillon MR, Montano PA: Effect of diuresis vs. therapeutic paracentesis on ascitic fluid opsonic activity and serum complement. *Gastroenterology* 97:158–162, 1989.

Peritoneovenous Shunting as Compared With Medical Treatment in Patients With Alcoholic Cirrhosis and Massive Ascites
Stanley MM, Ochi S, Lee KK, Nemchausky BA, Greenlee HB, Allen JI, Allen MJ, Baum RA, Gadacz TR, Camara DS, Caruana JA, Schiff ER, Livingstone AS, Samanta AK, Najem AZ, Glick ME, Juler GL, Adham N, Baker JD, Cain GD, Jordan PH, Wolf DC, Fulenwider JT, James KE, VA Cooperative Study on Treatment of Alcoholic Cirrhosis With Ascites, (VA Hosp, Hines, Ill; VA Med Ctrs, Albany, NY; Allen Park, Mich; Atlanta; Baltimore; et al)
N Engl J Med 321:1632–1638, Dec 14, 1989   45–2

The best management for patients with alcoholic cirrhosis who have marked ascites remains uncertain. A total of 299 men with alcoholic cirrhosis and persistent or recurrent severe ascites seen in a 5.5-year period were randomized to receive either intensive medical treatment or the LeVeen peritoneovenous shunt. Patients with normal or only mildly abnormal liver function were placed in risk group 1, those with more marked dysfunction or previous complications were placed in group 2, and those with severe prerenal azotemia without kidney disease were placed in group 3.

Twenty-five patients assigned to medical management eventually received shunts. The median time to resolution of ascites was 5.5 weeks in patients treated medically and 3 weeks in surgical patients. The median time to recurrence of ascites was prolonged in the surgical group (Fig 45–1). The median duration of hospitalization was longer for medically treated patients. The risk of infection, gastrointestinal bleeding, or encephalopathy was comparable in the medical and surgical groups.

The LeVeen shunt provides greater relief of ascites in a shorter time than

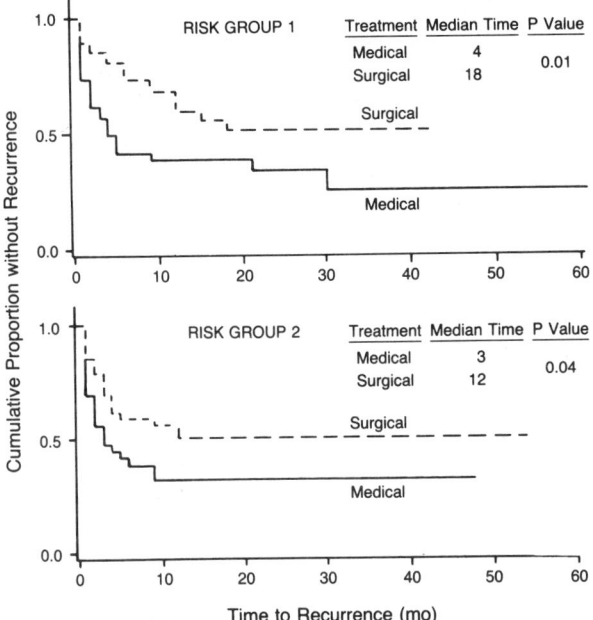

Fig 45–1.—Time to recurrence of grade 3+ or 4+ ascites after discharge from hospital. Surgical treatment significantly prolonged median time to recurrence in both groups. (Courtesy of Stanley MM, Ochi S, Lee KK, et al: *N Engl J Med* 321:1632–1638, Dec 14, 1989.)

does intensive medical care, and ascites recurs more rapidly in the latter patients. Overall mortality is similar with both approaches. Peritoneovenous shunting is indicated when ascites is not adequately managed medically.

▶ A large majority of patients with cirrhotic ascites respond well to diuretics as indicated by the data in this study. Of the 3,860 patients with ascites initially screened, 2,565 had grade 3+ or 4+ ascites and were eligible for this study. The standard medical treatment consisted of oral furosemide (40 mg/day), spironolactone (100 to 200 mg/day), and the restriction of sodium intake to 22 mmol/day. If a patient lost fewer than 0.45 to 1.8 kg (1 to 4 lb) a day (with peripheral edema) or 1.4 kg (3 lb) a week (without edema), the doses were increased to 80 mg of furosemide per day and 200 mg of spironolactone per day. Potassium intake was supplemented if serum levels of potassium fell below 3.6 mmol/L. If there was clinical evidence of fluid depletion or if the serum creatinine level increased to 130 μmol/Liter (1.5 mg/100 mL) or more, the administration of diuretic agents was decreased or stopped until these problems were corrected.

The patients who responded to standard medical treatment in the first 3 weeks with a reduction in the severity of ascites to grade 2+ or less and who had no complications were considered to have resolving ascites and when discharged were taking the smallest effective doses of diuretics that they could tolerate without ill effects. After discharge, they were followed up at 2- to 4-week intervals. The patients whose ascites remained at grade 3+ or 4+ after 3 weeks of standard medical treatment were said to have persistent ascites and were assigned randomly to treatment groups. Thus, of 2,565 initially eligible patients, only 299 (11.7%) were judged to have *resistant* ascites and were deemed candidates for this randomized trial of peritoneovenous shunting.—N.J. Greenberger, M.D.

Portal Hypertension, Bleeding Varices, Sclerotherapy, and Shunts

Effects of a Meal on Normal and Hypertensive Portal Venous System: A Quantitative Ultrasonographic Assessment

Goyal AK, Pokharna DS, Sharma SK (SMS Med College and Hosp, Jaipur, India)
Gastrointest Radiol 14:164–166, 1989   45–3

Many factors including food influence portal venous flow and, consequently, the dimensions of the portal vasculature. Real-time ultrasonography was performed in 72 healthy persons and 35 patients with portal hypertension. Studies were done in the fasted state with the subjects supine and again 45 minutes after a meal.

A significant increase in the diameter of the portal vein (PV), splenic vein (SV), and superior mesenteric vein (SMV) was seen in healthy persons after the meal (table). In contrast, no significant effect was noted in the hypertensive portal venous system.

A diminished meal-related caliber variation in the PV, SV, and SMV of less than 16%, 25%, and 20%, respectively, could be considered a sensitive ultrasound diagnostic index for patients with suspected portal hypertension.

▶ The investigators in this study convincingly show that ultrasonography can be used to distinguish between portal venous flow in healthy persons and that in patients with portal hypertension by observing failure of the PV, SMV, and SV to dilate after a meal. This observation emphasizes the normal physiology of portal vein dilatation after eating with a 65% increase in diameter. Although this is a potentially useful diagnostic test, in patients with portal hypertension the portal vein diameters appear large enough by themselves to make the diagnosis of portal hypertension without meal stimulation.—P.B. Miner, Jr., M.D.

Mean and Range of Postprandial Caliber Variation as Percentage of Fasting Value in Normal Subjects (N) and Patients With Portal Hypertension (P)

Vessels	Subjects	Mean (%)	Range (%)
PV	N	27.9	16.7–60.0
	P	1.4	0.0– 7.7
SV	N	46.5	25.0–83.3
	P	2.3	0.0–11.8
SMV	N	45.2	20.0–75.0
	P	3.1	0.0–15.4

(Courtesy of Goyal AK, Pokharna DS, Sharma SK: *Gastrointest Radiol* 14:164–166, 1989.)

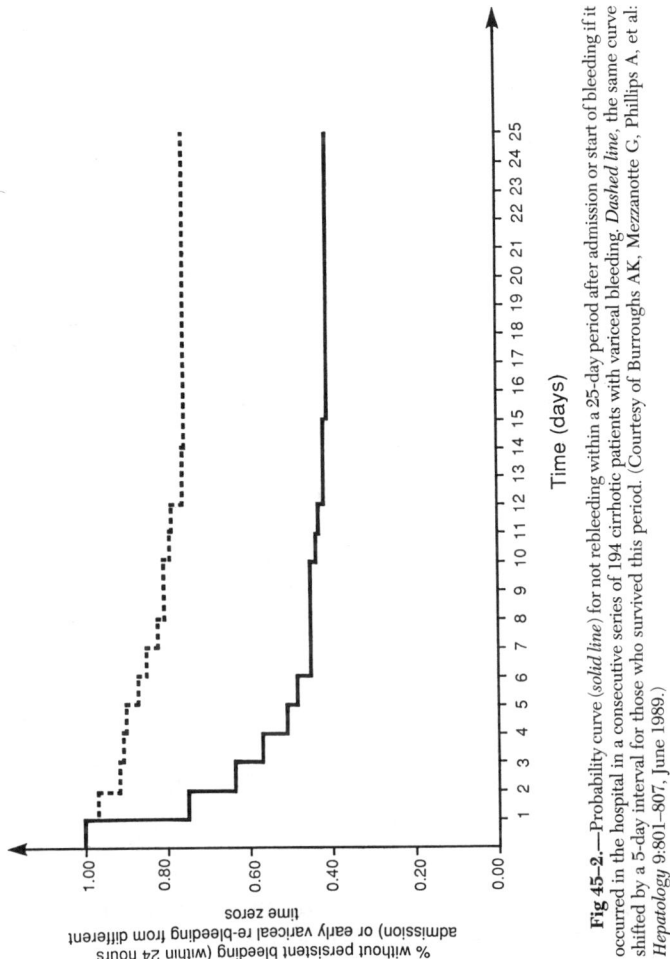

Fig 45-2.—Probability curve (*solid line*) for not rebleeding within a 25-day period after admission or start of bleeding if it occurred in the hospital in a consecutive series of 194 cirrhotic patients with variceal bleeding. *Dashed line*, the same curve shifted by a 5-day interval for those who survived this period. (Courtesy of Burroughs AK, Mezzanotte G, Phillips A, et al: *Hepatology* 9:801–807, June 1989.)

Cirrhotics With Variceal Hemorrhage: The Importance of the Time Interval Between Admission and the Start of Analysis for Survival and Rebleeding Rates

Burroughs AK, Mezzanotte G, Phillips A, McCormick PA, McIntyre N (Royal Free Hosp and School of Medicine, London)
Hepatology 9:801–807, June 1989

45–4

Reported early mortalities after emergency treatment for variceal bleeding vary widely. These differences have been attributed to differences in the severity of liver disease and hemorrhage at hospital admission. However, multivariate analysis indicates that most of the wide variation in mortality data remains after adjustment for these factors. Controversy exists regarding whether the time interval between hospital admission and the point used for the start of survival analysis is a major confounding variable. The importance of the time of entry into a trial after hospital admission for variceal bleeding was assessed as a confounding variable for analysis of survival data.

During a 40-month period, 194 cirrhotic patients were admitted to the hospital with bleeding varices. Three percent of the patients died within 2 days, 15% died within 2 weeks, 24% died within 30 days, and 27% died within 6 weeks of time zero.

Shifting the starting point for analysis of survival from time zero to 2 weeks after hospital admission and for analysis of rebleeding from time zero to 5 days after hospital admission yielded significant differences in both survival and rebleeding rates (Fig 45-2). Shifting the starting point affected rebleeding rates more than it affected survival rates. Any future clinical trials of variceal hemorrhage need to recognize that the interval between bleeding onset and point of entry into a trial is a confounding factor. Therefore, the time of entry point always should be standardized.

▶ The results of this study reinforce the message given by Graham and Smith (1,2) that variable time of entry into a study after admission for variceal bleeding is an important confounding variable when analyzing survival data. It is important that Burroughs and associates have shown that it also affects analysis of rebleeding statistics to a greater extent than those of survival.—N.J. Greenberger, M.D.

References

1. Graham DY, Smith JL: The cause of patients after variceal hemorrhage. *Gastroenterology* 80:800–809, 1981.
2. Smith JL, Graham DY: Variceal hemorrhage: A critical evaluation of survival analysis. *Gastroenterology* 82:968–973, 1982.

Schistosomal Versus Nonschistosomal Variceal Bleeders: Do They Respond Differently to Selective Shunt (DSRS)?
Ezzat FA, Abu-Elmagd KM, Sultan AA, Aly MA, Fathy OM, Bahgat OO, El-Fiky AM, El-Barbary MH, Mashhoor N (Mansoura Univ, Mansoura, Egypt)
Ann Surg 209:489–500, April 1989   45–5

The goal of a review of 125 patients with variceal bleeding who underwent distal splenorenal shunt was to compare the long-term effects of the procedure in patients with schistosomal, cirrhotic, and mixed forms of portal hypertension. The mean follow-up was 79 months. Forty-five patients had schistosomal hepatic fibrosis, 17 had nonalcoholic cirrhosis, and 23 had mixed patterns of disease.

Hospital mortality was 5%, and the current survival rate is 74%. Half the deaths were caused by liver-cell failure. Patients with schistosomal disease had a cumulative survival of 92%, compared with 76% for patients with cirrhosis and 65% for the group with mixed disease. Shunt occlusion was documented in 7 patients, and the same number had recurrent variceal bleeding. Ascites was much less frequent in schistosomal cases than in the other groups. Clinical encephalopathy developed in 15% of the patients, again much less often in those with schistosomal disease.

Distal splenorenal shunt is effective in variceal bleeding caused by schistosomal and other disease. Patients with schistosomal disease have a better survival rate than those with bleeding from other causes. The initial results of prospective comparative trials suggest that initial sclerotherapy and later selective shunting, if needed, is a good therapeutic approach for patients with cirrhosis. Selective shunting is the best initial management for patients with schistosomal hepatic fibrosis, in whom recurrent variceal bleeding is the leading cause of death.

▶ The distal splenorenal shunt as designed by Warren and his colleagues appears ideally suited for treating bleeding esophageal varices from portal hypertension secondary to hepatic fibrosis in such patients. As has been observed by others, the rate of encephalopathy is less than that among alcohol cirrhotic patients. A hospital mortality of 5% is commendable and serves as a testimony to the skills of the surgical team in the Mansoura University School of Medicine in Egypt.—F.G. Moody, M.D.

A Comparison of Sclerotherapy With Staple Transection of the Esophagus for the Emergency Control of Bleeding From Esophageal Varices
Burroughs AK, Hamilton G, Phillips A, Mezzanotte G, McIntyre N, Hobbs KEF (Royal Free Hosp and School of Med, London; Univ of Milan)
N Engl J Med 321:857–862, Sept 28, 1989   45–6

Emergency sclerotherapy in the treatment of acute esophageal variceal bleeding, with or without earlier balloon tamponade, is more effective than balloon tamponade alone. Sclerotherapy is now the treatment of choice in many centers, with operation a second-line treatment. Emergency esophageal transection with a staple gun effectively controls esophageal variceal bleeding and has an associated mortality similar to that of emergency sclerotherapy. Endoscopic sclerotherapy was compared with staple transection of the esophagus in the emergency treatment of esophageal variceal bleeding.

Of 101 patients with cirrhosis of the liver and bleeding esophageal varices, 50 were randomly assigned to emergency sclerotherapy and 51 to staple transection of the esophagus. Four patients assigned to sclerotherapy and 12 assigned to staple transection did not actually undergo those procedures, but all statistical analyses were made on an intention-to-treat basis.

Sclerotherapy controlled the variceal bleeding in 41 patients (82%) and failed in 9 (table). Transection controlled the bleeding in 49 patients (96%) and failed in 2. Twenty-two sclerotherapy patients (44%) and 18 transection patients (35%) died within 6 weeks of treatment. The difference was not statistically significant. However, blood and plasma requirements during the procedures and the first 5 days thereafter were substantially lower in the transection group, as was the incidence of rebleeding: a 5-day interval without bleeding was achieved in 88% of the patients assigned to staple transection,

Efficacy of Emergency Sclerotherapy vs. Staple Transection

Measure	Sclerotherapy Group (N = 50)*	Transection Group (N = 51)†
	number of patients	
Bleeding controlled after		
One session	31 (62%)‡	45 (88%)§
Two sessions	39 (78%)	49 (96%); ‖
Three sessions	41 (82%)	0
Failed procedures	9	2
Cause of rebleeding		
Esophageal varices	5	0
Esophageal ulcer	1	0
Gastric varices	2	0
Peptic ulcer	1	1
Gastrostomy site	0	1
Further procedures	7	0
Blood and plasma units used during procedures and for next five days	380	291
Death within six weeks	22 (44%)	18 (35%)
Discharged from hospital	28 (56%)	31 (61%)
Hospital stay (days) — median (range)	15 (1–48)	19 (1–96)

*Includes 2 patients who did not receive treatment because of rapidly fatal complications (intracerebral bleeding and cardiac arrest).
†Includes 3 patients who did not receive treatment because of rapidly fatal complications (septicemia with renal and cardiopulmonary failure).
‡Includes both patients who had transection as the primary procedure.
§Includes 5 of the 9 patients who received sclerotherapy as the primary procedure. $P < .01$ for the comparison with the sclerotherapy group.
‖Includes 4 of the 9 patients who received sclerotherapy as the primary procedure and required 2 sessions to achieve hemostasis. $P < .05$ for the comparison with the sclerotherapy group.
(Courtesy of Burroughs AK, Hamilton G, Phillips A, et al: N Engl J Med 321:857–862, Sept 28, 1989.)

whereas only 62% of the patients assigned to sclerotherapy stopped bleeding after a single injection.

Staple transection of the esophagus as an emergency treatment for variceal bleeding in patients with cirrhosis of the liver is as safe as sclerotherapy and more effective than a single sclerotherapy procedure.

▶ For a comprehensive review of controversies in the management of bleeding esophageal varices see the article by Terblanche, Burroughs, and Hobbs (1). Their summary recommendation for emergency management of variceal bleeding is cited below.

"Although controversial, pharmacologic therapy aimed at controlling acute variceal bleeding is widely used. A combination of intravenous vasopressin and nitroglycerin to lower portal pressure is currently recommended. Emergency endoscopy is mandatory to confirm that the patient is bleeding from varices. Once variceal bleeding is confirmed, the patient should immediately undergo sclerotherapy, if expert treatment is available, or have the bleeding controlled by balloon-tube tamponade or by pharmacologic means, with subsequent performance of sclerotherapy with use of a flexible endoscope within 6 to 24 hours. If the bleeding has stopped, sclerotherapy can be performed immediately, or the patient can be observed while the appropriate long-term management is planned. Patients who do not respond to immediate or delayed emergency sclerotherapy should be identified early, and their suitability for either a shunt insertion or a staple-gun transection should be assessed. Although sclerotherapy is currently the favored emergency treatment, esophageal transection with a staple-gun and portacaval shunting require further evaluation to determine whether they may be preferable therapeutic options in some patients."—N.J. Greenberger, M.D.

Reference

1. Terblanche J, Burroughs AK, Hobbs KEF: Controversies in the management of bleeding esophageal varices. N Engl J Med 320:1393–1398, 1469–1475, 1989.

Role of Endoscopic Variceal Sclerotherapy in the Long-Term Management of Variceal Bleeding: A Meta-Analysis
Infante-Rivard C, Esnaola S, Villeneuve J-P, (McGill Univ; Hôpital Saint-Luc, Montreal; Université de Montréal)
Gastroenterology 96:1087–1092, April 1989   45–7

A literature survey of randomized clinical trials was undertaken to evaluate the effect of repeated endoscopic variceal sclerotherapy on the long-term survival of patients with variceal hemorrhage. Findings from 7 clinical trials were combined using meta-analysis to draw an overall effect of serial sclerotherapy on long-term survival. In general, sclerotherapy was initiated soon after the bleeding episode in conjunction with some form of conventional medical treatment. Serial sclerotherapy was then performed at increasing intervals of 1–6 weeks. The results were compared with those of conventional medical treatment alone.

Repeated endoscopic variceal sclerotherapy was significantly associated with better survival than conventional medical treatment alone (Table 1). An

TABLE 1.—Total Mortality in Trials of Serial Endoscopic Variceal Sclerotherapy

Trial	Follow-up (mo)	Withdrawals (total/randomized)	Dead/total (%) Experimental	Dead/total (%) Control	Two-tailed p value
Barsoum	12–48	0/100	15/50 (30)	26/50 (52)	0.03
Terblanche	12–60	0/75	23/37 (62)	28/38 (63)	0.94
Copenhagen	9–52	0/187 *	60/93 (65)	74/94 (79)	0.03
Paquet	36†	4/43	7/21 (33)	17/22 (77)	0.01
Korula	13.6 †	26/120	21/63 (33)	19/57 (33)	1.00
Westaby	19–68	26/116	18/56 (32)	32/60 (53)	0.02
Soderlund	22†	0/117	32/57 (56)	35/50 (70)	0.14
Total		55/748	176/377 (47)	227/371 (61)	<0.0005 ‡

Note: Values in parentheses are 95% confidence limits.
*This total excludes 29 patients withdrawn because of violations of eligibilty criteria.
†Median or mean follow-up.
‡Mantel-Haenszel χ^2 = 16.81; test of homogeneity; Q_w = 10.14 (P = .12).
(Courtesy of Infante-Rivard C, Esnaola S, Villeneuve J-P: Gastroenterology 96:1087–1092, April 1989.)

TABLE 2.—Complications Associated With Endoscopic Variceal Sclerotherapy

	Observed/patients at risk* (%)
Esophageal stricture	27/229 (11.8)
Esophageal perforation	14/327 (4.3)
Bleeding due to ulceration	17/134 (12.7)
Pneumonia—aspiration pneumonitis	14/206 (6.8)

*Including trials explicitly reporting the observed frequencies.
(Courtesy of Infante-Rivard C, Esnaola S, Villeneuve J-P: *Gastroenterology* 96, 1087–1092, April 1989.)

overall risk difference of –0.15 (95% confidence limits, –0.21 to –0.08) was estimated, indicating that sclerotherapy reduced the number of deaths by 25%. The estimated risk difference remained significantly in favor of sclerotherapy even when all patients in the sclerotherapy group with unknown survival status were assumed dead. Complications associated with endoscopic variceal sclerotherapy included esophageal strictures, esophageal perforation, bleeding caused by ulceration, and aspiration pneumonia (Table 2).

Serial sclerotherapy should be included in the long-term management of patients with bleeding varices. Although the estimated reduction in mortality from sclerotherapy is only moderate, its clinical relevance is major, considering the high mortality associated with bleeding varices.

The results of this quantitative synthesis suggest that patients with bleeding esophageal varices benefit from inclusion of repeated sclerotherapy as part of their long-term management.

▶ All of the randomized controlled trials of long-term sclerotherapy, except one, have used emergency sclerosis in the sclerotherapy group but not in the control group, thus evaluating both acute and chronic injection versus none. Because acute injection reduces early rebleeding and mortality compared with conventional therapy, the beneficial effect of chronic injection in the trials may be overestimated. Accordingly, Burroughs and co-workers (1) randomized 204 cirrhotic patients with bleeding esophageal varices, entered into their study during a 62-month period, to weekly sclerotherapy (no. = 103) or no injection (no. = 103); the latter were given sucralfate, 1 g, 4 times daily. A standard protocol was used to treat all bleeds, and randomization took place after a 5-day bleed-free interval from admission stratified by the initial treatment used. Trial groups were matched for age, sex, etiology of cirrhosis, previous bleeding, treatment variables at index bleed, and Pugh's grades A, B, C, which were comparable in both groups. Separate episodes of rebleeding were defined by a bleed-free interval of 5 days, and were analyzed regardless of severity or source.

Deaths occurred in 55 sucralfate patients (53%) and 48 sclerotherapy patients (47%). Esophageal and gastric variceal rebleeding occurred in 59% of the sucralfate patients and in 55% of sclerotherapy patients. Total number of variceal rebleeds (unknown sources were considered variceal) were 183 among the sucralfate group and 130 among the sclerotherapy group. However, a rebleeding index, evaluating all sources and taking into account intervals without rebleeding, was not significantly different. In each trial group, 3% had transplants, 7% had shunts, and 1% had devascularization. Burroughs and associates conclude that long-term sclerotherapy does not significantly benefit patients when emergency treatment for bleeding is kept constant. In this study, the reduction in variceal bleeding episodes was marginal: 50 episodes for 100 patients treated over 5 years.—N.J. Greenberger, M.D.

Reference

1. Burroughs AK, McCormick PA, Sirings S, et al: Prospective randomized trial of long-term sclerotherapy for variceal rebleeding using the same protocol to treat rebleeding in all patients: Final report. *Hepatology* 10:579, 1989.

Distal Splenorenal Versus Lienorenal Shunt for Acute Variceal Haemorrhage: Is the Selective Shunt an Advance?
Lodge JPA, Mavor AID, Giles GR (St James's Univ Hosp, Leeds, England)
J R Coll Surg Edinb 34:59–62, April 1989

Data for 81 patients operated on between 1971 and 1986 for variceal bleeding were reviewed. Twenty-eight patients had lienorenal shunts, and 53 had distal splenorenal shunt (DSRS; Warren shunt) procedures. Twenty-seven percent of patients had Child's grade A disease, 49% had grade B disease, and 24% had grade C disease.

The rate of rebleeding within a month of surgery was 27%. Mortality was comparable between the 2 surgical groups. Only 32% of Child's class C patients were discharged from the hospital. Variceal bleeding occurred outside the immediate postoperative period in 7 patients. Twenty percent of long-term survivors had portasystemic encephalopathy; 8 of these 13 patients had had the DSRS operation.

Thirty-eight of 63 long-term survivors remained alive at last follow-up. Survivors of the lienorenal shunt operation had 3- and 5-year actuarial survival rates of 82% and 66%, respectively. The respective rates for patients who survived the DSRS operation were 64% and 43%.

The lienorenal shunt and DSRS operations are equally effective in controlling variceal bleeding in the short term. Surgery should be done when there is any indication that conservative management is failing. Long-term survival and subsequent morbidity probably are comparable after these operations.

▶ Not much is written these days about the effectiveness of portasystemic shunts in the treatment of bleeding esophageal varices. According to this report, the distal splenorenal shunt and the standard splenorenal shunt have about the same morbidity and effectiveness. In fact, the 5-year survival rates for the distal splenorenal shunt were somewhat less than for the lienorenal shunt, but the encephalopathy rate was the same (about 15%).—F.G. Moody, M.D.

Improved Results With Selective Distal Splenorenal Shunt in a Highly Selected Patient Population: A Prospective Study

Paquet K-J, Mercado MA, Koussouris P, Kalk J-F, Siemens F, Cuan-Orozco F (Heinz-Kalk Hosp, Bad Kissingen, West Germany)
Ann Surg 210:184–189, August 1989

The selective distal splenorenal shunt is the preferred treatment for many patients with variceal bleeding from portal hypertension. Acute bleeding is managed with endoscopic sclerotherapy. Among 299 patients with bleeding varices seen in a 5-year period, 121 patients with Child-Pugh class A or B conditions were considered for shunts. Thirty-two of them had a liver volume of 1,000–2,500 mL determined by ultrasound, portal perfusion exceeding 30%, and no progression or activity of liver disease proved by biopsy. In addition, stenosis of the hepatic arteries was excluded and the anatomy was suitable for a Warren shunt.

A shunt was technically not possible in 7 instances. There were 2 postoperative deaths (8%). No patient had encephalopathy, and none had recurrent variceal bleeding. Splenic angiography done 2 weeks and 6 months after surgery showed that all shunts were patent and ruled out portal vein thrombosis. Survival was 88% at 1 year and 75% at 5 years.

The Warren shunt is the preferred approach to hemorrhagic portal hypertension. The results can be improved through careful patient selection, although the number of candidates is lowered. Preoperative sclerotherapy enhances the outcome of the selective distal splenorenal shunt procedure.

▶ Paquet and his associates in Bad Kissingen, West Germany, describe their experience with the distal splenorenal (Warren) shunt. Their report reveals what can be accomplished with this operation in carefully selected patients. A mortality of 8%, a demonstrated shunt patency of 100%, and a survival of 75% at 5 years is commendable. Preoperative sclerotherapy was a helpful adjunct.—F.G. Moody, M.D.

Portal Systemic Encephalopathy

Effects of the Benzodiazepine Receptor Antagonist Flumazenil in Hepatic Encephalopathy in Humans

Bansky G, Meier PJ, Riederer E, Walser H, Ziegler WH, Schmid M (Univ Hosp; City Hosp Waid, Zurich)
Gastroenterology 97:744–750, September 1989

Increased γ-aminobutyric acid (GABA)-mediated inhibitory neurotransmission may contribute to the manifestations of hepatic encephalopathy. Therefore, it may be possible to induce ameliorations of this syndrome by pharmacologically antagonizing a component of the GABA/benzodiazepine receptor complex.

The benzodiazepine receptor antagonist flumazenil was given intravenously to 14 patients with hepatic encephalopathy complicating cirrhosis. Flumazenil administration induced variable, transient, yet distinct improvements in the mental status of 71% of the patients. In 4 patients the degree of encephalopathy improved from stage IV to stage II, and in 2 patients it improved from stage IV to stage III. The mental status of patients with less advanced encephalopathy also improved, although less dramatically. The arousal effect was noted within minutes after the injection and persisted for 1–2 hours. It was associated with a significant increase in the mean electroencephalographic frequency. Of the 8 patients ultimately discharged from the hospital, 7 responded to flumazenil. None of those who died within 48 hours of flumazenil injection showed any arousal effect (table).

Flumazenil induced transient but distinct arousal effects of variable magnitude in 10 of 14 patients with stage II–IV hepatic encephalopathy caused by chronic liver disease. A positive response to flumazenil might be of prognostic value in predicting short-term survival in these patients.

▶ The effect of benzodiazepine receptor antagonists in hepatic encephalopathy remains controversial. This controversy is underscored by the above study as well as the following comments, which describe 2 studies, 1 positive and 1 negative.

Grimm and co-workers (1) studied the effects of the benzodiazepine antagonist flumazenil in 20 episodes of hepatic encephalopathy (HE) in 17 patients with acute (no. = 9) or chronic (no. = 8) liver failure who had not responded to conventional therapy. Patients with histories of benzodiazepine intake were excluded. Changes in HE stage, in Glasgow coma scale, and in somatosensory-evoked potentials were measured. In 12 of 20 episodes, HE stage improved. The response to treatment occurred rapidly, within 3–60 minutes. In 8 of these 12 episodes HE worsened 0.5–4 hours after treatment. In 5 of the 8 episodes that did not respond to flumazenil, patients had clinical evidence of brain edema. Grimm and co-workers conclude that flumazenil may be valuable in the treatment of HE in acute and chronic liver failure.

Van der Rijt (2) performed a double-blind crossover study on the effect of flumazenil in 8 patients with HE unresponsive to conventional therapy for at least 24 hours. Other nonhepatic causes of encephalopathy could not be detected before entrance into the study, and screening for benzodiazepines in the plasma was negative. The immediate effect of a single injection (1.0 mg) of flumazenil and that during a 3-day infusion regimen (0.25 mg/hr) were assessed by clinical grading of HE, electroencephalographic (EEG) grading, and spectral analysis, measuring the mean dominant frequency (MDF) of the EEG. Fifteen minutes after injection the clinical grade of HE was decreased in 3 patients given flumazenil and increased in 2 patients given placebo. However, the EEG grade did not change in any of the patients, and the changes in MDF did not differ between flumazenil and placebo. Furthermore, clinical and EEG grades of HE did not differ between the 3-day infusion periods of flumazenil and the placebo.

Nine patients excluded from the controlled trial were studied for the immediate effect of 1.0 mg of flumazenil in an open study. Both the clinical and the EEG grade of HE decreased in 2 patients. The responders had used benzodiazepines previously. Van der Rijt and associates could not demonstrate a major effect of flumazenil in HE unresponsive to standard therapy. Flumazenil may be worthwhile in treating HE precipitated by benzodiazepines.

These 3 studies are all consistent with the view that flumazenil treatment can result in transient improvement in HE. However, the patients studied were not

Effects of Flumazenil in Cirrhotic Patients With Hepatic Encephalopathy

Patient no.	Age (yr)	Sex	Etiology of cirrhosis*	Dose of flumazenil MED	Dose of flumazenil Total	Stage of encephalopathy Before flumazenil	Stage of encephalopathy After flumazenil	Remarks and outcome†
1	38	M	Alcoholic (A) HB$_s$+ve	0.4	0.4	II	II (I)	Hepatorenal syndrome with anuria. Died of refractory hypotension and shock (after 7 days).
2	44	M	Alcoholic (V)	0.4	4.5	III	II	Splenorenal shunt. Discharge.
3	51	M	Alcoholic (SM)	0.8	1.6	III	II	Died of miliary tuberculosis in uremia (after 8 days).
4	67	F	Alcoholic (A)	0.4	9.6	III	II	Flumazenil effect only seen after infusion of 10% mannitol. Discharge.
5	58	F	Alcoholic (A, V)	0.2	0.2	IV	II	Discharge.
6	51	F	Alcoholic (A, V)	0.4	1.6	IV	II	Discharge.
7	49	F	Unknown (V)	0.4	0.4	IV	II	Accidental injection of midazolam (1 mg) 4 days before the flumazenil trial. Discharge.
8	43	F	Alcoholic (V)	0.4	0.4	IV	II	Chlordiazepoxide in serum: 0.3 μg/ml. Discharge.
9	37	F	Alcoholic (A)	0.2	2.9	IV	III	Klebsiella pneumoniae sepsis. Discharge.
10	75	M	Alcoholic (V)	0.4	8.2	IV	III	Died in hepatic coma (after 13 days).
11	51	M	Alcoholic (V)	0.4	4.0	IV	IV	Died in hepatic coma (after 1 day).
12	67	M	CAH (V) HB$_s$+ve	0.4	4.0	IV	IV	Administration of oxazepam (15 mg) and chlordiazepoxide (50 mg) 4 and 2 days before the

							flumazenil trial, respectively. Discharge.
13	52	F	Alcoholic (V)	0.4	3.6	IV	Died in hepatic coma with refractory hypotension and renal failure (after 1 day).
14	66	M	CAH (A, V) HB$_s$+ve	0.4	1.6	IV	Died of advanced hepatocellular carcinoma (after 2 days). No brain metastasis.

Abbreviations: CAH, chronic active hepatitis; *HB$_s$+ve*, hepatitis B surface positive; *MED*, minimal effective dose.
*Portal hypertension was suspected from the presence of splenomegaly (*SM*), ascites (*A*), and/or esophageal varices (*V*).
†In patients with fatal outcome, the time of death is indicated in parentheses (days after flumazenil testing).
(Courtesy of Bansky G, Meir PJ, Reiderer E, et al: *Gastroenterology* 97:744–750, September 1989.)

comparable. In future studies, a distinction should be made between patients with acute HE and those with chronic portal systemic encephalopathy.—N.J. Greenberger, M.D.

References

1. Grimm G, Katzenschlager R, Schneeweiss B, et al: Improvement of hepatic encephalopathy treated with flumazenil. *Lancet* 2:1392–1394, 1988.
2. Van der Rijt CCD, Schalm SW, Mecilstee J, et al: Flumazenil therapy for hepatic encephalopathy: A double-blind cross-over study. *Hepatology* 10:590, 1989 (abstract).

46 Drug-Associated Hepatic Injury

Amiodarone Hepatotoxicity: Prevalence and Clinicopathologic Correlations Among 104 Patients
Lewis JH, Ranard RC, Caruso A, Jackson LK, Mullick F, Ishak KG, Seeff LB, Zimmerman HJ (Georgetown Univ; Armed Forces Inst of Pathology; VA Med Ctr, Washington, DC)
Hepatology 9:679–685, May 1989

Amiodarone, an iodine-containing benzofuran derivative structurally related to thyroxine, is effective in the treatment of refractory supraventricular and ventricular tachyarrhythmias. However, its use has been tempered by reports of significant adverse effects, forcing discontinuation in up to 26% of patients. The most commonly reported serious effect is pulmonary toxicity, but hepatic injury has also been described. Experience with amiodarone-associated liver disease was evaluated.

The prevalence of apparent amiodarone-related hepatic injury in 104 patients was compared with that reported in the literature. An asymptomatic increase of serum aminotransferase levels was found in about 25% of the patients, comparable to that in previous reports. The frequency of extrahepatic organ toxicity was higher in patients with increased serum levels of aminotransferases. Symptomatic hepatitis developed in 3% of these patients, compared with less than 1% of reported patients (table).

Hepatic phospholipidosis and the development of pseudoalcoholic liver injury is probably a result of the biochemical effects of the drug and possible metabolic idiosyncrasy, respectively. Serial blood enzyme measurements might offer some protection against more serious liver injury. However, amiodarone levels may persist in various tissues for weeks to months after withdrawal. Stopping the drug does not guarantee timely reversal of organ toxicity. Therefore, the risks and benefits of amiodarone must be carefully weighed before the drug is continued, as the risk of sudden cardiac death may outweigh the hazards of ongoing hepatic, pulmonary, or other toxicity.

▶ As the authors point out in their discussion, asymptomatic minor elevations in aminotransferase values have preceded symptomatic hepatotoxicity with cirrhosis by as long as 18 months. These minor elevations may be a precursor of more severe liver damage, may remain unchanged, or may even resolve despite continued therapy. The manufacturer recommends (1) monitoring hepatic enzymes on a regular basis for patients receiving more than 400 mg/day as a maintenance dose, and (2) reducing or stopping the drug in patients whose aminotransferase levels rise

Comparison of Patients With and Without Elevated Hepatic Enzymes Among 104 Patients on Oral Amiodarone Longer Than 2 Weeks

	Patients with elevated hepatic enzymes *	Patients without elevated hepatic enzymes
Number	25	79
Mean age	62	64
(Range)	(41–79)	(26–82)
Sex (M:F)	20:5	55:24
Mean dose (mg)	400	339
(Range)	(200–800)	(100–800)
Mean cumulative dose (gm)	104 †	155
(Range)	(17–470)	(10–412)
Duration (mo)	10.4 †	18
(Range)	(1–28)	
Mean peak AST (IU/liter)	89	
(Range)	(44–230)	
(Normal = 10–42)		
Mean peak ALT (IU/liter)	104	
(Range)	(56–337)	
(Normal = 10–40)		
Mean peak alkaline phosphatase (IU/liter)	117	
(Range)	(36–337)	
(Normal = 76–100)		
Mean peak total bilirubin (mg/dl)	0.8	
(Range)	(0.1–4.4)	
(Normal = 0.2–1.5)		
Significant extrahepatic organ toxicity	19 (76%)	29 (37%) ‡

*Elevated alanine aminotransferase (ALT), aspartate aminotransferase (AST), or alkaline phosphatase in excess of twice baseline or in excess of the upper limit of normal.
†From onset of therapy until elevated hepatic enzymes were recognized.
‡$P < .001$.
(Courtesy of Lewis JH, Ranard RC, Caruso A, et al: *Hepatology* 9:679–685, May 1989.)

to more than 3 times the upper limit of normal or in a patient with an elevated baseline level with risk more than twofold. These guidelines seem reasonable, but Lewis and colleagues recommend that if aminotransferase level remains elevated, a liver biopsy should be considered to help characterize the type and degree of hepatic injury.—N.J. Greenberger, M.D.

47 Liver Neoplasms

Primary Liver Cancer

Primary Hepatic Malignancy: Surgical Management and Determinants of Survival
Nagorney DM, van Heerden JA, Ilstrup DM, Adson MA (Mayo Clinic and Mayo Found, Rochester, Minn)
Surgery 106:740–749, October 1989

Data were reviewed on 110 patients who had surgical treatment for primary hepatic malignancy between January 1975 and June 1986. Twenty-six patients had chronic liver disease with cirrhosis, and 13 had histories of hepatitis.

Half the patients had multicentric malignancies; these were especially prevalent in patients with cirrhosis. Fifteen patients had extrahepatic invasion, and 11 had gross intraluminal tumor in the portal and hepatic veins. Hepatocarcinoma was diagnosed in 72% of cases.

Curative resection was undertaken in 67% of patients (Fig 47–1), and palliative resection was done in 6%; 27% had biopsy only. Hospital mortality was 9%, including 3 intraoperative deaths, and serious morbidity was 22%. The 5-year survival was 18%, with a median survival of 12.6 months. The 5-year survival of patients who had resection with curative intent was 27%. On multivariate analysis curative resection, normal performance status, and well-differentiated tumor predicted longer survival, and prolonged prothrombin time and hypocalcemia were adverse prognostic factors.

Further studies of host and tumor factors in relation to survival will help refine the management of primary hepatic malignancy.

▶ Primary hepatic malignancies are uncommon in America, as evidenced by the relatively small experience at the Mayo Clinic than at centers in the Orient. Nagorney and his colleagues, in spite of being expert in the management of liver tumors,

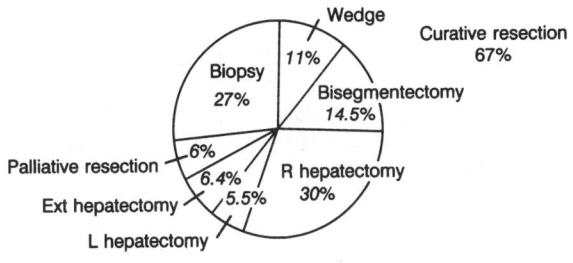

Fig 47–1.—Frequency distribution of hepatic resections in patients with primary hepatic malignant conditions. (Courtesy of Nagorney DM, van Heerden JA, Ilstrup DM, et al: Surgery 106:740–749, October 1989.)

encountered 3 deaths on the table and a hospital mortality of 9%. The median survival of a year and a 5-year survival of only 18% is indicative of the complex and as yet not well defined selection process for this disease in the United States. The occurrence of a hepatoma in a patient with cirrhosis should be approached with caution in view of the multicentricity of such lesions and the relatively high morbidity associated with postoperative liver dysfunction.—F.G. Moody, M.D.

Metastatic Liver Disease

Repeat Hepatectomy for Recurrent Malignant Tumors of the Liver
Lange JF, Leese T, Castaing D, Bismuth H (Hôpital Paul Brousse; Université Paris-Sud, Villejuif, France)
Surg Gynecol Obstet 169:119–126, August 1989

Between 1972 and 1987, 34 repeat hepatectomies were performed for recurrent malignant tumors of the liver in 28 patients. There was no operative mortality. The morbidity was 15%, and none of the patients had postoperative hepatic insufficiency. Only 5 of the repeat hepatectomies involved 3 or more hepatic segments.

Thirteen repeat hepatectomies were performed on 11 patients with hepatocellular carcinoma. The interval between primary and repeat hepatectomy was less than 1 year in 7 patients. Serial measurements of serum alpha-fetoprotein levels and ultrasound were valuable adjuncts to management. Four patients are alive during a mean follow-up of 33 months (range, 4–54), and only 1 has tumor recurrence. Ten repeat hepatectomies were performed for 9 patients with colorectal metastases. All but 1 of the recurrent tumors was discovered during the first 2 years after the primary hepatectomy. Five patients are alive, 1 having a recurrent disease, with a mean follow-up of 13 months (range, 1–35). Three of four patients who died had multiple hepatic metastases at the initial hepatectomy. Eleven resections were performed on 8 patients with recurrent miscellaneous malignant tumors. Four are alive with a mean follow-up of 28 months (range, 20–36), including 3 with recurrent disease. Two patients who underwent repeat hepatectomy for endocrine hepatic metastases are both alive.

Repeat hepatectomies for recurrent malignant tumors of the liver are technically highly feasible. Segmentectomy is the operation of choice. The results are beneficial in a minority of patients, particularly in those with hepatocellular carcinoma, colorectal metastases, and endocrine tumor metastases.

▶ The Bismuth Liver Surgery Unit at the Hôpital Paul Brousse in Paris-Sud describes the feasibility of segmental liver resection for recurrent malignancies. There were no deaths in this select group of patients with hepatomas, colon metastases, or endocrine tumors, most of which recurred within a few years after the initial hepatectomies. The study does not prove that the patients were benefited by this approach, but it is likely that at least a few were offered a chance for longer survival.—F.G. Moody, M.D.

Imaging Studies

Prospective Comparison of Preoperative Imaging and Intraoperative Ultrasonography in the Detection of Liver Tumors
Clarke MP, Kane RA, Steele G Jr, Hamilton ES, Ravikumar TS, Onik G, Clouse ME (New England Deaconess Hosp, Boston)
Surgery 106:849–855, November 1989   47–3

In prospective comparison of preoperative CT, ultrasonography (US), and angiography 54 patients undergoing resection of hepatic tumors were studied. The findings were compared with those of operative exploration and intraoperative US.

A total of 167 lesions were observed with intraoperative US. With preoperative US, 127 (76%) of those lesions were detected. With CT, 91 of 150 lesions were detected in 48 patients, and with angiography 56 of 105 lesions were demonstrated in 35 patients. Ultrasonography was much better for detection of lesions in the lateral segment of the left lobe of the liver than the other methods. In addition, more lesions less than 2 cm in size were detected with US than with CT. With combined CT and US, 81% of right-lobe lesions and 76% of left-lobe tumors were detected. In contrast, 66% of right-lobe lesions and 23.5% of left-lobe lesions were detected with angiography.

Because intraoperative US resulted in demonstration of at least 25% more lesions than preoperative US and CT and many of those lesions are not visible or palpable at surgery, intraoperative US should be considered whenever resection of a liver tumor is planned.

48 Liver Transplantation

FK 506 For Liver, Kidney, and Pancreas Transplantation
Starzl TE, Todo S, Fung J, Demetris AJ, Venkataramman R, Jain A (Univ Health Ctr of Pittsburgh; Univ of Pittsburgh; VA Med Ctr, Pittsburgh)
Lancet 2:1000–1004, October 28, 1989   48–1

A macrolide produced by *Streptomyces tsukubaensis* (FK 506) is a new immunosuppressive and cancer chemotherapeutic agent. It was given for both salvage and primary immunosuppression in 14 liver recipients at high risk.

Because conventional immunosuppression was deemed to have failed, FK 506 was used in the first 10 liver recipients. This salvage therapy was successful in 7 patients, and improvements in liver function were prompt. On biopsy, findings of liver rejection were either ameliorated or eliminated. Except for 1 patient, renal function remained almost unchanged after FK 506. Two patients who had graft losses after salvage therapy with FK 506, and 4 new patients underwent fresh orthotopic liver transplantation under FK 506 plus low-dose steroids. None of these 6 patients had rejection, although 1 with preexisting cor pulmonale and coronary atherosclerosis died of myocardial infarction.

Postoperative biopsy specimen of the 2 livers inserted at retransplantation showed no evidence of rejection, and all 6 patients showed no signs of nephrotoxicity. Two of the 14 liver recipients were given cadaveric kidneys, either from the same donor or from a different donor. A third recipient received a pancreas as well as kidney from the liver donor. None of these recipients had evidence of rejections of the kidney and pancreas, and no serious side effects were observed.

These findings demonstrate the impressive performance of FK 506 both for salvage and for primary immunosuppression for liver, kidney, and pancreas transplantation in high-risk patients. It is remarkably free from unwanted effects.

▶ Cyclosporine has been a vital factor in the expansion of liver transplantation services during the past decade. However, its nephrotoxicity and other limitations have stimulated a continuing search for other agents. Starzl and his associates now report the first clinical trials in liver recipients of a new drug that is not related chemically to cyclosporine or to other standard immunosuppressive drugs. The performance of FK 506 both for salvage and for primary immunosuppression in high-risk patients was impressive. Further observations in a larger number of patients will be awaited with interest.—N.J. Greenberger, M.D.

The Role of Liver Transplantation in Hepatobiliary Malignancy: A Retrospective Analysis of 95 Patients With Particular Regard to Tumor Stage and Recurrence

Ringe B, Wittekind C, Bechstein WO, Bunzendahl H, Pichlmayr R (Medizinische Hochshule Hannover; Klinik für Abdominal und Transplantationschirurgie; Pathologisches Institut, Hannover, West Germany)
Ann Surg 209:88–98, January 1989

The role of hepatic transplantation in patients with nonresectable liver or bile duct cancer remains controversial. In a retrospective analysis of 95 consecutively treated patients who underwent liver transplantations for hepatobiliary malignancy, the various prognostic factors, particularly the pathologic tumor stage according to the TNM classification, were correlated with the outcome after transplantation. Hepatocellular carcinoma was present in 52 patients, cholangiocellular carcinoma in 10, hepatoblastoma in 2, hemangiosarcoma in 2, bile duct carcinoma in 20, and hepatic metastasis from different primary tumors in 9.

The overall actuarial survival rate at 5 years was 20.4%. The median mortality was reduced significantly from 29.2% during 1975–1983 (median survival, 4 months) to 17% during 1984–1987 (median survival, 18.06 months), reflecting improvement in perioperative management and patient selection with regard to tumor stage. Currently, 27 patients are alive with the longest follow-up more than 12 years. Overall incidences of residual or recurrent tumor were 27 and 28, respectively.

Median survival times were significantly better in patients with hepatocellular (median, 120 months) or bile duct carcinoma (median, 35 months). Prognoses were poor for patients with cholangiocellular carcinoma; either residual tumor or early and mostly widespread recurrence precluded tumor-free survival of those patients. In patients with hepatocellular carcinoma, those with T2 N0 M0, stage II or III, respectively, had better prognoses than those with T4 or with extrahepatic growth (N1 and/or M1).

A normal or slightly raised preoperative serum alpha-fetoprotein level, as well as normalization postoperatively, was a leading prognostic factor after resection for hepatocellular carcinoma. Tumor recurrence was associated with failure to decline or early reappearance of alpha-fetoprotein. Among patients with bile duct carcinoma, actuarial survival rates were significantly better in patients without tumor-infiltrated regional lymph nodes. None of the patients who underwent liver transplantation for metastases survived beyond 10 months.

Hepatobiliary malignancy should not be regarded as a contraindication for liver transplantation per se. On the contrary, liver transplantation is justified on the premise of careful patient selection by adequate tumor staging.

▶ The liver transplant group in Hannover, West Germany, reports long-term results of its experience with liver transplantation for malignancy. In spite of few long-term survivors, the group remains enthusiastic for transplantation in selected patients whose tumors cannot otherwise be removed. I tend to agree with the group's philosophy, especially for those patients with hepatomas confined to the liver. Patients with cholangiocellular carcinoma and metastatic liver disease obviously should not be transplanted because they do not benefit from the procedure.—F.G. Moody, M.D.

Change in Hepatic Function, Hemodynamics, and Morphology After Liver Transplant: Physiological Effect of Therapy
Millikan WJ Jr, Henderson JM, Stewart MT, Warren WD, Marsh JW, Galloway JR, Jennings H, Kawasaki S, Dodson TF, Perlino CA, Hertzler GL, Hooks MA, Smith SL, Moore PB (Emory Univ; Pittsburgh School of Medicine)
Ann Surg 209:513–525, May 1989   48–3

Patients with acute hepatic necrosis and end-stage liver disease now commonly have orthotopic liver transplantation (OLT). The physiologic response after OLT was measured and compared with that after selective shunt and sclerotherapy to determine which patients should receive which therapy.

Thirty-seven patients underwent OLT in a 2-year period. The operative mortality was 18%, comparable to that of selective shunt in patients with Child's class C cirrhosis. Changes in hepatic function, liver blood flow, hepatic volume, and morphologic findings after OLT were measured. Galactose elimination capacity (GEC) and hepatic volume were lower in transplant recipients than in patients with cirrhosis who were treated with selective shunt or sclerotherapy. Galactose elimination capacity, flow, and volume normalized after OLT. After selective shunt and sclerotherapy, GEC was preserved, but hepatic volume dropped.

Three preoperative patterns were identified that can help in the selection of candidates for OLT: patients with chronic cirrhosis need OLT when GEC is 225 mg/min or less and volume is 50% normal or less; patients with Budd-Chiari syndrome need OLT if cirrhosis has evolved; and patients with sclerosing cholangitis and primary biliary cirrhosis need transplants when complications of the portal hypertensive syndrome develop. Selective shunt is indicated for patients with stable disease when their GECs are 300 mg/min or more and liver volume is greater than 75% of normal. Orthotopic liver transplantation is indicated for patients with cirrhosis whose GECs are less than 225 mg/min and liver volumes are less than 50% predicted normal.

▶ The surgical groups at Emory University and the University of Pittsburgh have teamed up to address when patients with the complications of portal hypertension should be transplanted. Quantitation of liver function and mass appear to be useful in treating cirrhosis. The use of a selective shunt buys time and may offer definitive therapy for Child's class C cirrhotic patients. Only time will tell whether the dry alcoholic patient will stay dry with a new liver.—F.G. Moody, M.D.

Abdominal Organ Cluster Transplantation for the Treatment of Upper Abdominal Malignancies
Starzl TE, Todo S, Tzakis A, Podesta L, Mieles L, Demetris A, Teperman L, Selby R, Stevenson W, Stieber A, Gordon R, Iwatsuki S (Univ Health Ctr of Pittsburgh; Univ of Pittsburgh; VA Med Ctr, Pittsburgh)
Ann Surg 210:374–386, September 1989   48–4

The liver, pancreas, and duodenum are closely related in fetal development and remain anatomically interconnected. As a result, malignant tumors originating in one of those organs often metastasize to the others and create an unresectable condition. In the radical treatment presented, 10 patients with such malignancies underwent removal of the liver, stomach, spleen, pancreas, duodenum, proximal jejunum, terminal ileum, and ascending and transverse colon.

Ages of the patients ranged from 27 to 46 years. Only 1 had received chemotherapy; 5 had undergone some previous operative procedure. Six patients had duct cell carcinomas, and all had liver involvement. Organ clusters from 11 donors were transplanted into the 10 recipients. In 8 procurements, 10 to 20 mg of OKT3 was given in an attempt to prevent graft-vs.-host-disease; in 6, 200 µg of Sandozstatin was given to minimize the risk of pancreatitis. The composite grafts consisted of the liver, pancreas, and duodenum, plus small segments of the proximal jejunum (Fig 48–1). Immunosuppressive therapy consisted of OKT3, cyclosporine, and prednisone. No adjuvant cancer therapy was given.

One patient died at 9 days after nonfunction of the liver and severe graft pancreatitis necessitated retransplantation 3 days after the first operation. A second patient died of multiple infections after 112 days. The remaining 8 patients were alive 3 to almost 9 months after transplantation. All were able to eat well and began to gain weight. None have required insulin, although 2 had significant complications of pancreatitis. Liver function was normal or nearly normal in all 8 survivors. In the first few weeks, mild rejection occurred in 5 patients. The current average dose of cyclosporine is equivalent to that given liver transplant recipients.

One concern is that the drugs given to prevent graft rejection might enhance the growth of microscopic metastases. If that does not occur in these patients, the value of foregut resection will be confirmed.

▶ Starzl and his colleagues have tested the concept of foregut multivisceral transplantation in 10 patients with unresectable tumors within the organ cluster. Eight patients were alive without evidence of recurrence at the time of the report. A longer follow-up that should be available next year will clarify whether immunosuppression has unmasked the growth of microscopic metastases. Graft-vs.-host disease apparently was controlled by the monoclonal antibody OKT3.—F.G. Moody, M.D.

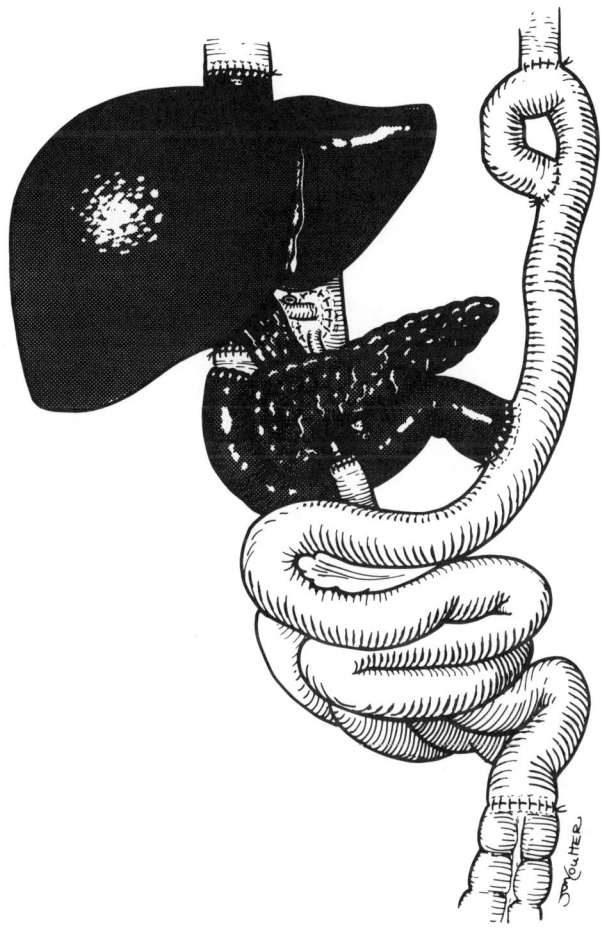

Fig 48–1.—Completed superior mesenteric vein reconstruction and usual gastrointestinal reconstruction. (Courtesy of Starzl TE, Todo S, Tzakis A, et al: *Ann Surg* 210:374–386, September 1989.)

49 Primary Biliary Cirrhosis

Detection of Autoantibodies to Recombinant Mitochondrial Proteins in Patients With Primary Biliary Cirrhosis
Van de Water J, Cooper A, Surh CD, Coppel R, Danner D, Ansari A, Dickson R, Gershwin ME (Univ of California, Davis; Emory Univ; Mayo Clinic, Rochester, Minn; Walter and Eliza Hall Inst for Med Research, Melbourne)
N Engl J Med 320:1377–1380, May 25, 1989

Primary biliary cirrhosis (PBC) is an autoimmune disease characterized by the presence of antibodies reactive against mitochondrial proteins of 74 kilodaltons (kd) and 52 kd. Detection procedures for these antibodies all have certain limitations, and an enzyme-linked immunosorbent assay (ELISA) is not currently available. Given the recently cloned genes encoding both the 74- and 52-kd proteins, the study was designed to develop and evaluate ELISA and immunoblot assays for their corresponding antibodies. In all, 217 serum samples from 93 patients confirmed as having biliary cirrhosis and 124 controls (healthy volunteers or patients with primary sclerosing cholangitis) were screened for reactive antibodies by these methods. The results were compared with those obtained from immunofluorescence testing.

Based on the ELISA, 89 of 93 serum samples from patients with PBC were positive, compared with none of 86 control samples (table). Immunoblotting showed 84 of 93 patient samples with positive results, compared with none of 86 control samples. Samples from patients with PBC that were negative on immunoblotting and ELISA were also negative on immunofluorescence testing.

These results indicate that the use of recombinant, cloned autoantigens provides a simple, accurate, and rapid method of quantifying and monitoring the levels of specific mitochondrial antibodies in serum from patients with PBC. The cost of this test should be similar to that of other ELISAs.

▶ Interest in the treatment of PBC is considerable. Three agents under active clinical investigation are colchicine, ursodeoxycholic acid (UDCA), and methotrexate. I will comment specifically about UDCA. At the 1989 meeting of the American Association for the Study of Liver Diseases (AASLD) there were 4 presentations on the efficacy of UDCA in PBC. Hadziyannis and colleagues evaluated over a 2-year period 50 PBC patients given either placebo or UDCA. They presented evidence supporting the following conclusions: (1) long-term UDCA therapy of PBC is associated with an early, striking improvement of clinical and biochemical features of

Reactivity of Serum Samples in Testing With Mitrochondrial
Antigens, According to Study Group

ASSAY	PATIENTS WITH BILIARY CIRRHOSIS (N = 93)	CONTROL GROUPS*	
		HEALTHY VOLUNTEERS (N = 86)	PATIENTS WITH CHOLANGITIS (N = 38)
	no. of subjects with positive serum samples		
ELISA (cloned autoantigen)			
Total reactive	89	0	0
74 kd only	36	0	0
74 kd and 52 kd	46	0	0
52 kd only	7	0	0
Nonreactive	4	86	38
Immunoblotting (rat-liver mitochondria)			
Total reactive	84	0	0
74 kd only	35	0	0
74 kd and 52 kd	44	0	0
52 kd only	5	0	0
Nonreactive	11	86	38
Immunofluorescence testing (HEp-2 cells)	87	ND	ND

*ND, not done.
(Courtesy of Van de Water J, Cooper A, Surh CD, et al: *N Engl J Med* 320:1377–1380, May 25, 1989.)

cholestasis; (2) this effect cannot be maintained for long, particularly in patients with stage 3 and 4 disease; and (3) there seems to be no beneficial effect on liver histology and on the final outcome of the disease.

Poupon and colleagues (2,3) reported on 70 PBC patients given either placebo or UDCA. They concluded that placebo or UDCA therapy not only provides clinical and biochemical improvement but also has marked beneficial effects on histologic features and progression of PBC. The results of this interim analysis, in patients having early as well as advanced PBC, confirm and extend the biologic data provided by their previous pilot study. However, the analysis of the trial, according to the defined end points, must be awaited to assess definitively the safety and efficacy of UDCA in PBC.

Podda and co-workers reported on 86 PBC patients given either UDCA or placebo. They report preliminary data for patients with symptomatic PBC that indicate an improvement of pruritus during treatment with UDCA, but failed to detect any difference with placebo. Nevertheless, the fall in serum bilirubin levels, the most important prognostic factor in PBC, and the increase in serum prealbumin, an index of liver synthesis, suggest a favorable effect of UDCA on the outcome of the disease. These 4 trials, although incomplete, suggest that UDCA may well prove to be effective in the treatment of PBC.—N.J. Greenberger, M.D.

References

1. Hadziyannis SJ, Hadziyannis ES, Makris A: A randomized controlled trial of ursodeoxycholic acid (UDCA) in primary biliary cirrhosis (PBC). Hepatology 10:580, 1989.

2. Poupon R, Balkan B, Legendre C: Ursodeoxycholic acid improves histologic features and progression of primary biliary cirrhosis. Hepatology 10:637, 1989.
3. Poupon RE, Poupon R, The UDCA-PBC Group: Ursodeoxycholic acid (UDCA) for treatment of primary biliary cirrhosis (PBC): Interim analysis of a double-blind multicenter trial. Hepatology 10:639, 1989.
4. Podda M, Battezzat PM, Crosignani A, et al: Ursodeoxycholic acid (UDCA) for symptomatic primary biliary cirrhosis: A double blind multicenter trial. Hepatology 10:639, 1989.

Antimitochondrial Autoantibodies in Primary Biliary Cirrhosis Recognize Cross-Reactive Epitope(s) on Protein X and Dihydrolipoamide Acetyltransferase of Pyruvate Dehydrogenase Complex
Surh CD, Roche TE, Danner DJ, Ansari A, Coppel RL, Prindiville T, Dickson ER, Gershwin ME (Univ of California, Davis; Kansas State Univ, Manhattan; Emory Univ; Royal Melbourne Hosp; Mayo Clinic, Rochester, Minn)
Hepatology 10:127–133, August 1989   49–2

Primary biliary cirrhosis (PBC) is considered an autoimmune disorder involving either T cells or disease-specific antimitochondrial autoantibodies. Such autoantibodies typically are present in the sera of affected patients. They recognize 4 major antigens of beef heart mitochondria at relative molecular weights of 74, 56, 52, and 48 kilodaltons (kd). The 56-kd antigen was shown to be the protein X of pyruvate dehydrogenase complex and has cross-reactive epitopes with the 74-kd antigen, the acetyltransferase (E2) of the pyruvate dehydrogenase complex.

In 2-dimensional gel analysis, both PBC sera and protein X-specific rabbit antiserum reacted to the same 2 isoelectric point polypeptides at 56 kd. Absorption of PBC sera with human recombinant pyruvate dehydrogenase-E2 removed reactivity to both the 74-kd and 56-kd antigens. Immunoblot analysis of 82 antimitochondrial autoantibody-positive PBC sera showed no serum that reacted solely against either the 74-kd or the 56-kd antigen (table). The PBC

Frequencies of PBC Sera Reactive Against 4 Antimitochondrial Autoantibody-Specific Antigens in Beef Heart Mitochondria

M_r of reactive antigens (kD)				No. positive/ total	% of total
74	56	52	40		
+	+			30/82	37
+	+	+	+	21/82	26
+	+		+	15/82	18
+	+	+		14/82	17
			+	2/82	2

Note: A group of 82 antimitochondrial autoantibody-positive PCB sera tested against beef heart mitochondrial proteins by immunoblotting at 1/1,000 dilution. Control sera from progressive sclerosing cholangitis, chronic active hepatitis, and normal healthy persons were negative against the 4 antigens recognized by PCB sera.
(Courtesy of Surh CD, Roche TE, Danner DJ, et al: *Hepatology* 10:127–133, August 1989.)

sera recognized protein X from human, bovine, and porcine sources, but not that of rat or mouse origin.

If protein X is a major target of the autoimmune response in PBC, the pyruvate dehydrogenase complex could have a central role in its origin. Chronic infection might activate T cell clones that recognize cross-reactive determinants on bile duct epithelial cell membranes and lead to destruction of intrahepatic bile ducts.

▶ The above article reflects the increasing knowledge of the biochemical nature and structure of the M_2 autoantigens in PBC. It seems clear that molecular or enzyme-linked specific serologic tests of greater sensitivity and specificity will be developed. Equally important, there is the promise of developing an experimental model of PBC and gaining a better understanding of this autoimmune disease.

The Mayo Clinic group has developed an accurate model to predict survival of PBC (1) that should enhance a clinician's decision-making process in the management of PBC. The comment after the following article provides up-to-date information on current treatment of PBC.—N.J. Greenberger, M.D.

Reference

1. Dickson ER, Grambsch PM, Fleming TR, et al: Prognosis in primary biliary cirrhosis: Model for decision making. Hepatology 10:1–7, July 1989.

Ursodeoxycholic Acid in Primary Biliary Cirrhosis: Results of a Controlled Double-Blind Trial
Leuschner U, Fischer H, Kurtz W, Güldütuna S, Hübner K, Hellstern A, Gatzen M, Leuschner M (Johann Wolfgang Goethe-Universität, Frankfurt/Main, West Germany)
Gastroenterology 97:1268–1274, November 1989   49-3

The effects of ursodeoxycholic acid (UDCA) on primary biliary cirrhosis were evaluated in a prospective, double-blind, controlled study. After a 3-month observation period, 18 women and 2 men with histologically proved primary biliary cirrhosis received treatment for 9 months with either UDCA, 10 mg/kg/day, or placebo.

After 18–24 weeks, all 10 patients given UDCA showed significant reductions (48% to 79%) in mean serum levels of glutamate dehydrogenase, aspartate and alanine aminotransferases, alkaline phosphatase, and g-glutamyl transpeptidase. Prothrombin time, serum bilirubin level, albumin level, results of the antipyrin breath test, and plasma disappearance of indocyanine green, which were normal, initially did not change during UDCA therapy. Concentrations of total serum bile acid increased, with UDCA being the predominant bile acid. In contrast, no significant changes occurred in the placebo group.

Liver biopsy specimens showed histologic improvement in 6 patients given UDCA, whereas 4 patients receiving placebo had deterioration. In vitro studies of bile acid toxicity to erythrocyte membranes showed that UDCA was less toxic than chenodeoxycholic or deoxycholic acid, and that addition of UDCA abolished the toxic effects of the latter 2 bile acids. Therapy was well tolerated, and no serious side effects were reported.

These favorable results warrant further trials of UDCA in larger groups of patients with primary biliary cirrhosis, including those with more advanced disease complicated by cirrhosis and portal hypertension.

▶ At the November 1989 meeting of the American Association for the Study of Liver Diseases, 4 presentations described controlled trials of the efficacy of UDCA in primary biliary cirrhosis (1–4). Hadziyannis and associates reported on 50 PBC patients, 25 randomized to receive UDCA and 25 to receive no treatment. Improvement in symptoms (pruritus) and liver tests occurred during the first 3–12 months, but was not sustained during the second year of UDCA therapy as pruritus increased in several patients and biochemical changes deteriorated compared with the 6 and 12 data. Two other trials (2,3) involving 70 and 86 patients, respectively, both reported significant improvement in symptoms and liver tests after 6 months of UDCA therapy. A fourth report (4), utilizing serial liver biopsies documented improvement in histologic features in 12 PBC patients, but not in untreated controls.

It seems clear that longer-term (perhaps 2–4 years) trials of UDCA in a larger number of PBC patients are needed to establish whether UDCA is an effective therapy. It is possible that UDCA will prove to be more effective in patients with less advanced disease and in whom serum bilirubin levels are less than 5.0 mg/dL.— N.J. Greenberger, M.D.

References

1. Hadziyannis SJ, Hadziyannis ES, Makris A: A randomized controlled trial of ursodeoxycholic acid (UDCA) in primary biliary cirrhosis. Hepatology 10:580, 1989 (abstract).
2. Poupon RE, Poupon R: Ursodeoxycholic acid (UDCA) for treatment of primary biliary cirrhosis (PBC): Interim analysis of a double-blind multicenter randomized trial. Hepatology 10:639, 1989 (abstract).
3. Podda M, Batezatti PM, Crosignani A, et al: Ursodeoxycholic acid (UDCA) for symptomatic primary biliary cirrhosis (PBC): A double-blind multicenter trial. Hepatology 10:639, 1989 (abstract).
4. Poupon R, Balkau B, Legendre C, et al: Ursodeoxycholic acid improves histologic features and progression of primary biliary cirrhosis. Hepatology 10:637, 1990 (abstract).

Efficacy of Liver Transplantation in Patients With Primary Biliary Cirrhosis
Markus BH, Dickson ER, Grambsch PM, Fleming TR, Mazzaferro V, Klintmalm GBG, Wiesner RH, Van Thiel DH, Starzl TE (Univ of Pittsburgh; Mayo Clinic and Mayo Found, Rochester, Minn; Univ of Washington, Seattle; Baylor Univ Med Ctr, Dallas)
N Engl J Med 320:1709–1713, June 29, 1989

The efficacy of liver transplantation was examined in 161 patients who survived transplantation and in controls not having transplantation. The patients underwent liver transplantation between 1980 and 1987 and were followed up for a median of 25 months. The primary indication for liver transplantation was poor liver function in 132 cases.

Analysis using the Mayo model indicated a substantially higher probability of survival in the recipients 3 months after liver transplantation than in the controls. At 2 years the Kaplan-Meier survival probability was 0.74, whereas the mean Mayo-model survival probability was 0.31. Patients at all risk levels were more likely to survive after liver transplantation. At last follow-up two thirds of the transplant recipients were working full-time and another 27% part-time. Only 3% of the patients were hospitalized.

Liver transplantation demonstrably improves long-term survival in patients with primary biliary cirrhosis. Survival recently has improved further with the use of OKT3 treatment for transplant rejection. More than 90% of patients who survive transplantation can expect to return to work at least part-time.

▶ The value of liver transplantation for primary biliary cirrhosis is firmly established in this report. Furthermore, the quality of life is remarkably good: more than two thirds of surviving patients were able to work full-time. This represents a remarkable advance in the treatment of this previously uniformly fatal disease.—F.G. Moody, M.D.

50 Miscellaneous Topics

Major Hepatic Resection

Major Hepatic Resection Under Total Vascular Exclusion
Bismuth H, Castaing D, Garden OJ (Hôpital Paul Brousse, Villejuif, France)
Ann Surg 210:13–19, July 1989   50–1

Blood loss is a major problem during liver resection, especially in those cases in which the lesion is located close to or involves the hepatic veins and the inferior vena cava. Total vascular exclusion is one method of establishing control of the major vascular structures. The technique was examined in 51 resections performed during a 9-year period.

Most (62%) of the patients were undergoing treatment for liver metastases. After a vascular clamp was applied to the hepatic pedicle to occlude inflow, the vena cava was clamped below and above the liver. The mean operating time was 5.8 hours; average time of vascular exclusion was 46.5 minutes. Patients received 4.5 units of blood and 8.2 units of plasma, on average, generally before the start of total vascular exclusion. During the latter procedure, 2,631 mL of crystalloid fluid was infused. Mean systolic blood pressure, mean central venous pressure, and urinary output all fell temporarily but returned at least to preexclusion values after declamping.

There were 8 (16%) complications, including respiratory infection and biliary fistula. One patient died of sepsis and multiorgan failure on the 45th postoperative day. The low mortality indicates that total vascular exclusion is a safe and useful technique in resection of hepatic lesions that involve the hepatic veins. The technique may not be well tolerated, however, in hypovolemic patients because of a significant reduction in venous return to the heart. Preoperative ultrasonography is essential in evaluating the hepatic lesion and tumor invasion of the hepatic veins and portal venous branches.

▶ Bismuth and his associates add another useful technique to the armamentarium of the liver surgeon. The effects of total hepatic vascular exclusion are well documented and should be carefully noted by those who plan to adopt the approach. The key appears to be preloading the cardiovascular system. Possibly a venovenous bypass of the vena cava and portal venous system also would be of some value, although it is difficult to see how the results could be improved significantly.—F.G. Moody, M.D.

Vascular Occlusions for Liver Resections: Operative Management and Tolerance to Hepatic Ischemia: 142 Cases

Delva E, Camus Y, Nordlinger B, Hannoun L, Parc R, Deriaz H, Lienhart A, Huguet C (St-Antoine Hosp, Paris; Princess Grace Hosp, Monaco)
Ann Surg 209:211–218, February 1989   50–2

Intraoperative bleeding is the chief risk of liver resection. Temporary portal triad clamping can minimize bleeding from the liver surface during transection, but it does not counter bleeding from hepatic vein branches. Hepatic vascular exclusion totally isolates the liver and retrohepatic vena cava from the rest of the circulation. Both types of occlusion lead to liver ischemia. In this study, 142 patients who underwent liver resection with the use of vascular occlusion were reviewed. Eighty-five had major liver resections. Portal triad clamping alone was used in 107 cases, and hepatic vascular exclusion was used for 35 major resections.

The overall operative mortality was 5.6%, and the complication rate, including postoperative deaths, was 32%. More blood transfusions prolonged the hospital stay and were associated with a higher complication rate. The duration of liver ischemia up to 90 minutes did not correlate with the postoperative hospital stay. Mortality and morbidity after major liver resections were similar with the use of hepatic vascular exclusion and with portal triad clamping alone, despite larger lesions in the former group.

Most liver resections may be done with portal triad clamping alone for vascular control. Hepatic vascular exclusion lowers the risk of massive bleeding or air embolism if the vena cava or a hepatic vein is torn during resection; it should be reserved for large or posterior tumors. The human liver can tolerate up to 90 minutes of normothermic ischemia.

▶ The authors provide further evidence that total hepatic vascular exclusion is well tolerated for up to 90 minutes. It should be reserved for posterior bulky lesions or those in which the hepatic veins or cava are at risk.—F.G. Moody, M.D.

Wilson's Disease

Wilson's Disease Presenting With Features of Hepatic Dysfunction: A Clinical Analysis of Eighty-Seven Patients

Walshe JM (Univ of Cambridge, England)
Q J Med 70:253–263, March 1989   50–3

The neurologic signs and symptoms of Wilson's disease have been well described, but symptoms of hepatic Wilson's disease have received less attention. The findings for 87 patients with hepatic Wilson's disease were reviewed. Of the 87, hepatic Wilson's disease was diagnosed in 30 patients before CNS signs or symptoms developed. In 22 patients, hepatic Wilson's disease was not diagnosed until CNS signs and symptoms developed. In another 22 patients who died, hepatic Wilson's disease was not diagnosed until very late in the course or at death, and 13 patients probably had incorrect diagnoses because after they died, hepatic Wilson's disease was diagnosed in a younger sibling.

TABLE 1.—Analysis of Clinical Symptoms

	Group 1 Hepatic disease with recovery	Group 2 Hepatic to neurological syndrome	Group 3 Patients who died of liver disease	Group 4 'Sibling biopsy'
Number of patients				
M	14	11	12	5
F	16	11	10	8
Mean age of onset				
M	10	10	13	9
F	12	11	13	11
Symptom				
Jaundice, anorexia, nausea, vomiting	11	9	13	6
Abdominal pain	1	4	7	3
Ascites/oedema	3	8	8	4
Bleeding diathesis	4	2	1	
Bleeding varices	2	2	1	
Haemolysis	4	7	4	2
Hepatosplenomegaly	5	6	3	
Diarrhoea/vomiting	2	0	0	
Itching	0	1	1	
Amenorrhoea	2	2	0	
Kayser-Fleischer rings				
Seen	17	22	11	0
Not seen	6	0	3	0
Not recorded	7	0	8	13
Reducing compound in urine	6	0	1	1
Mean duration of symptoms to death (years)		10	1.7	0.7
Number who died	0	4	22	13

Abbreviations: M, male; F, female.
(Courtesy of Walshe JM, Q J Med 70:753–263, March 1989.)

The 30 patients for whom the diagnosis was made early responded well to treatment with chelating agents and remained in full remission after 1–23 years of follow-up. Although symptoms were common to other forms of liver disease, a lack of response to standard therapy usually raised the suspicion of Wilson's disease (Tables 1 and 2).

Signs and symptoms of liver damage had disappeared in 20 of 22 patients for whom Wilson's disease was not diagnosed until after CNS symptoms developed. The interval between recovery from liver disease and the development of CNS abnormalities ranged from 1 to 8 years. Of the 22 patients who died of hepatic Wilson's disease before onset of any CNS signs or symptoms, 19 had been ill for a mean of only 4 months.

Despite recent advances in the treatment of hepatic Wilson's disease, the mortality among these patients remains high. Early diagnosis appears to be the key to improving survival.

▶ The 3 tests usually employed to screen patients for Wilson's disease include (1) slit lamp examination for Kayser-Fleischer rings, (2) serum ceruloplasmin, and (3)

TABLE 2.—Initial Copper Values (Median and Range)

	Plasma Cu (µg/dl)	Caeruloplasmin (mg/dl)	Plasma 'free copper' (µg/dl)	Urine Cu µg/24-h	Liver Cu (µg/g w/w)
Group 1 (n=30)	42	6.5	28	200	164
Range	7–181	0–23	7–139	70–8050	57–266
Group 2 (n=22)	28	<1.0	25	242	159
Range	7–56	0–14	7–55	45–830	56–292
Group 3 (n=22)	74.5	10.0	33	614	197
Range	17–180	0–19	10–123	62–2142	17–330
Normal range	80–150	25–45	<10	<30	<10

Courtesy of Walshe JM, *Q J Med* 70:753–263, March 1989.)

24-hour urine copper excretion. In a classic study (1) of Wilson's disease presenting as chronic active hepatitis, only one third of the patients had all 3 of the above abnormalities. Thus, all 3 tests must be used when Wilson's disease is a serious diagnostic consideration. In this regard, the possibility of Wilson's disease should be excluded from all patients with chronic active liver disease who are aged less than 35 years. Sternlieb (2) has estimated that in patients with a diagnosis of chronic active hepatitis, after excluding those with chronic hepatitis of known etiology, the yield of screening for Wilson's disease in patients aged less than 35 years is probably on the order of 5%. Although this disease is relatively rare, therapy with D-penicillamine or trientine can save lives.

Scheinberg and Sternlieb (3) have provided important insight into Wilson's disease from their extensive experiences with more than 320 patients with the disorder. A key finding in that study bears emphasis. If a patient discontinued penicillamine therapy even after having been free of any manifestation of the disease for more than a decade, he or she was likely to be dead within 3 years.—N.J. Greenberger, M.D.

References

1. Scott J, Gollan JL, Samourian S, et al: Wilson's disease presenting as chronic active hepatitis. *Gastroenterology* 74:645–651, 1978.
2. Sternlieb I: Diagnosis of Wilson's disease. *Gastroenterology* 74:787–789, 1978.
3. Scheinberg IH, Joffe ME, Sternlieb I: The use of trientine in preventing the effects of interrupting penicillamine therapy in Wilson's disease. *N Engl J Med* 317:209–213, 1987.

Hepatic Hemangiomas

Giant Cavernous Hemangioma of the Liver: CT and MR Imaging in 10 Cases
Choi BI, Han MC, Park JH, Kim SH, Han MH, Kim C-W (Seoul Natl Univ, Seoul, Korea)
AJR 152:1221–1226, June 1989

A giant cavernous hemangioma of the liver can be confused with primary or metastatic malignancy. A definitive noninvasive assessment can avoid invasive procedures including exploration, but the specificity of CT diagnosis is in doubt. Ten giant cavernous hemangiomas in 8 patients were examined with both magnetic resonance (MR) imaging and dynamic bolus CT. At least 1 dimension of these tumors exceeded 6 cm, and the mean largest diameter was 11 cm.

All 10 hemangiomas had a heterogeneous appearance and consisted of a main tumor with cleftlike areas and in 5 cases internal septa (Fig 50–1,A). The cleftlike regions were well defined and of lower intensity than the main tumor. The latter was of high intensity on T_2-weighted MR images. Low-density areas were present consistently in unenhanced CT scans. In characterizing the internal architecture of the hemangiomas MR imaging was superior to dynamic bolus CT studies (Fig 50–1,B).

The hemorrhage, thrombosis, hyalinization, liquefaction, and fibrosis found in giant hemangiomas explain their heterogeneous intensity on MR imaging. Early peripheral enhancement and centripetal filling are characteristic findings on CT examination, but the cleftlike areas seen on MR images do not have contrast enhancement on delayed imaging. The finding of a capsule, target, or halo sign will help distinguish hepatoma or metastasis from hemangioma.

▶ Computed tomographic criteria for the diagnosis of giant hemangioma are controversial. This study allows the improved vascular imaging MR to be used in identifying these lesions. All the MR images showed heterogenous intensity with diverse internal components paralleling the known histopathologic findings of giant hemangioma. Cleftlike areas in the hemangiomas are of unclear origin, but may be caused by areas of cystic degeneration containing a gelatinous-like material on pathologic exam. The use of MR in identifying these lesions may be important in their long-term management and in distinguishing them from other, more serious lesions.—P.B. Miner, Jr., M.D.

Hydatid Cysts

Comparison of the Results of Different Surgical Techniques in the Management of Hydatid Cysts of the Liver
Demirci S, Eraslan S, Anadol E, Bozatli L (Ankara Univ, Ankara, Turkey)
World J Surg 13:88–91, January–February 1989   50–5

The surgical management of hydatid disease of the liver has changed markedly in the past 2 decades. A total of 260 patients with hydatid cysts of the liver were operated on between 1980 and 1985; patients with disseminated disease or cysts in organs other than the liver were excluded. Nearly all patients had pain or an abdominal mass. Diaphragmatic elevation was a frequent finding. Radionuclide scanning of the liver confirmed hepatic lesions in 97% of cases. Results of ultrasonography also were nearly always positive. A single cyst was present in 170 patients.

Eighty-seven patients had management by cystectomy, lobectomy, primary closure, and capitonnage. The other 173 patients had either simple external

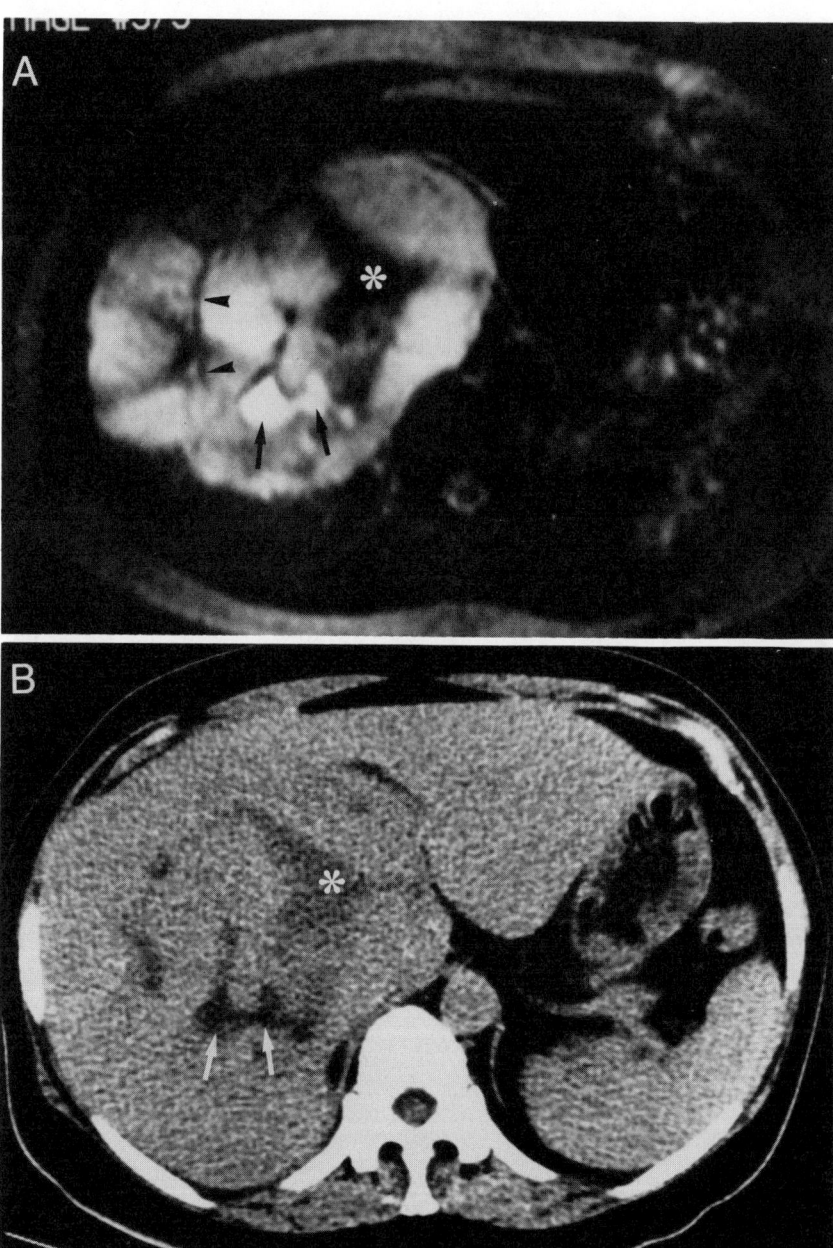

Fig 50–1.—Giant cavernous hemangioma of liver in woman aged 43 years with epigastric discomfort. **A,** spin-echo 2,000/180 MR image shows 3 different parts of hemangioma: main part of tumor, cleftlike part (*arrows*), and internal septa (*arrowheads, asterisk*). **B,** delayed CT scan 30 minutes after injection shows isodense filling that spares cleftlike areas (*arrows*) and central part (*asterisk*), which correspond to central low-density zone on MR images. However, delineation of fine internal septa, which are visualized clearly on MR images, is poor. (Courtesy of Choi BI, Han MC, Park JH, et al: *AJR* 152:1221–1226, June 1989.)

drainage or marsupialization. Cysts tended to be larger in the latter group. The overall mortality was 2.8%. Complications, such as intra-abdominal abscess, infection of the cyst cavity, and biliary fistula, were much more frequent in the patients with external drainage. Symptoms recurred in 23% of patients after 1 to 6 years, but the actual confirmed cyst recurrence rate was 10.5%.

Resection or hepatic lobectomy should be reserved for peripherally located hydatid cysts, pedunculated lesions, and small cysts in the left lobe of the liver. External drainage promotes postoperative morbidity in patients with uncomplicated cysts and should be avoided if possible.

▶ The authors provide an up-to-date review from a large experience of how to diagnose and manage hydatid cysts of the liver.—F.G. Moody, M.D.

Blunt Trauma

Patterns of Organ Injury in Blunt Hepatic Trauma and Their Significance for Management and Outcome
Rivkind AI, Siegel JH, Dunham CM (Univ of Maryland)
J Trauma 29:1398–1415, October 1989

Data for 185 patients consecutively admitted to a trauma center in 1983–1986 with blunt traumatic liver injuries were reviewed. Seventy percent of the group were male; the mean age was 30 years. Motor vehicle accidents were the most frequent cause of blunt liver trauma.

The pattern of associated organ injuries was a major determinant of immediate resuscitation needs, complications, and the ultimate outcome. Brain and chest trauma together were significantly related to death among patients with all classes of blunt liver injury. Of patients who survived initial surgery, sepsis and adult respiratory distress syndrome were correlated significantly with death. The only significant direct causes of death in all patient groups were brain deterioration and exsanguinating hemorrhage. Injuries of the bowel, spleen, stomach, and pancreas did not differ significantly in frequency between survivors and patients who died. The most prominent single injury determining the ultimate outcome was blunt injury to the brain.

Reintroduction of liver packing for major injuries where parenchymal bleeding is poorly controlled seems justified, especially if disseminated intravascular coagulation or hypothermia-related coagulopathy is present. In comparison with anatomical lobectomy, limited hepatectomy or débridement is likely to be associated with a reasonable chance of survival. Prophylactic perihepatic drainage for less marked hepatic injuries remains controversial.

▶ The outcome of blunt hepatic trauma is dependent on the extent of liver damage and associated injuries, especially the brain. Exsanguinating hemorrhage represented a major intraoperative challenge; we agree with the value of packing when bleeding cannot be controlled promptly.—F.G. Moody, M.D.

The Gallbladder and Biliary Tract

Chapter 51. Physiology and Pathophysiology
  Bile Acid Kinetics After Cholecystectomy
  Cholecystokinin and Analogues

Chapter 52. Radiographic and Imaging Considerations

Chapter 53. Gallstones and Related Problems
  Pathophysiology
  Gallstone Dissolution and Fragmentation
  Gallstone Recurrence After Dissolution
  Percutaneous Cholecystostomy

Chapter 54. Sphincter of Oddi Dysfunction and Sphincterotomy

Chapter 55. Bile Duct Problems
  Common Duct Stones
  Sclerosing Cholangitis
  AIDS-Related Cholangiopathies
  Bile Duct Strictures and Atresia

Chapter 56. Carcinoma of the Gallbladder

51 Physiology and Pathophysiology

Bile Acid Kinetics After Cholecystectomy

Effects of Cholecystectomy on the Kinetics of Primary and Secondary Bile Acids
Berr F, Stellaard F, Pratschke E, Paumgartner G (Univ of Munich, West Germany)
J Clin Invest 83:1541–1550, May 1989   51–1

The effects of cholecystectomy on the composition and kinetics of cholic acid (CA), deoxycholic acid (DCA), and chenodeoxycholic acid are of interest because of concern over the possible changes in formation and size of the bile acid pool after surgery. These effects were studied in 9 women with well-functioning gallbladders before and after cholecystectomy.

Gallbladder surgery increased the level and output of bile acids in relation to bilirubin in fasting duodenal bile. This increase caused a significant 27% decrease in cholesterol saturation. The turnover and pool size of chenodeoxycholic acid remained steady (Fig 51–1). A significant decrease of 37% occurred in synthesis of CA, the precursor of DCA. As a result, although the fraction of CA transferred to the DCA pool increased significantly (table), the input and size of the DCA pool stayed the same.

Enterohepatic cycling of bile acids in the fasting state is intensified by cholecystectomy. Their loss from the enterohepatic circulation is not increased, but CA synthesis, which apparently is regulated by transhepatic flux of bile acids, is diminished. Earlier 7α-dehydroxylation of CA and the in-

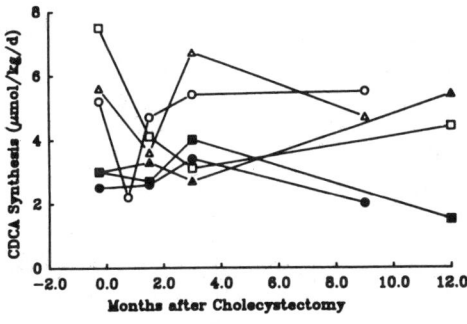

Fig 51–1.—Time-related changes in chenodeoxycholic acid (*CDCA*) synthesis of 6 patients after cholecystectomy. Chenodeoxycholic acid synthesis returned to steady rates at 3 months after surgery. (Courtesy of Berr F, Stellary F, Pratschke E, et al: *J Clin Invest* 83:1541–1550, May 1989.)

Fraction of Cholic Acid Transferred to the Deoxycholic Acid Pool*

		Mo after cholecystectomy		
Subject	Before	1.5	3	12
		%		
A.N.	54	71	89	90
C.S.	49	71	88	—
E.B.	40	57	36	99
C.V.	67	37	100	—
K.F.	19	6	22	9
A.E.	45	68	63	—
$\bar{x}$	46	52	66†	—
SD	±16	±26	±32	—

*Calculated from bile acid kinetics as DCA input rate divided by CA synthesis rate times 100.
†$P < .05$ as compated with preoperative percentage (paired t = test.).
(Courtesy of Berr F, Stellaard F, Pratschke E, et al: *J Clin Invest* 83:1541–1550, May 1989.)

creased absorption of DCA result from continuous exposure of CA to intestinal anaerobic bacteria. These changes allow the DCA pool size and turnover to remain the same after surgery.

Role of Primary and Secondary Bile Acids as Feedback Inhibitors of Bile Acid Synthesis in the Rat In Vivo
Stange EF, Scheibner J, Ditschuneit H (Univ of Ulm, West Germany)
J Clin Invest 84:173–180, July 1989   51-2

Numerous earlier studies support the classic view that the bile acid synthesis rate is controlled by the bile acids that are returned to the liver via the portal vein. However, the existence of such a feedback regulation mechanism has not been accepted universally, as the findings of several more recent in vivo studies failed to support the feedback concept. The effects of various primary and secondary bile acids on the rate of bile acid synthesis in rats with an extracorporeal bile duct were assessed.

The rats were infused with labeled solutions of taurocholic acid, cholic acid, deoxycholic acid, taurodeoxycholic acid, taurochenodeoxycholic acid, whole bile, or combinations thereof for 54 hours. Bile acid synthesis was assessed after 30–54 hours of continuous infusion. In a second set of experiments, bile acids were infused for 54 hours, after which a tracer dose was infused during the final 54–78 hours to allow direct measurement of bile acid synthesis after the infused bile acid pool had been depleted. The various bile acid concentrations were measured with high-performance liquid chromatography.

During the derepression phase, bile acid synthesis was inhibited only by infusion of taurocholic acid at supraphysiologic doses, but not by infusion of

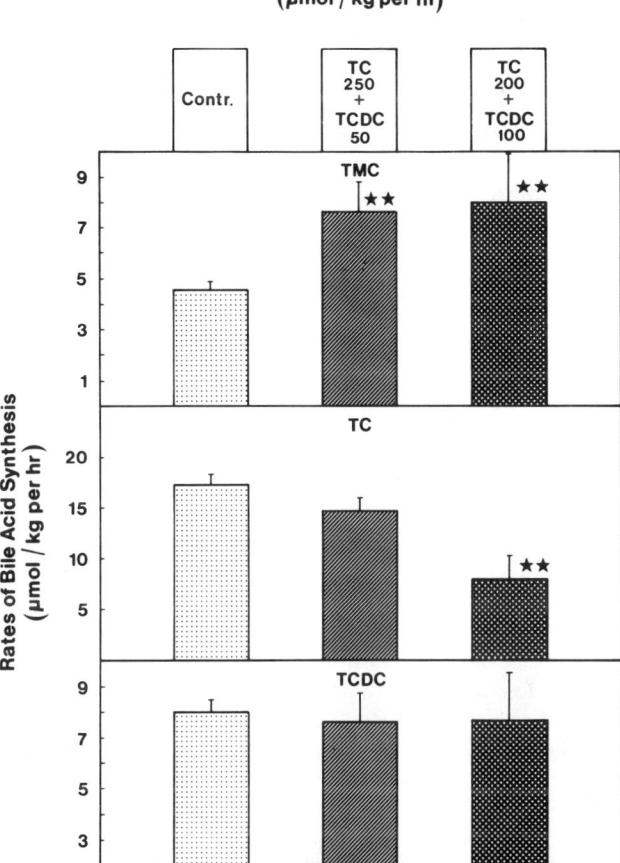

Fig 51-2.—Rates of tauromuricholic (*TMC*), taurocholic (*TC*), and taurochenodeoxycholic acid (*TCDC*) synthesis at 30–54 hours during the infusions of taurocholic acid plus taurochenodeoxycholic acid. Values represent the means ± 1 SEM. °°P < .01 vs. controls. (Courtesy of Stange EF, Scheibner J, Ditschuneit H: *J Clin Invest* 84:173–180, July 1989.)

lower doses of taurocholic acid approximating normal, initial bile acid secretion. Administration of a high dose of taurochenodeoxycholic acid combined with taurocholic acid inhibited taurocholic acid synthesis, but not synthesis of tauromuricholic acid or taurochenodeoxycholic acid (Fig 51–2). Deoxycholic or taurodeoxycholic acid, when infused at rates close to normal portal flux, were the only bile acids suppressing formation of taurocholic and taurochenodeoxycholic acid. Therefore, deoxycholic and perhaps some of the other secondary bile acids appear to be much more potent inhibitors of bile acid synthesis than the primary bile acids.

► These studies suggest that deoxycholic acid is a major determinant of synthesis of taurocholic and taurochenodeoxycholic acid in the rat and possibly in other species as well. Deoxycholic acid and other secondary bile acids appear to be much more potent inhibitors of bile acid synthesis than primary bile acids in this setting.—N.J. Greenberger, M.D.

Cholecystokinin and Analogues

CCK Receptor Antagonism by Loxiglumide and Gall Bladder Contractions in Response to Cholecystokinin, Sham Feeding, and Ordinary Feeding in Man
Konturek JW, Konturek SJ, Kurek A, Bogdal J, Olesksy J, Rovati L (Academy of Medicine, Krakow, Poland; Rotta Research Laboratorium, Milan, Italy)
Gut 30:1136–1142, 1989   51–3

The interaction of various neurohormonal factors in producing postprandial contractions of the gallbladder is not well understood. The role of cholecystokinin (CCK) was examined using loxiglumide (CR-1505), a highly selective and potent CCK receptor antagonist. Twenty healthy men (mean age, 24 years) were either infused with graded doses of up to 50 pmol/kg/hour of CCK or underwent modified sham feeding and ordinary feeding tests. Gallbladder volume was measured by real-time ultrasonography.

A dose-dependent decrease in gallbladder volume followed infusion of CCK8. Contraction amounted to about 15% at an infusion rate of 1.6 pmol/kg/hour and 91% at 50 pmol/kg/hour. The decrease in volume correlated closely with the dose of CCK or the increase in plasma CCK bioactivity. Bioactivity persisted after pretreatment with loxiglumide, but gallbladder volume was less affected. Modified sham feeding lowered the gallbladder volume by 20%. Real feeding reduced it by 70%, and loxiglumide decreased the value to 30%.

Endogenous CCK may have an important role in postprandial gallbladder contractions. It has a tonic effect on the gallbladder basally and is the chief factor responsible for postprandial contractions.

► Liddle and his associates (1) also have explored the physiology of CCK in human beings by investigating the effect on gallbladder contraction and gastric emptying of a recently developed CCK receptor antagonist, MK-329. In a double-blind, 4-period crossover study 8 persons received single doses of MK-329, 0.5, 2, or 10 mg or placebo, followed by an intravenous infusion of CCK-8. In placebo-treated persons, gallbladder volumes decreased on average to 43% of initial volumes after 2 hours of CCK infusion. A dose-dependent inhibition of CCK-stimulated gallbladder contraction was caused by MK-329; 10 mg produced complete blockade. Rates of gallbladder contraction and gastric emptying after a mixed meal then were measured in a 2-period crossover study. Placebo or 10 mg of MK-329 was given to each person 2 hours before eating. Gastric emptying of both solids and liquids was measured simultaneously by gamma scintigraphy. In placebo-treated persons plasma CCK levels *increased* postprandially to 2.3 pM, gallbladder volumes decreased 68.4 ± 3.8% (SE), and the times for 50% emptying of liquids and solids from the stomach were 58 ± 10 and 128 ± 8 minutes, respectively. Persons given MK-329 had marked elevation in peak CCK levels to 13.8 pM, and gallbladder contraction was inhibited completely.

These findings demonstrate that (1) MK-329 is a potent, orally active antagonist of CCK in humans and (2) CCK is the major regulator of postprandial gallbladder contraction. These data also support the concept of negative feedback regulation of CCK secretion and suggest that mechanisms other than CCK play a dominant role in the regulation of postprandial gastric emptying rates.—N.J. Greenberger, M.D.

Reference

1. Liddle RA, et al: Effects of a novel cholecystokinin (CCK) receptor antagonist, MK-329, on gallbladder contraction and gastric emptying in humans. *J Clin Invest* 84:1220–1225, 1989.

Role of Cholecystokinin in Regulation of Gastrointestinal Motor Functions
Meyer BM, Werth BA, Beglinger C, Hildebrand P, Jansen JBMJ, Zach D, Rovati LC, Stalder GA (Univ Hosp, Basle, Switzerland; Univ Hosp, Leiden, The Netherlands; Rotta Research Laboratorium, Monza, Italy)
Lancet 2:12–15, July 1, 1989   51-4

The possibility of a physiologic role for cholecystokinin (CCK) in regulating gastrointestinal motility has been suggested. The availability of loxiglumide, a potent, specific antagonist of CCK, allowed the effects of blocking CCK receptors on gallbladder contraction and gastrointestinal motility to be studied in 37 healthy men aged 21–39 years.

When loxiglumide was given orally 30 minutes before a liquid test meal, gallbladder contraction was abolished completely. After loxiglumide, radiopaque markers ingested with a liquid test meal emptied out of the stomach significantly faster than after placebo. Loxiglumide had no significantly greater effect on small bowel transit time than placebo, but when 800 mg of loxiglumide was given orally 3 times a day for 1 week, colonic transit time was significantly accelerated.

This study demonstrates that CCK has an important role in regulating postprandial gallbladder contraction. It also appears to be involved in the regulation of gastric emptying and colonic transit. The possibility that loxiglumide may have a pharmacologic role awaits further exploration.

▶ That CCK receptor antagonists also may inhibit pancreatic exocrine secretion has been demonstrated in elegant studies by Konturek and associates.

Exocrine pancreatic response to food is believed to result from the interaction of neural and hormonal factors, but their contribution in the net postprandial secretion is unknown. Recent description of a highly specific and potent CCK-receptor antagonist (known as CR-1409, compound 53, proglumide analogue 10) permitted Konturek and associates to evaluate the physiologic role of CCK in postprandial pancreatic secretion. In dogs with chronic pancreatic fistula, CCK antagonism caused little alteration in pancreatic protein secretion induced by sham feeding or urecholine, but reduced by approximately 60% the pancreatic protein response to a gastrointestinal meal and virtually abolished the pancreatic responses to duodenal perfusion with amino acids or oleate and to exogenous CCK, but not to secretin or neurotensin. The pancreatic protein responses, particularly to lower doses of gastrin, also were reduced by CCK-receptor antagonist, but no changes in the responses to secretin or neurotensin were detected. Cholecystokinin antagonism also significantly reduced the pancreatic polypeptide responses to CCK, gastrin, and the gastrointestinal meal, possibly because of removal of the CCK-mediated release of pancreatic polypeptide. Konturek and associates conclude that CCK plays a crucial role in the mediation of the gastrointestinal phase, but not the cephalic phase, of pancreatic secretion.—N.J. Greenberger, M.D.

Reference

1. Konturek SJ, Tasler J, Cieskowski M, et al: Effect of cholecystokinin receptor antagonist on pancreatic responses to exogenous gastrin and cholecystokinin and to meal stimuli. *Gastroenterology* 94:1014–1023, 1989.

52 Radiographic and Imaging Considerations

Simultaneous Measurement of Gallbladder Emptying With Cholescintigraphy and US During Infusion of Physiologic Doses of Cholecystokinin: A Comparison
Masclee AAM, Hopman WPM, Corstens FHM, Rosenbusch G, Jansen JBMJ, Lamers CBHW (Univ Hosp Nijmegen; Univ Hosp, Leiden, The Netherlands)
Radiology 173:407–410, November 1989 52–1

Cholecystography is a questionable method of quantifying gallbladder emptying because it measures volume change in 2 dimensions. The information obtained on gallbladder emptying at real-time ultrasonography was compared with that obtained at cholescintigraphy in 6 healthy volunteers with a mean age of 40 years. Cholecystokinin-33 (CCK-33) served as a stimulus for gallbladder contraction. For scintigraphy ^{99m}Tc-labeled HIDA was used.

The amount of CCK infused was correlated closely with the rise in plasma level of CCK. There was no significant difference in the percentage of gallbladder emptying as measured with ultrasound or cholescintigraphy, and the results of the 2 methods were correlated to a significant degree (Fig 52–1). A decrease in gallbladder volume of 1% corresponded to a 1% decline in counts over the gallbladder region.

Ultrasonography gives a true estimate of gallbladder volume, whereas cholescintigraphy, a nongeometric method, allows calculation of relative changes in gallbladder content. Real-time ultrasonography avoids the problem of radiation exposure.

▶ The importance of gallbladder emptying has been emphasized as we progress to medical treatment of gallstones with lithotripsy or ursodeoxycholic acid. This study eliminates the concern over the differences between cholescintigraphy and ultrasonography for evaluating gallbladder emptying. The percentage of emptying when measured by radioisotope or by changes in measured gallbladder volume with ultrasonography correlate with an extraordinarily low P value of less than 0.0005. Ultrasound examination may be more useful because changes in gallbladder volume as well as relative emptying of the gallbladder can be determined. With either test the measurement of gallbladder kinetic activity can be evaluated. This important paper will allow correlation of studies looking at the physiology of gallbladder kinetics in various disease states.—P.B. Miner, M.D.

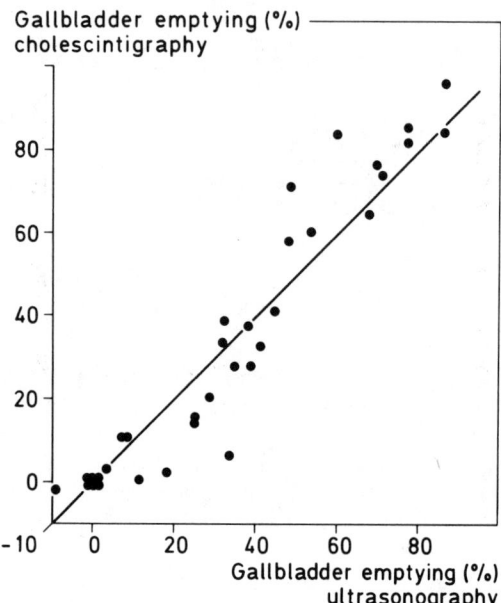

Fig 52–1.—Correlation between gallbladder emptying measured with ultrasound and with cholescintigraphy during infusion of stepwise increasing doses of CCK-33 ($y = 1.03x - 1.5$, $r = .95$; $P < .005$). (Courtesy of Masclee AAM, Hopman WPM, Corstens FHM, et al: *Radiology* 173:407–410, November 1989.)

Diagnosis of Acute Cholecystitis by Cholescintigraphy: Significance of Pericholecystic Hepatic Uptake

Swayne LC, Ginsberg HN (Morristown Mem Hosp, Morristown, NJ)
AJR 152:1211–1213, June 1989   52–2

Increased pericholecystic activity in the liver parenchyma of the gallbladder fossa is considered useful as a secondary cholescintigraphic sign of acute gallbladder disease. It is frequently associated with both gangrenous cholecystitis and gallbladder perforation. The positive predictive value of the sign was determined with 780 consecutive cholescintigrams done for patients aged 8–96 years.

Acute cholecystitis was seen in 135 of 141 patients without scintigraphic gallbladder visualization. Forty-six of the patients also had evidence of gangrenous cholecystitis, perforation of the gallbladder, or both. Increased pericholecystic uptake of nuclide was present in 34% of the patients with nonvisualization (table). The sign was always seen within 1 hour (Fig 52–2). Three of the 48 patients had chronic rather than acute cholecystitis. Increased uptake was present in 57% of 46 patients with gangrenous cholecystitis and in 4 of 13 patients with perforation. The sign was highly specific for acute cholecystitis and had a positive predictive value of 94%, but its sensitivity was only 33%.

Increased pericholecystic activity may increase the specificity of early cholescintigraphic images and preclude pharmacologic intervention or delayed imaging. Visual assessments of uptake do not correlate with the degree of inflammation.

Relationship of Gallbladder Nonvisualization to Increased
Pericholecystic Activity on Cholescintigraphy

Pathologic Changes	Results of Cholescintigraphy	
	Gallbladder Nonvisualization	Increased Pericholecystic Uptake
Acute (n = 135)	128 *	45
Gangrene †(n = 46)	44*	26
Perforation‡ (n = 13)	11 *	4
Chronic (n = 91)	13	3
Total (n = 226)	141 *	48

*Two other patients had no cholescintigraphic evidence of perforation.
†Cases of gangrenous cholecystitis are included in the cases of acute cholecystitis.
‡Cases of gallbladder perforation are included in the cases of gangrenous cholecystitis.
(Courtesy of Swayne LC, Ginsberg HN: AJR 152:1211–1213, June 1989.)

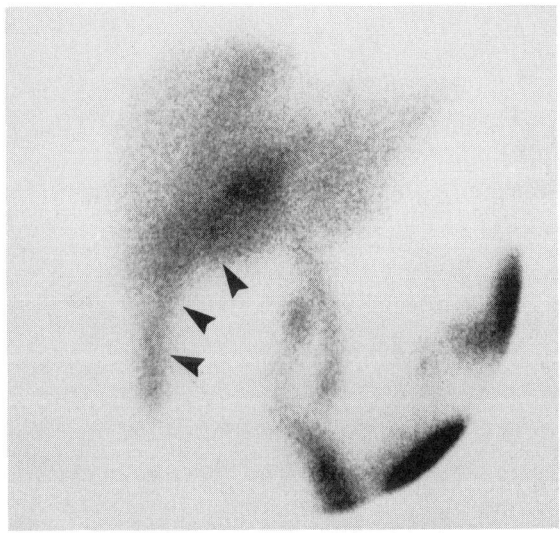

Fig 52–2.—Grade 4 pericholecystic hepatic uptake in a 64-year-old man with acute right-upper-quadrant pain. Scintigram (anterior view) at 1 hour does not visualize gallbladder but shows diffuse intense increased activity (*arrowheads*) involving entire inferior border of right lobe or liver and extending medially to porta hepatis. Surgery, performed same day, revealed acute gangrenous cholcystitis and cholelithiasis. (Courtesy of Swayne LC, Ginsberg HN: AJR 152: 1211–1213, June 1989.)

▶ Failure to visualize the gallbladder has been an important test for diagnosis of acute cholecystitis. This paper emphasizes the presence of a pericholecystic halo of radionuclide activity as a second sign for diagnosing acute cholecystitis. This finding was highly specific (97%) with a very high positive predictive value (94%), making it a useful observation for patients in whom acute cholecystitis may be suspected.—P.B. Miner, M.D.

53 Gallstones and Related Problems

Pathophysiology

Weight, Diet, and the Risk of Symptomatic Gallstones in Middle-Aged Women
Maclure KM, Hayes KC, Colditz GA, Stampfer MJ, Speizer FE, Willett WC (Harvard School of Public Health; Brandeis Univ, Waltham, Mass)
N Engl J Med 321:563–569, Aug 31, 1989   53–1

Obesity is a known risk factor for cholesterol gallstones, and dietary composition has been a suspected risk factor for many years. To assess risk factors for symptomatic gallstones, obesity, total energy intake, and alcohol intake were analyzed using data on 88,837 women, all United States residents, aged 34–59 years, in the Nurses' Health Study cohort. The women were followed for 4 years after completing a detailed questionnaire about food and alcohol consumption in 1980.

During follow-up, 433 cholecystectomies were performed and 179 patients with newly symptomatic, unremoved gallstones, diagnosed by ultrasonography or radiographically, were reported. The age-adjusted relative risk for very obese women, with a Quetelet index of relative weight of more than 32 kg/m^2 was 6.0 compared with those whose relative weight was less than 20 kg/m^2 (Fig 53–1). Slightly overweight women had a relative risk of 1.7.

Overall, there was a roughly linear relationship between relative weight and gallstone risk. Of the 59,306 women whose relative weight was less than 25 kg/m^2, those with a high energy intake had an increased incidence of symptomatic gallstones, and women who consumed at least 5 gm of alcohol daily had a reduced risk compared with those who abstained. Parity was not an important risk factor after adjustment for weight.

These results, when added to those of others, indicate a strong association between obesity and symptomatic gallstones. Even a slight excess of weight may be an important determinant of the increased risk of gallstones in middle-aged women.

▶ Two recent studies (1,2) have noted that the incidence of cholesterol gallstones increases even more when obese patients begin to lose weight. Liddle and Goldstein (1) investigated the development of gallstones over 8 weeks of dieting among 51 obese men and women and in 26 nondieting controls. Gallbladder examinations were done with abdominal real-time ultrasonography to detect gallstones. Sonography initially was done before dieting, and only those subjects for whom initial sonograms

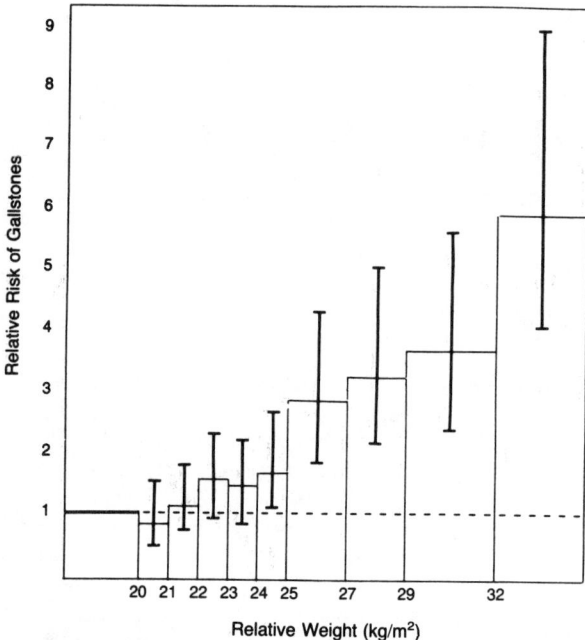

Fig 53-1.—Relationship of relative weight to age-adjusted relative risk of newly symptomatic gallstones, 1980–1984, in a cohort of 88,837 women aged 34–59 years in 1980. *Error bars* represent 95% confidence intervals. Quetelet's index, the weight in kilograms divided by the square of the height in meters, was used as a measure of relative weight. (Courtesy of Maclure KM, Hayes KC, Colditz GA, et al: *N Engl J Med* 321:563–569, Aug 31, 1989.)

showed no gallstones or sludge were included in the study. Sonography was repeated at 4-week intervals for 8 weeks while subjects remained on daily diets of 2,100 kJ.

Initial weights before dieting averaged 105.9 ± 3.8 kg (162% of ideal body weight) and decreased to 89.4 ± 3.2 kg (137.3% of ideal body weight) after 8 weeks of dieting. Sonography performed after 4 weeks of dieting revealed new sludge in the gallbladder of 1 person and gallstones in 4 persons. After 8 weeks of dieting sludge was detected in 3 persons, and gallstones, in 13 (25.5%). By contrast, none of the nondieting controls had development of any detectable gallbladder abnormalities. During dieting and thereafter 3 of 51 persons had symptoms of biliary colic, necessitating cholecystectomy. Eleven of the 13 patients with gallstones were followed up for 6 months after discontinuation of the diet. Besides the 3 undergoing cholecystectomy, 4 persons had gallstones on follow-up ultrasound examination, whereas sonographically detectable gallstones had disappeared in 4 persons.

Lithogenic changes in bile that form gallstones may be prevented with aspirin, a prostaglandin synthetase inhibitor, which affects gallbladder glycoprotein mucus production. Ursodeoxycholic acid, which decreases bile cholesterol saturation, also may prevent formation of gallstones. Broomfield and co-workers (2) evaluated these 2 agents in a group of obese patients enrolled in a weight loss program. Of 51 patients without gallstones who completed the study, 19 received a placebo, 18 received ursodeoxycholic acid, and 14 took aspirin. After the end of a monthlong weight loss program, *no patient taking ursodeoxycholic acid had gallstones, microstones, or crystals.* By contrast, in the placebo group, 5 had gallstones, 2 had microstones and crystals, and 4 had only crystals. Gallstones developed in only 2 patients receiving aspirin. These findings indicate that ursodeoxycholic acid prevents lithogenic change in bile and the formation of gallstones in obese persons during weight loss. The data obtained for aspirin are provocative, and with either a larger number of patients or larger doses of aspirin, similar protective effects of aspirin might well be demonstrable.—N.J. Greenberger, M.D.

References

1. Liddle RA, Goldstein RB: Gallstone formation during weight reduction dieting. *Arch Intern Med* 140:1750–1753, 1988.
2. Broomfield, PH, et al: Effects of ursodeoxycholic acid and aspirin on the formation of lithogenic bile and gallstones during loss of weight. *N Engl J Med* 319:1567–1572, 1988.

Estrogen-Induced Gallstone Formation in Males: Relation to Changes in Serum and Biliary Lipids During Hormonal Treatment of Prostatic Carcinoma
Henriksson P, Einarsson K, Eriksson A, Kelter U, Angelin B (Karolinska Inst at Huddinge Univ Hosp, Huddinge, Sweden)
J Clin Invest 84:811–816, September 1989   53–2

Cholesterol gallstones are more common among women than men in every population studied. Estrogens may be an important factor in the formation of gallstones. To learn whether and by what mechanisms pharmacologic estrogen treatment induces gallstone disease, 72 patients with recently diagnosed prostatic cancer were studied. By random assignment, 37 received estrogen therapy and 35, orchidectomy. Estrogen was given as polyestradiol phosphate, 160 mg intramuscularly monthly for the first 3 months, followed by 80 mg intramuscularly every month. In addition, the patients were given ethinyl estradiol, 1 mg orally daily for the first 2 weeks and then 150 mg daily.

After 1 year, new gallstones were diagnosed with ultrasonography in 5 of 28 estrogen-treated patients, compared with none in 26 orchidectomized patients. Estrogen treatment for 3 months increased the relative concentration of cholesterol and cholesterol saturation of bile by about 30%. Serum low-density lipoprotein cholesterol dropped by about 40%, and its relative change was inversely related to that of bile cholesterol. No changes occurred in biliary or serum lipids after orchidectomy. Biliary lipid secretion rates were determined with a duodenal perfusion method. Patients given long-term estrogen treatment had about 40% higher biliary excretion rates of cholesterol than age-matched controls (table). Phospholipid secretion also was higher, but there was no difference in bile secretion.

Increased hepatic secretion of cholesterol results in increased cholesterol saturation of bile and a higher rate of gallstone formation during estrogen therapy. The changes in bile cholesterol appear to be associated with the induced changes in serum lipoprotein metabolism.

Results of Biliary Lipid Analysis Before and 3 Months After Onset of Therapy (Means ± SEM)

	Study group			
	Estrogen (n = 10)		Orchidectomy (n = 9)	
	Before	During	Before	After
Biliary lipid classes				
Cholesterol (M%)	5.4±0.6	7.2±0.9*†	5.6±0.6	5.2±0.6
Bile acids (M%)	74.7±1.5	71.2±2.0	73.3±1.8	75.9±2.7
Phospholipids (M%)	19.8±1.3	21.6±1.9	21.2±1.3	18.9±2.2
Cholesterol saturation (%)	80±9	110±11*†	80±7	80±7
Biliary bile acid composition ‡				
Cholic acid (%)	39±4	43±5	35±4	36±3
Chenodeoxycholic acid (%)	36±4	29±2 †	41±3	43±2
Deoxycholic acid (%)	25±4	28±5	25±6	21±5

*$P < .01$ compared with pretreatment value.
†$P < .05$ compared with orchidectomy group.
‡Trace amounts (< 1%) of lithocholic acid and ursodeoxycholic acid were observed.
(Courtesy of Henrikkson P, Einarsson K, Eriksson A, et al: *J Clin Invest* 84:811–816, September 1989.)

▶ Before treatment, the prevalence of gallstone disease was similar in both groups. In the group randomized to receive estrogens, 4 patients (11%) had had cholecystectomy and 5 (14%) had gallstones. Similarly, in the group randomized to undergo orchidectomy, 5 patients (14%) had had cholecystectomy and 4 (11%) had gallstones. One year after treatment a significantly higher incidence of formation of new gallstones was found only in estrogen-treated patients (5 of 28, or 18%) compared with patients undergoing orchidectomy (0 of 26). Further, size or number of gallstones or both were increased in estrogen-treated patients who previously had had gallstones (4 of 5 patients). In addition to the clear-cut changes in biliary lipids, other (additive) effects on gallstone formation may have been induced by the pharmacologic doses of estrogen used in this study. Such mechanisms theoretically might include estrogen-mediated effects on the rate of nucleation of cholesterol crystals, gallbladder emptying, and production of mucous glycoproteins.—N.J. Greenberger, M.D.

Effect of Ursodeoxycholic Acid Administration on Nucleation Time in Human Gallbladder Bile

Tazuma S, Sasaki H, Mizuno S, Sagawa H, Hashiba S, Horiuchi I, Kajiyama G (Hiroshima Univ)
Gastroenterology 97:173–178, July 1989

Ursodeoxycholic acid (UDCA) is not always successful in dissolving cholesterol gallstones. To determine whether cholesterol crystal nucleation is influenced by UDCA therapy, and whether the effect is related to altered lipid metabolism, gallbladder bile was sampled from 21 patients with cholesterol stones, 15 with noncholesterol stones, and 24 without stones.

In the patients with cholesterol gallstones, preoperative UDCA treatment was associated with a significantly longer nucleation time compared with untreated patients; the respective median times were 16 days and 4 days. Patients with noncholesterol stones had a median nucleation time of 15 days, and those without gallstones, 14 days. Treatment with UDCA for 3 months significantly increased the serum level of apolipoproADHbtein A-I, an antinucleating factor.

Administration of UDCA to patients with cholesterol gallstone disease prolongs cholesterol crystal nucleation and retards crystal growth. However, it does not lead to cholesterol desaturation in the bile. Recurrent formation of cholesterol stones may be inhibited by UDCA after dissolution or cholecystectomy. Changes in lipoprotein metabolism may be involved in this effect.

▶ These findings suggest that UDCA retards cholesterol crystal nucleation, thereby inhibiting formation of cholesterol gallstones. Further, it is possible that apolipoprotein A-I plays a role in this process. It is anticipated that research now in progress will clarify the role of several factors that may either accelerate or retard cholesterol crystal nucleation, processes that are obviously important in the pathogenesis of cholesterol gallstones.—N.J. Greenberger, M.D.

Canine Common Duct and Gallbladder Bile Contain Antinucleating Factors That Inhibit $CaCO_3$ Precipitation
Rege RV, Dawes LG, Moore EW (Northwestern Univ; Med College of Virginia, Richmond)
J Lab Clin Med 113:642–650, May 1989   53–4

Calcium precipitation in the bile may be critically important in the initiation of cholesterol stones, which consistently contain calcium in their central regions. Large incremental additions of calcium were made to canine bile to determine how much $CaCO_3$ supersaturation is possible, compared with that in simple saline-$NaHCO_3$ solutions. Common duct bile and gallbladder bile both were sampled.

Addition of $CaCl_2$ to bile increased total and free ionized calcium levels by fourfold to 12-fold. The final concentrations were 2–3 times greater than the peak levels encountered in vivo. The saturation index of bile increased fourfold to 12-fold (Fig 53–2). Nevertheless, evidence of $CaCO_3$ precipitation was not found in either common duct or gallbladder bile for 24 hours. When calcium was added to saline-$NaHCO_3$ solution, $CaCO_3$ precipitated within 4 hours if the saturation index exceeded 12. Indices as high as 73 were reached in common duct bile.

Native bile contains potent antinucleating factors that inhibit precipitation of $CaCO_3$. Acidification of bile by the gallbladder is important, regardless of

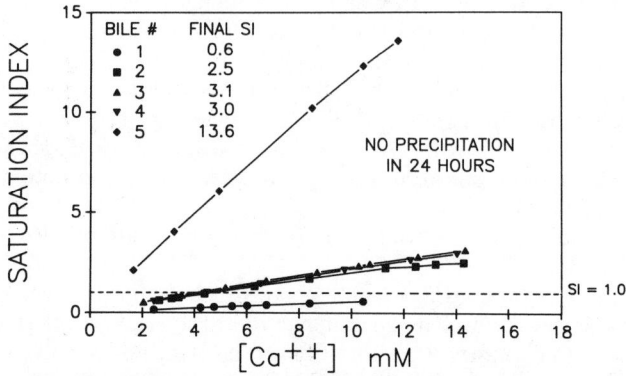

Fig 53-2.—Effect of $CaCl_2$ addition on $CaCO_3$ saturation indices of gallbladder bile. Each symbol represents a different bile sample. Despite a fourfold increase in (CA^{++}), gallbladder bile no. 1 never became supersaturated. In other samples, degree of $CaCO_3$ saturation increased from initial SI of 0.6, 0.5, 0.6, and 2.1 to final values of 2.5, 3.1, 3.0, and 13.6, respectively. These samples demonstrate the protective value of bile acidification; if pH is low, it is impossible to reach $CaCO_3$ saturation at normal values of bile (Ca^{++}). As with common duct samples, no precipitation was observed in any gallbladder sample. (Courtesy of Rage RV, Dawes LG, Moore EW: *J Lab Clin Med* 113:642–650, May 1989.)

the presence or absence of nucleating and antinucleating agents. Precipitation of $CaCO_3$ in the gallbladder probably requires both defective acidification of bile and an imbalance between nucleating and antinucleating agents.

▶ In seeking to identify nucleating and antinucleating proteins involved in the pathogenesis of cholesterol gallstones, Shimizu and colleagues (1) isolated a major acidic protein from each of 13 samples of cholesterol gallstones. After the stones were extracted with methyl *tert*-butyl ether to remove cholesterol and methanol to remove bile salts and other lipids, they were demineralized with ethylenediamine tetraacetic acid. The extracts were desalted with Sephadex-G25, and the proteins separated by PAGE. A protein was isolated, of molecular weight below 10 kilodaltons, which included firmly bound diazo-positive yellow pigments and contained 24% acidic, but only 7% basic, amino acid residues. The presence of N-acetyl glucosamine suggested that this was a *glycoprotein*. This protein at concentrations as low as 2 mg/mL, but neither human serum albumin nor its complex with bilirubin, inhibited calcium carbonate precipitation from a supersaturated solution in vitro. This protein could be precipitated from 0.15-M NaCl solution by the addition of 0.5 M calcium chloride. Considering that cholesterol gallstones contain calcium and pigment at their centers, and that small acidic proteins are important regulators in other biomineralization systems, this protein seems likely to play a role in the pathogenesis of cholesterol gallstones.—N.J. Greenberger, M.D.

Reference

1. Shimizu S, Sabsay B, Veis A, et al: Isolation of an acidic protein from cholesterol gallstones, which inhibits the precipitation of calcium carbonate in vitro. *J Clin Invest* 84:1990–1996, 1989.

The Role of Bacteria in Gallbladder and Common Duct Stone Formation
Kaufman HS, Magnuson TH, Lillemoe KD, Frasca P, Pitt HA (Johns Hopkins Med Inst, VA Med Ctr, Baltimore)
Ann Surg 209:584–592, May 1989   53–5

The role of bacteria in the pathogenesis of gallstones in Western countries has not been established definitely. Gallbladder and common duct stones from consecutively seen patients undergoing cholecystectomy, common bile duct exploration, or both were examined.

Stones from 67 patients were studied for bacteria with scanning electron microscopy (SEM). Bile was cultured, and stone cholesterol content was determined. Windowless energy-dispersive x-ray microanalysis was used to classify individual calcium salts (Fig 53–3). Gallbladder stones from 65 patients were cholesterol in 71% of the cases, black pigment in 26%, and brown pigment in 3%. Common bile duct stones from 10 patients were cholesterol in 4, brown pigment in 4, and black pigment in 2. The patients with brown pigment stones were significantly older, more likely to be male, and more likely to have bile duct obstruction than other patients.

Thirteen percent of patients with cholesterol stones, 14% with black pigment stones, and all with brown pigment stones had positive results of bile cultures. Bacteria were seen only in the calcium bilirubinate-protein matrix of brown pigment stones, according to SEM. Brown stones were more likely than black stones to contain calcium palmitate and cholesterol.

Black and brown pigment stones appear to have different pathogenic mechanisms. Bacterial infection seems to be an initiating or promoting factor, or both, in brown pigment stones, but not in black or cholesterol gallstones.

Gallstone Dissolution and Fragmentation

Use of External Shock-Wave Lithotripsy and Adjuvant Ursodiol for Treatment of Radiolucent Gallstones: A National Multicenter Study
Burnett D, Ertan A, Jones R, O'Leary JP, Mackie R, Robinson JE Jr, Salen G, Stahlgren L, Van Thiel DH, Vassy L, Greenberger N, Hofmann AF (Univ of Nebraska Med Ctr/Bishop Clarkson Hosp, Omaha; Tulane Univ; Louisiana State Univ; Abbott-Northwestern Hosp, Minneapolis; Baptist Mem Hosp, Memphis; et al.)
Dig Dis Sci 34:1011–1015, July 1989   53–6

Use of external shock-wave lithotripsy (ESWL) is an effective, safe treatment for kidney stones. Extensive clinical experience with ESWL for gallstones has been limited to water-bath machines made by a single manufacturer, with most patients treated at 1 or 2 sites. A non-water-bath machine was approved in 1988 for use in kidney stone therapy. A prospective multicenter study was done to assess the use of ESWL and adjuvant medical therapy in gallstone treatment.

Using the non-water-bath machine (Medstone STS lithotriptor) with ursodiol, 223 patients were treated. Seventy-five percent were given general anesthesia and 25%, intravenous analgesia. The initial treatments were done on an inpatient basis. As experience was gained, outpatient treatments became

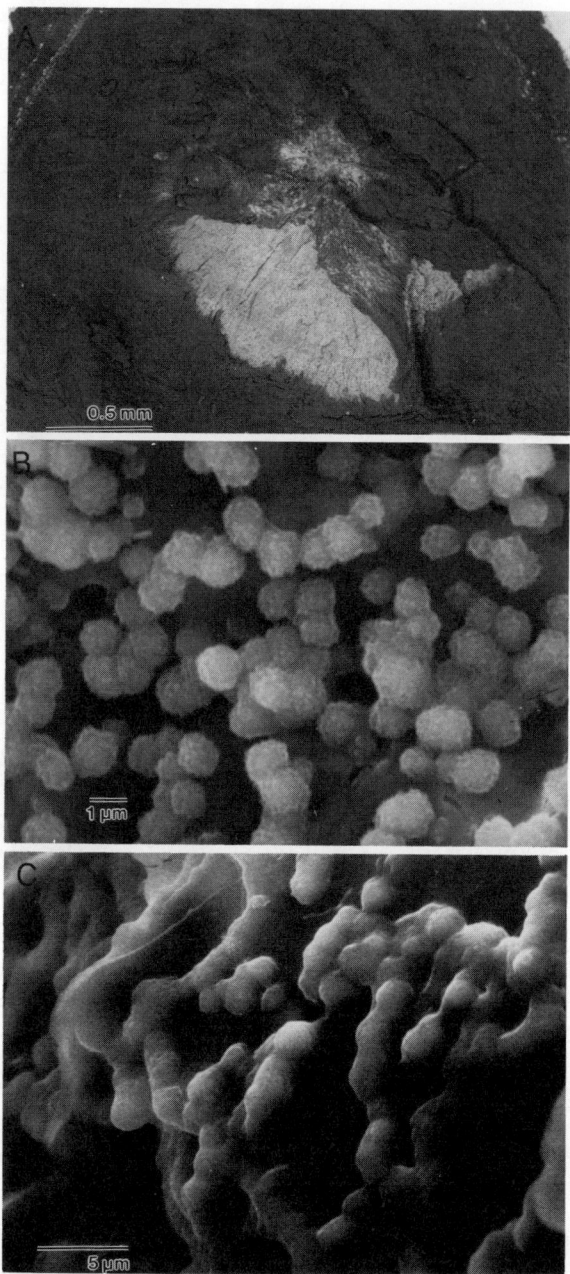

Fig 53–3.—A, low magnification backscattered electron imaging (BEI) of cholesterol gallstone cross section demonstrating the localization of calcium salts in the core of this gallstone. **B,** high magnification BEI of the core of this same stone showing calcium-containing microspheres. **C,** high magnification secondary electron imaging of similar microspheres. (*Continued.*)

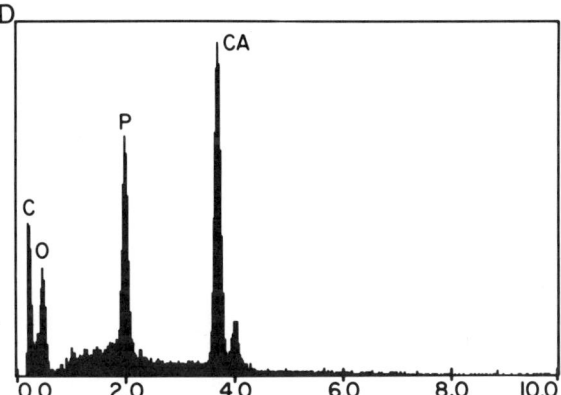

Fig 53-3 (cont.).—D, windowless energy-dispersive X-ray microanalysis spectrum identifying microsphere composition as calcium phosphate. (Courtesy of Kaufman HS, Magnuson TH, Lillemoe KD, et al: *Ann Surg* 209:584–592, May 1989.)

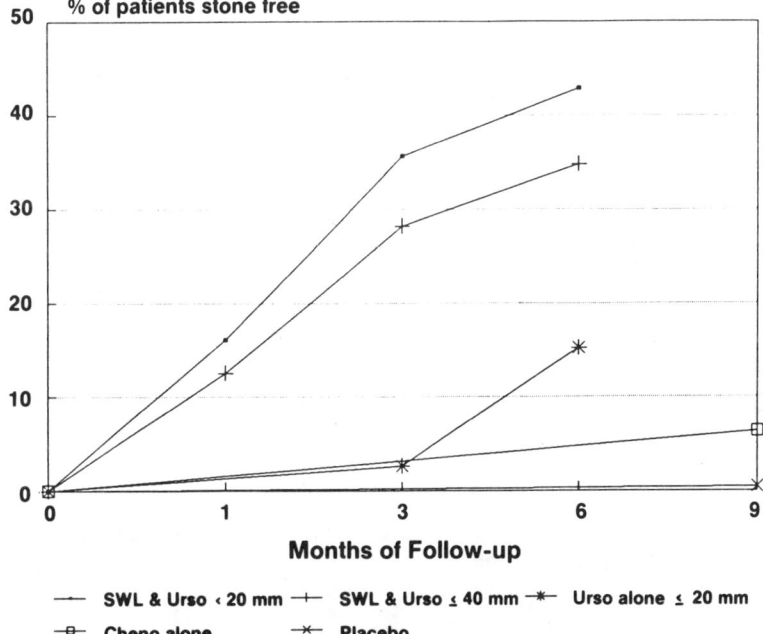

Fig 53-4.—Life-table estimates of stone-free rates: lithotripsy/ursodiol combination vs. ursodiol alone; chenodiol alone; and placebo. (Courtesy of Burnett D, Ertan A, Jones R, et al: *Dig Dis Sci* 34:1011–1015, July 1989.)

more common. Stone fragmentation and clearance were the greatest in patients who had solitary gallstones less than 2 cm in diameter. Stone fragmentation occurred in 97% of these patients. The 6-month follow-up data on 206 patients included 67 who had solitary stones ≤ 20 mm and 34 (51%) were free of stones and fragments. This is in reasonable agreement with the life-table estimates (Fig 53–4), indicating a stone-free rate of 42%.

Fragmentation of gallstones can be achieved with a dry shock-wave lithotriptor. Stone clearance is induced faster with ESWL and adjuvant ursodiol treatment than with ursodiol treatment alone.

▶ The preliminary studies under way at several medical centers in the United States, utilizing several different types of lithotripsies, indicate that gallstone lithotripsy followed by dissolution treatment of residual fragments with ursodeoxycholic acid is safe and effective treatment in *selected* patients. Several important questions remain, including the following:

1. Of the very large number of patients in the United States with symptomatic gallstones, what proportion meet the inclusion criteria for gallstone lithotripsy? From both retrospective as well as prospective studies it appears that only 15% to 20% meet these criteria.

2. Who are the best candidates for gallstone lithotripsy? The best candidates are patients with solitary gallstones no larger than 20 mm in diameter.

3. Why are the results with gallstone lithotripsy in the United States, that is, stone-free rates at 6 months, lower than those reported from West Germany? This is a complex issue, but contributing factors would include patient selection, operative expertise and the resultant learning curve, assessment of stone- and fragment-free state, type and power of lithotriptors employed, and site-to-site variations. The emerging data, however, do suggest that 40% to 50% of patients with solitary stones will be stone- and fragment-free at 6 months and that higher rates can be expected after 12 months.

4. What is the recurrence rate after gallstone lithotripsy and dissolution treatment of fragments with ursodeoxycholic acid? Early data suggest that the recurrence rate after 1 year is about 12%; for further details on recurrences see the following article.

5. Is the treatment cost-effective? Currently, the costs are equivalent to those for a cholecystectomy but without the associated morbidity, mortality, and time lost from work. However, that does not include patients who ultimately will need cholecystectomy (? 5% to 8%). Finally, treatment with ursodeoxycholic acid is expensive (about $1,500/yr), and it is hoped that less expensive ursodeoxycholic acid products will become available in the United States.—N.J. Greenberger, M.D.

Extracorporeal Shock-Wave Lithotripsy and Methyl *tert*-Butyl Ether for Partially Calcified Gallstones

Peine CJ, Petersen BT, Williams HJ, Bender CE, Patterson DE, Segura JW, Nagorney DM, Warner MA, Thistle JL (Mayo Clinic)
Gastroenterology 97:1229–1235, November 1989

To explore the possibility that gallbladder stone fragments might be safely dissolved by using methyl *tert*-butyl ether (MTBE) immediately after extracorporeal shock-wave lithotripsy, a pilot study was undertaken in 8 patients with 1 to 4 partially calcified gallbladder stones that averaged 2.2 cm in diameter and contained layered or diffuse calcium.

Lithotripsy was carried out with a renal stone lithotriptor after percutaneous placement of a 5F pigtail catheter into the gallbladder. General anesthesia was used. Then MTBE was infused and aspirated via the catheter until no further stone material was detected radiologically. Further treatment was given to enhance the dissolution of residual material not apparent by catheter cholecystogram.

No detectable fragments remained in 6 of the 8 patients after 8 to 26 hours of MTBE treatment. Patients tolerated the treatment well, but 3 had bile leakage after catheter removal and 1 underwent cholecystectomy.

Predissolution gallstone lithotripsy does not likely predispose the patient to side effects from MTBE when it is used immediately after lithotripsy.

▶ This is a new wrinkle in the attempt to develop an effective alternative to cholecystectomy for partially calcified gallstones. Dissolution with MTBE immediately after extracorporeal fragmentation appeared to be well tolerated. However, the morbidity (50%), which included bile leakage in 3 patients and a cholecystectomy in a fourth, must be reduced to make this a safe alternative. In addition, the treatment time, which may exceed 24 hours, must be shortened if a cost-effective method is desired.—F.G. Moody, M.D.

Dissolution of Cholesterol Gallbladder Stones by Methyl *Tert*-Butyl Ether Administered by Percutaneous Transhepatic Catheter
Thistle JL, May GR, Bender CE, Williams HJ, LeRoy AJ, Nelson PE, Peine CJ, Petersen BT, McCullough JE (Mayo Clinic and Found, Rochester, Minn)
N Engl J Med 320:633–639, March 9, 1989   53–8

The efficacy and safety of methyl *tert*-butyl ether (MTBE) in dissolving cholesterol gallstones was investigated in 75 patients with symptomatic radiolucent gallstones. This substance, in volumes of 2–15 mL (mean volume, 4 mL) was continuously infused and aspirated manually 4–6 times per minute through a percutaneous transhepatic catheter, for an average of 5 hours per day for 1–3 days. Treatment was monitored with fluoroscopy.

Dissolution of more than 95% of stone mass was achieved in all but 3 patients (Fig 53–5). Of the 21 patients who were completely free of stones after treatment, 4 had stone recurrence 6–16 months later. The remaining 51 patients had residual debris; 15 were stone free within 6–35 months, and 7 had persisting symptoms. Five of the initial 6 patients, but only 1 of the next 69, needed surgery during follow-up periods of 6–42 months.

The total treatment time averaged 12.5 hours. Solitary stones dissolved within an average of 8.4 hours, whereas multiple stones required an average of 13.8 hours. Placement of the catheter was generally not difficult, and in no patient was the catheter completely dislodged. Side effects were few and included transient nausea, mild sedation, abdominal pain, and transient elevations of hepatic enzymes. Overflow of MTBE resulting in superficial ulcerative duodenitis and transient intravascular hemolysis occurred in 1 patient; these side effects did not warrant discontinuance of MTBE treatment, however.

Dissolution of gallstones by MTBE through a percutaneous transhepatic catheter is an attractive alternative to surgery in selected patients with symptomatic cholesterol gallstones.

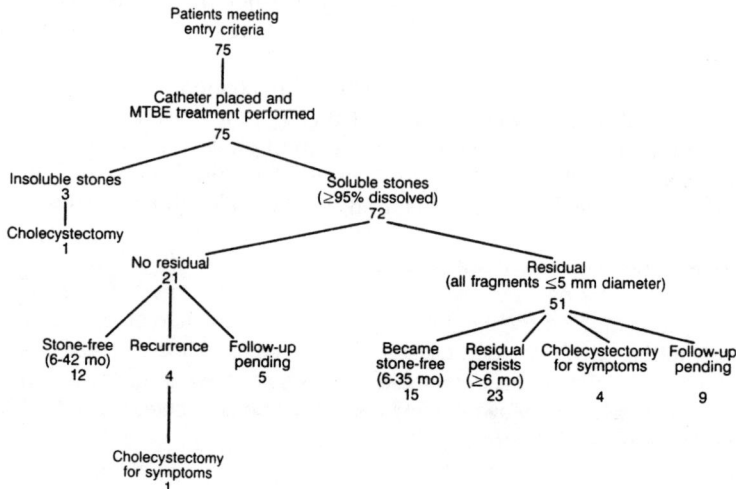

Fig 53-5.—Outcome of treatment with MTBE and initial follow-up of 75 patients entering the study. (Courtesy of Thistle JL, May GR, Bender CE, et al: *N Engl J Med* 320: 633–639, March 9, 1989.)

▶ Currently, there are 4 alternatives to cholecystectomy in patients with cholesterol gallstones:

1. *Expectant management* is indicated for patients with asymptomatic gallstones or with gallstones and gastrointestinal symptoms but not biliary colic (nonspecific pain, dyspepsia, flatulence, etc.).

2. *Treatment with oral dissolution agents such as ursodeoxycholic acid* is indicated for symptomatic, multiple, small (5–10 mm) cholesterol-rich stones, especially floating stones, in patients who wish to avoid cholecystectomy.

3. *Treatment with gallstone lithotripsy followed by oral dissolution therapy with ursodeoxycholic acid or a combination of ursodeoxycholic acid and chenodeoxycholic acid* is indicated for solitary cholesterol gallstones 20 mm or less in diameter or at most 3 stones, none larger than 20 mm, in patients who wish to avoid surgery or who are at higher risk for surgery (see preceding article).

4. *Treatment with MTBE* would seem to have its application for patients with solitary or especially multiple cholesterol gallstones who wish to avoid surgery. However, further study will be necessary to establish the long-term effectiveness of this treatment in the management of the various types of gallstones. As noted in the discussion above on gallstone lithotripsy, a key issue will be the recurrence of gallstones. In this regard, 4 of 21 patients rendered stone free by MTBE treatment had recurrence of stones 6 to 16 months later.—N.J. Greenberger, M.D.

Gallbladder Motility Before and After Extracorporeal Shock-Wave Lithotripsy

Spengler U, Sackmann M, Sauerbruch T, Holl J, Paumgartner G (Univ of Munich,

West Germany)
Gastroenterology 96:860–863, March 1989

Extracorporeal shock-wave lithotripsy (ESWL) of gallbladder stones may cause damage to the tissue of the gallbladder wall that could decrease gallbladder motility. Because ultrasonography is useful in the investigation of gallbladder motility, it was used to assess gallbladder contraction induced by intravenous cholecystokinin before and after ESWL for gallbladder stones in 21 patients with radiolucent gallbladder stones. Twelve patients aged 18–60 years underwent gallbladder motility tests on the day before and the day after ESWL (group A). All 12 patients were receiving oral litholytic therapy that had been initiated 3 weeks before gallbladder motility was assessed. In the other 9 patients, aged 28–64 years, gallbladder motility was assessed the day before ESWL and 212–503 days after ESWL when all stone fragments had completely disappeared (group B). None of these 9 patients were taking oral litholytic therapy. All patients were given intravenous infusions of cholecystokinin to induce gallbladder contractions. Gallbladder volumes were assessed with ultrasonography.

No difference was noted between the fasting gallbladder volumes of patients with gallstones who were not receiving oral bile acid therapy and healthy controls. However, patients with gallstones who were receiving oral litholytic therapy had significantly larger fasting gallbladder volumes than did healthy controls. After cholecystokinin infusion had been initiated, gallbladder contraction was slower and less complete in both groups of patients with gallstones as compared with controls. The difference in gallbladder volume was statistically significant for each measurement taken more than 20 minutes after the start of cholecystokinin infusion.

One day or 1 year after ESWL, gallbladder contractility was similar to pretreatment contractility in both groups of patients. No correlation was found between gallbladder motility and the time required for complete stone disappearance. Thus ESWL does not appear to affect gallbladder motility adversely or damage the gallbladder wall.

▶ Recent studies have suggested that gallstones do recur after initially successful therapy with ESWL and oral dissolution treatment of fragments with agents such as ursodeoxycholic acid. The rate of gallstone recurrence is approximately 10% after 1 year and 16% to 18% after 2 years, with higher rates observed if multiple gallstones were present initially. The reasons for gallstone recurrence are largely unknown. However, it has been suggested that patients with impaired gallbladder motility would be more likely to have recurrent gallstones after successful lithotripsy. The studies of Spengler and co-workers fail to support this hypothesis. Their studies indicate that ESWL has no immediate or long-term effects on gallbladder motility and that the defect of gallbladder motility associated with gallstone disease is not abolished by stone removal.—N.J. Greenberger, M.D.

Gallstone Recurrence After Dissolution

Gallstone Recurrence After Successful Oral Bile Acid Treatment: A 12-Year Follow-Up Study and Evaluation of Long-Term Postdissolution Treatment

Villanova N, Bazzoli F, Taroni F, Frabboni R, Mazzella G, Festi D, Barbara L, Roda E (Univ of Bologna, Italy; Istituto Superiore di Sanita', Rome)
Gastroenterology 97:726–731, September 1989   53-10

Recurrence is a major problem in the medical management of gallstones. To assess the magnitude of recurrence and the efficacy of postdissolution treatment in preventing it, the recurrence rate after 96 confirmed dissolutions in 86 patients during a 12-year period was determined. A low-dose postdissolution treatment—ursodeoxycholic acid (UDCA), 300 mg/day—was given to 36 patients; the remaining 60 received no treatment.

By actuarial life-table analysis, the cumulative proportion of gallstone recurrence in the first year was 12.5%, increasing to 61% at year 11. Postdissolution therapy reduced the frequency of gallstone recurrence, but this was primarily because of its effect on younger patients. The recurrence rate was unaffected by treatment in patients aged more than 50 years. The probability of recurrence was significantly higher in patients with multiple stones before dissolution therapy than in those with solitary stones. No other factor predicted recurrence (Figs 53–6 and 53–7).

▶ The recurrence of gallstones after dissolution treatment alone or lithotripsy plus dissolution therapy remains a vexing problem. The results of this trial, that more than 50% of patients remain stone free after dissolution treatment *without* prophylactic postdissolution treatment, are in accord with the previously reported British-Belgian study (1). In the latter study a recurrence rate of approximately 10% per year for the first 3–5 years with virtually no recurrence thereafter was reported. It is important that the study by Villanova and colleagues indicates a significantly lower probability of gallstone recurrence for patients with *solitary* stones than for those with multiple stones (Figs 53–6 and 53–7). This key finding fits with emerging data from Paumgartner's group suggesting that the recurrence rate after lithotripsy plus ursodeoxycholic acid is lower than that found for ursodeoxycholic acid, and in these studies, a majority of the patients had solitary stones.

The factors predictive of a low recurrence rate after either dissolution treatment alone or lithotripsy plus dissolution therapy are especially important if these therapies are to be cost-effective. Further, it will be necessary to determine whether agents such as aspirin and nonsteroidal anti-inflammatory drugs actually do reduce gallstone recurrence, presumably by interfering with gallbladder production of mucous glycoproteins.—N.J. Greenberger, M.D.

Reference

1. Hood K, Gluson D, Ruppen DC, et al: The British/Belgian gallstone study group's (BBGSC) postdissolution trial. *Gut* 28:1359, 1987 (abstract).

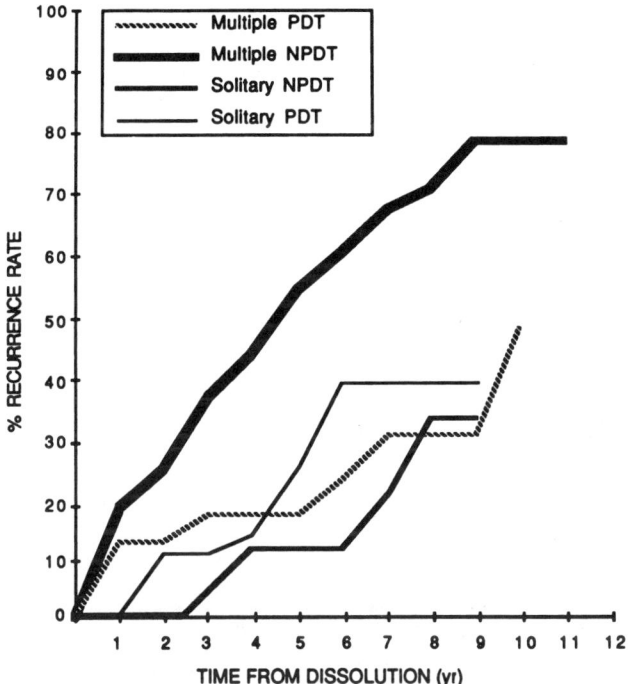

Fig 53-6.—Cumulative proportion of gallstone recurrence by pretreatment gallstone number (multiple vs. solitary stones) and postdissolution treatment with 300 mg/day of ursodeoxycholic acid. (Courtesy of Villanova N, Bazzoli F, Taroni F, et al: *Gastroenterology* 97:726–731, September 1989.)

Percutaneous Cholecystostomy

Percutaneous Cholecystostomy in the Diagnosis and Treatment of Acute Cholecystitis in the High-Risk Patient
Werbel GB, Nahrwold DL, Joehl RJ, Vogelzang RL, Rege RV (Northwestern Univ; VA Lakeside Med Ctr, Chicago)
Arch Surg 124:782–786, July 1989   53-11

Percutaneous cholecystostomy is a bedside procedure that requires only local anesthesia and does not produce significant intraperitoneal adhesions. Twenty-three percutaneous cholecystostomies were performed in 22 high-risk patients who were critically ill and suspected of having acute cholecystitis. All patients received broad-spectrum antibiotics before the procedure.

Acute cholecystitis was accurately diagnosed in 17 cases and ruled out in 5. Cholecystotomy stabilized the condition of 16 of the 17 patients, allowing elective surgery in 8 of them. Eight other patients did not become candidates for surgery. There were no operative deaths in the patients who required surgery. Catheters were dislodged 5 times, and bile leaked 3 times. There was a single duodenal puncture. No deaths were ascribed directly to percutaneous cholecystostomy or to persistent biliary tract disease.

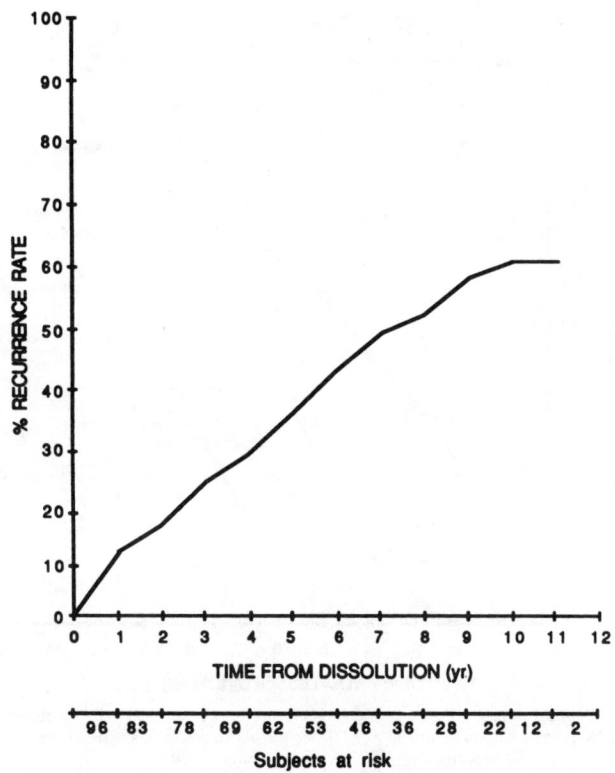

Fig 53–7.—Cumulative proportion of gallstone recurrence rate after 96 occasions of dissolution. (Courtesy of Villanova N, Bazzoli F, Taroni F, et al: *Gastroenterology* 97:726–731, September 1989.)

Percutaneous cholecystostomy is a safe, easily performed procedure that is preferable to abdominal operation in patients suspected of having acute cholecystitis. Critically ill patients should have percutaneous cholecystostomy early. This approach may be most helpful to patients who have acute acalculous cholecystitis, who can be treated definitively without surgery.

▶ The simplicity and effectiveness of percutaneous catheter drainage in treating acute cholecystitis should make it an attractive initial approach to such a complication in the elderly. I like the idea of stabilizing such patients before operative therapy and agree that percutaneous drainage may be definitive in the acalculous state.—F.G. Moody, M.D.

Percutaneous Cholecystostomy: An Alternative to Surgical Cholecystostomy for Acute Cholecystitis?
McGahan JP, Lindfors KK (Univ of California, Davis, Med Ctr, Sacramento)
Radiology 173:481–483, November 1989   53–12

Treating acute cholecystitis can be problematic. Cholecystectomy is the accepted procedure, with cholecystostomy reserved for patients too ill to tolerate cholecystectomy. Emergency surgical cholecystostomy is associated with both fatal and nonfatal complications. Thus, percutaneous cholecystostomy has been proposed as an alternative. The efficacy of this procedure was reviewed for a series of patients.

Emergency percutaneous cholecystostomy, attempted 40 times in 37 hospitalized patients with possible acute cholecystitis, was successful in 39 cases (Fig 53–8). All cholecystostomies were done with ultrasound guidance preferentially using the transhepatic route. All except 4 of the procedures were performed at the patient's bedside. The patients had been in the hospital an average of 27 days before undergoing the procedure. Twenty-two patients (59%) eventually died in the hospital; these deaths were caused by other medical or surgical problems. Only minor complications were associated with percutaneous cholecystostomy: catheter dislodgment without sequelae in 2 patients and significant abdominal pain in another 2. Technical problems occurred twice, including buckling of a guide wire during catheter insertion and a failed attempt at cholecystostomy.

These and other published results are encouraging. Emergency percutaneous cholecystostomy is a safe alternative to emergency surgery for patients with possible acute cholecystitis.

▶ The authors provide further confirmation that bedside percutaneous cholecystostomy is a safe and effective procedure.—F.G. Moody, M.D.

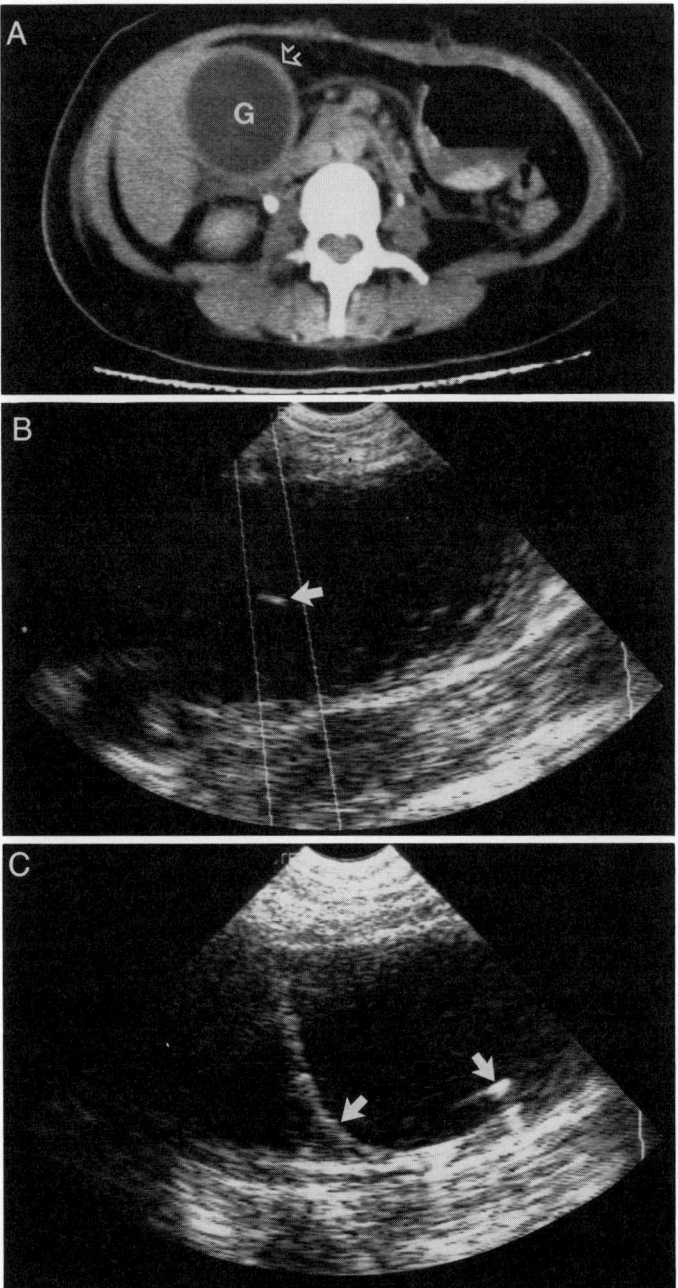

Fig 53–8.—A, CT scan of the upper abdomen demonstrates an enlarged gallbladder (*G*) with a thickened wall (*arrow*). **B,** ultrasonographic scan of cholecystostomy performed with the Seldinger technique demonstrates initial needle puncture (*arrow*). **C,** final position of the cholecystostomy catheter (*arrows*) within the gallbladder. (Courtesy of McGahan JP, Lindfors KK: *Radiology* 173:481–485, November 1989.)

54 Sphincter of Oddi Dysfunction and Sphincterotomy

Transduodenal Sphincteroplasty and Transampullary Septotomy for Primary Sphincter of Oddi Dysfunction
Nussbaum MS, Warner BW, Sax HC, Fischer JE (Univ of Cincinnati)
Am J Surg 157:38–43, January 1989

Sphincter of Oddi dysfunction has been difficult to define and to diagnose accurately. To determine which patients would most benefit from sphincteroplasty, historical, clinical, diagnostic, and follow-up information was reviewed for a consecutive group of 29 patients who had undergone transduodenal sphincteroplasty with transampullary septotomy for symptoms of biliary colic or recurrent pancreatitis attributed to isolated sphincter of Oddi dysfunction between October 1979 and November 1987. Twenty-four of the 29 patients had had endoscopic retrograde cholangiopancreatography.

Surgical outcome was excellent in 9, good in 9, fair in 4, and poor in 7. Fifteen of 20 patients with sphincter fibrosis had an excellent or good result, and only 3 of 9 patients with inflammation or neither inflammation nor fibrosis had an excellent or good outcome. Of the 17 patients with underlying pancreatitis, 7 (41%) had excellent or good outcomes. When performed for biliary symptoms, however, sphincteroplasty resulted in excellent or good outcomes for 92% of patients. Five (63%) of 8 postcholecystectomy patients who had pancreatitis had excellent or good outcomes. Four (80%) of 5 postcholecystectomy patients had good or excellent outcomes when sphincteroplasty was performed for biliary symptoms.

Poor results occurred primarily because of preexisting pancreatitis with continued pain, despite adequate sphincteroplasty and transampullary septotomy. When pancreatitis is associated with obvious stenosis and fibrosis of the sphincter of Oddi, the best results occur in postcholecystectomy patients, although unfavorable outcome can be expected 40% of the time. In contrast with those having pancreatitis, most patients with symptoms of biliary colic or dyskinesia and evidence of ampullary fibrosis can expect to have a favorable outcome from sphincteroplasty and transampullary septotomy.

▶ Nussbaum and colleagues describe their experience with a transduodenal sphincteroplasty that includes enlargement of the ostium of the duct of Wirsung. Patients with obvious fibrosis of the papilla had good outcomes. Those with preexisting pancreatitis were not relieved of pain. This experience mirrors that of my own: patients with chronic episodic pain after cholecystectomy and with stenosing papillitis are likely to have a favorable outcome from sphincteroplasty with septotomy.—F.G. Moody, M.D.

The Efficacy of Endoscopic Sphincterotomy After Cholecystectomy in Patients With Sphincter-of-Oddi Dysfunction
Geenen JE, Hogan WJ, Dodds WJ, Toouli J, Venu RP (Med College of Wisconsin, Milwaukee; St Luke's Hosp, Racine, Wis)
N Engl J Med 320:82–87, Jan 12, 1989   54–2

Upper abdominal pain after cholecystectomy that cannot be explained with conventional diagnostic studies often is attributed to obstructive dysfunction of the sphincter of Oddi. In a prospective, double-blind study of 47 patients who had undergone cholecystectomy and had pain resembling biliary pain and clinical characteristics suggesting biliary obstruction, 23 were assigned randomly to undergo endoscopic sphincterotomy and 24 were assigned to undergo sham sphincterotomy. Manometric examination of the sphincter of Oddi was performed before treatment.

Among the patients with elevated basal sphincter pressures, improvement in pain scores at 1-year follow-up was noted in 10 of 11 patients who underwent sphincterotomy compared with only 3 of 12 patients who underwent the sham procedure. In contrast, clinical improvement was similar regardless of treatment in patients with normal basal sphincter pressure. Twelve symptomatic patients who had undergone sham therapy, including 7 with increased sphincter pressure and 5 with normal sphincter pressure, subsequently underwent sphincterotomy. Forty patients were followed for 4 years. Among the 23 patients with increased sphincter pressures, 10 of the original 11 who underwent sphincterotomy and all of the patients who subsequently underwent sphincterotomy were virtually free of symptoms. Thus, 17 of 18 patients with sphincter of Oddi dysfunction verified by manometry benefited from sphincterotomy (Fig 54–1). In contrast, sphincterotomy was no more beneficial than sham therapy in patients with normal sphincter pressure.

Endoscopic sphincterotomy offers long-term relief of pain in patients with verified sphincter of Oddi dysfunction. Manometric examination of the sphincter of Oddi is useful in determining whether patients thought to have sphincter of Oddi dysfunction will benefit from sphincterotomy.

▶ Symptomatic sphincter of Oddi (SO) dysfunction associated with persistent or intermittent partial common bile duct obstruction may be caused by mechanical narrowing (stenosis) or by abnormal motility (dyskinesia). The 47 patients in this trial (45 women and 2 men) fulfilled the following criteria for SO dysfunction: (1) unexplained pain resembling biliary pain and lasting for more than 6 months after cholecystectomy and (2) either 1 or 2 of 3 objective findings suggesting partial common duct obstruction: (a) common duct dilatation to more than 12 mm as determined with endoscopic retrograde cholangiopancreatography (ERCP); (b) delayed emptying of contrast medium during ERCP; and (c) abnormal liver tests

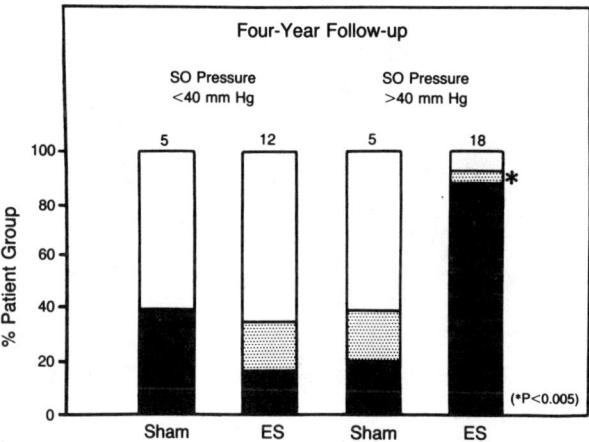

Fig 54-1.—Symptom score (graded good, fair, or poor) at 4-year follow-up after endoscopic sphincterotomy (ES) or the sham procedure, in relation to normal basal sphincter-of-Oddi (SO) pressure (< 40 mm Hg) as compared with elevated basal SO pressure (> 40 mm Hg). Courtesy of Geenen JE, Hogan WJ, Dodds WJ, et al: N Engl J Med 320:82–87, Jan 12, 1989.)

(elevation of concentration of serum alkaline phosphatase and aspartate transaminase to twice their normal levels) documented on at least 2 occasions. Patients in whom ERCP revealed a specific cause of biliary pain (i.e., common bile duct stones, bile duct stricture, or papillary tumor) were excluded, as were patients who fulfilled *all* of the above criteria. The 47 patients remaining were classified as having probable SO dysfunction and underwent manometric studies of the SO. It is interesting that the morphine Prostigmin test, performed for 35 of the 47 patients, yielded positive results for only 7 patients.

The key finding in this study is that 17 of 18 patients with SO dysfunction verified with manometry benefited from sphincterotomy. In patients with normal sphincter pressure, sphincterotomy was no more beneficial than sham therapy. These observations suggest that endoscopic sphincterotomy offers long-term relief of pain in a group of patients with verified SO dysfunction.—N.J. Greenberger, M.D.

Complications of Endoscopic Retrograde Sphincterotomy: Computed Tomographic Evaluation

Kuhlman HE, Fishman EK, Milligan FD, Siegelman SS (Johns Hopkins Med Institutions)
Gastrointest Radiol 14:127–132, 1989   54–3

Complications have been reported to occur in up to 12% of patients who have endoscopic retrograde cholangiopancreatography (ERCP) with sphincterotomy and range from a mild elevation of amylase to hemorrhagic pancreatitis, septic shock, and death. Thirty-six patients had CT evaluation for possible procedure-related complications of sphincterotomy. The sphincterotomies

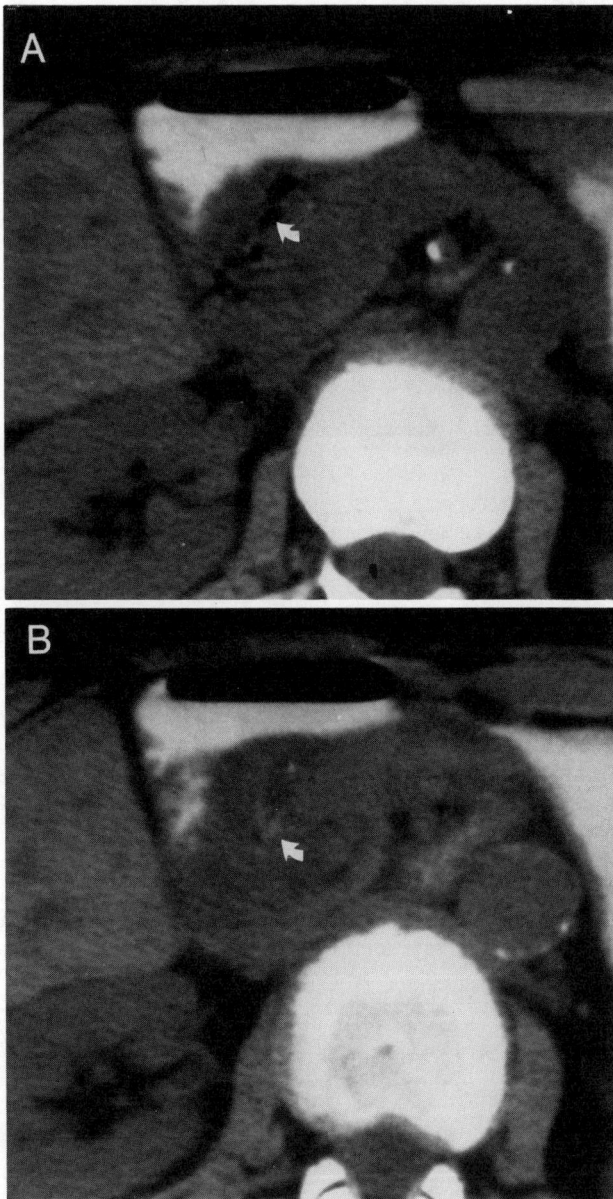

Fig 54-2.—Duodenal perforation after ERCP with sphincterotomy. **A,** air bubbles (*arrow*), and **B,** small amount of contrast (*arrowhead*) have tracked between duodenal wall and pancreatic head after perforation of duodenum at sphincterotomy. Duodenal wall is thickened from adjacent pancreatic inflammation. Patient responded to conservative management and was followed up with serial CT scans. (Courtesy of Kuhlman JE, Fishman EK, Milligan, FD, et al: *Gastrointest Radiol* 14:127–132, 1989.)

	Computed Tomography Findings in 38 Patients With Postsphincterotomy Complications							
	Day							
	1*	2	3	4	5	6	7	Total (%)
Patients examined	19	9	4	1	1		2	36 (100)
CT findings								
Pancreatitis	12	5	2	1	1		2	23 (64)
Duodenal perforation	2	4	4				1	11 (31)
Retroperitoneal dissection of air	1	1	2					4 (11)
Pneumoperitoneum	2	1	1					4 (11)
Air or contrast in biliary tree	15	6	3	1	1		1	27 (75)

*Day 1, initial CT obtained within 24 hours of procedure.
(Courtesy of Kuhlman JE, Fishman EK, Milligan FD, et al: *Gastrointest Radiol* 14:127–132, 1989.)

ranged from 10 to 15 mm in length and the most frequent indications for the procedure were retained common duct stones, recurrent biliary colic or pancreatitis, and papillary stenosis.

Computed tomography demonstrated acute pancreatitis in 23 cases, duodenal perforation in 11, retroperitoneal dissection of air in 4, and pneumoperitoneum in 4 (table). Six patients had both pancreatitis and duodenal perforation. Eight patients with pain after sphincterotomy had normal findings at CT study. Perforation was characterized by pneumoperitoneum, retroperitoneal dissection of air, and localized collections of air between the duodenum and pancreatic head (Fig 54–2). Most perforations occurred posteriorly, behind the pancreatic head or uncinate process.

Conservative management sufficed in all but 2 of the 11 patients with duodenal perforation. In all, 31 patients had conservative treatment with antibiotics, intravenous hydration, and restricted oral intake. Four patients needed surgery.

Computed tomography is the best means of evaluating postspherincterotomy patients suspected of having complications. If the sphincterotomy is too long or is directed too obliquely, and extends beyond the choledochoduodenal junction, the lumina of the duodenum and common bile duct are perforated into the retroperitoneum.

▶ This article emphasizes the frequency and importance of complications related to endoscopic retrograde sphincterotomy. Computed tomography is effective in identifying specific postsphincterotomy abnormalities. Pancreatitis is the most frequently identified complication, but CT is most useful in providing evidence of duodenal perforation or air in the retroperitoneum or biliary tree. Indications for the CT scan included persistent pain, fever, or technical difficulties with the sphincterotomy, which place the patient at risk for perforation. The authors stress the role of conservative management, with improvement by restriction of oral intake and hydration and intravenous antibiotics.—PB Miner, M.D.

Endoscopic Sphincterotomy in 1,000 Consecutive Patients
Vaira D, D'Anna L, Ainley C, Dowsett J, Williams S, Baillie J, Cairns S, Croker J, Salmon P, Cotton P, Russell C, Hatfield A (Middlesex Hosp, London)
Lancet 2:431–434, Aug 19, 1989   54–4

Endoscopic sphincterotomy now is used routinely for the clearance of common bile duct stones. Reported complication rates range from 5% to 20%, and mortality, from 0.3% to 5%. Various techniques have been developed to improve the results, including administration of prophylactic antibiotics, needle-knife sphincterotomy, and a combined percutaneous and endoscopic technique. An attempt was made to determine whether the new techniques have improved the overall outcome of endoscopic sphincterotomy.

During a 5-year study period, endoscopic sphincterotomy was attempted on 1,000 patients with clinical diagnoses of common bile duct stones. The patients ranged in age from 20 to 100 years (mean, 70.6 years). Among the patients, 714 had intact gallbladders and 286 had undergone cholecystectomy. Endoscopic cholangiography demonstrated common bile duct stones in 782 patients and a dilated bile duct without visible stones in 203 patients, but was unsuccessful in the remaining 15 patients, all of whom underwent operation. All patients were given prophylactic antibiotics intravenously before and after sphincterotomy.

Two of the 15 patients operated on died during surgery. Both were elderly, aged 85 and 89 years. Endoscopic sphincterotomy was successful in 975 of the 985 patients (97.5%) in whom it was attempted. The bile duct was cleared at the first attempt in 611 of 772 patients with visible stones in whom sphincterotomy was successful and in an additional 63 of 161 patients at a subsequent attempt after temporary bile duct drainage. Thus the overall success rate of bile duct clearance was 674 (84.5%) of 797 patients with stones (Fig 54–3).

Early complications, which included hemorrhage, cholangitis, pyrexia, acute pancreatitis, and duodenal perforation, occurred in 69 patients (6.9%). Twelve patients died within 30 days of surgery, but 6 deaths were unrelated to the procedure. Thus the mortality associated with endoscopic sphincterotomy was 0.6%.

Endoscopic sphincterotomy is a safe procedure for clearing stones from the bile duct. However, because immediate bile duct clearance is not always achieved, endoscopic bile duct drainage remains an important adjunct.

▶ These results are truly impressive, especially for elderly ill patients. Other reports also have indicated that in such high-risk patients with intact gallbladders and common bile duct stones, endoscopic sphincterotomy alone is sufficient if a cholangiogram reveals gallbladder filling and biliary symptoms are resolved promptly after the procedure (1). However, for patients with nonvisualization of the gallbladder,

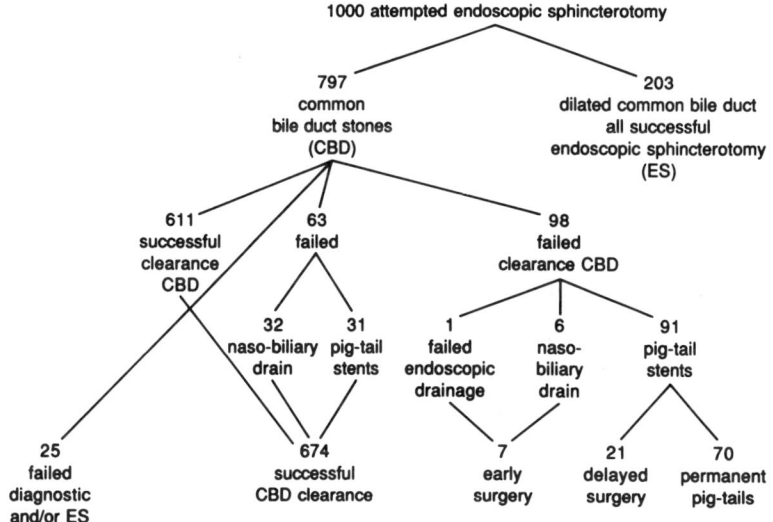

Fig 54-3.—Outcome of attempted endoscopic sphincterotomy in 1,000 patients. (Courtesy of Varia D, D'Anna L, Ainley C, et al: *Lancet* 2:431–434, Aug 19, 1989.)

early cholecystectomy should be considered. Further, as noted by Vaira and colleagues, if prompt bile duct clearance of stone is not achieved, endoscopic bile duct drainage will be an important adjunct.—N.J. Greenberger, M.D.

Reference

1. Worthly CS, Tauli J: Gallbladder non-filling: An indication for cholecystectomy after endoscopic sphincterotomy. *Br J Surg* 75:796, 1988.

55 Bile Duct Problems

Common Duct Stones

Pernasal Catheter Perfusion Without Dissolution Agents Following Endoscopic Sphincterotomy for Common Duct Stones
Martin DF, McGregor JC, Lambert ME, Tweedle DEF (Univ Hosp of South Manchester, Manchester, England)
Br J Surg 76:410–411, April 1989   55–1

Complications are more likely to occur if stones remain after endoscopic sphincterotomy in the common duct. It is not clear whether dissolution agents are required in this setting or whether flushing or drainage per se is effective. Stones remained in 74 of 315 patients after endoscopic sphincterotomy in 1981 through 1985.

A 7F wire-guided pigtail catheter was positioned above the stones in the bile duct and perfused with 2–3 liters of 5% dextrose solution daily for 3–4 days before cholangiography was performed. If stones remained, perfusion continued for 4–7 more days and, if necessary, endoscopic retrograde cholangiopancreatography was repeated with attempted extraction.

Pernasal catheterization succeeded in all patients but 1; however, 16 catheters were dislodged before cholangiography could be done. Two other catheters were blocked, and acute cholangitis developed. Eighteen patients had their ducts cleared of stones. Subsequently 40 patients had stones removed at endoscopic retrograde cholangiopancreatography and 12 underwent surgery.

Pernasal perfusion with a nondissolving solution was effective in one third of the patients in this study when the catheter remained in place. This approach may be effective if single small stones remain in the common duct after endoscopic sphincterotomy. If, however, multiple larger stones are present, dissolution therapy may be preferable. Lithotripsy may offer a less toxic alternative.

▶ The authors address the issue of clearing the bile duct of stones after endoscopic sphincterotomy. Perfusion of the bile duct with 5% dextrose was effective in flushing out small residual stones, but was ineffective with larger stones. Extracorporeal shock-wave lithotripsy appears to be the best way to assist in removing the latter.—F.G. Moody, M.D.

A Multivariate Analysis of Preoperative Risk Factors in Patients With Common Bile Duct Stones: Implications for Treatment

Neoptolemos JP, Shaw DE, Carr-Locke DL (Leicester Royal Infirmary, Leicester, England)
Ann Surg 209:157–161, February 1989

Preoperative risk factors were studied in 240 patients who had surgery alone for common bile duct stones and in 190 others who underwent endoscopic sphincterotomy (ES). Seventy-seven of the latter patients subsequently were operated on. Eighty-three patients had complications after surgery, and in 32 cases these were major.

On univariate analysis an increased risk of postprocedural-postoperative complications was associated with male sex; fever; jaundice; acute cholangitis; high serum levels of urea, creatinine, and bilirubin; and a low serum level of albumin. On multivariate analysis the only factors that predicted postsphincterotomy complications were the serum levels of albumin and bilirubin. In the patient population as a whole postprocedural-postoperative complications were associated with high serum levels of bilirubin and urea.

High-risk patients are reasonably managed with ES alone, but patients who are fit for surgery should not routinely have preoperative ES. Exceptions include patients who have severe acute pancreatitis or acute cholangitis, or both.

▶ Neoptolemas and his associates in Leicester have defined risk factors for either a surgical or an endoscopic approach to choledocholithotomy. It should come as no surprise that the degree of cholestasis and impaired renal or hepatic function were associated with the highest complication rates. The clinical signs of cholangitis are especially ominous.—F.G. Moody, M.D.

Choledochoscopic Electrohydraulic Lithotripsy and Lithotomy for Stones in the Common Bile Duct, Intrahepatic Ducts, and Gallbladder

Yoshimoto H, Ikeda S, Tanaka M, Matsumoto S, Kuroda Y (Fukuoka Univ; Kyushu Univ, Fukuoka, Japan)
Ann Surg 210:576–582, November 1989

A variety of nonsurgical treatments for cholelithiasis exists. Electrohydraulic lithotripsy under direct visual control during choledochoscopy has been used to remove intrahepatic stones. Choledochoscopic electrohydraulic lithotripsy and lithotomy were performed in 40 patients: 16 with choledocholithiasis, 15 with hepatolithiasis, and 9 with cholecystolithiasis.

Percutaneous transhepatic biliary drainage followed by dilatation of the track was established in 31 cases. Stone size, as measured on direct cholangiograms, was greater than 30 mm in diameter in 9 patients, was 20–30 mm in 10, and was 7–20 mm in 21. The stones were removed completely from 38 patients. In 1 patient with hepatolithiasis, small stones deep in inaccessible branches of the intrahepatic duct could not be removed. There were no serious, but some minor, complications, including bleeding from the bile duct mucosa in 4 cases and chills and fever after the procedure in 3.

Choledochoscopic lithotomy with electrohydraulic lithotripsy is an efficient, useful procedure for removing biliary calculi in patients who are poor surgical risks. The success or failure of the technique does not depend on the nature of the stones. Even hard, calcified cholesterol stones can be fragmented.

▶ Access to the biliary tree by a percutaneous transhepatic route has become a standardized, relatively safe procedure. This report demonstrates the effectiveness of bile duct and gallstone removal through the percutaneous tract after fragmentation by electrohydraulic lithotripsy. The large incidence of hepatic stones in the Orient should lead to a continual evolution of this technique.—F.G. Moody, M.D.

Lithotripsy for Bile Duct Stones
Moody FG, Amerson JR, Berci G, Bland KL, Cotton PB, Graham JB, Jones RS, Maher JW, Munson JL, Pennell TC, Way LW (Univ of Texas, Houston; Emory Clinic, Atlanta; Cedars Sinai Med Ctr, Los Angeles; Univ of Florida; Duke Univ; et al)
Am J Surg 158:241–247, September 1989   55–4

The use of extracorporeal shock wave lithotripsy (ESWL) for bile duct stones was first reported in 1986 by Sauerbruch et al. in 1986 from Munich, West Germany. When the early results were encouraging, the multihospital Dornier study was initiated in the United States in 1987. A preliminary report of the first 42 patients in this trial indicated a stone fragmentation rate of 95%; 74% of patients were stone free at discharge.

At the end of the American trial in December 1988 there were 56 participants, including 31 men and 25 women aged 25 to 98 years. Stone fragmentation occurred in 91% of patients and duct clearance occurred in 79%. Adjunctive procedures were used in 54% of patients. Two ESWL treatments were required for fragmentation in 28%.

Complications were mild and relatively infrequent, with hemobilia (8%), gross hematuria (6%), and biliary sepsis (4%) occurring less often than expected. There were no deaths during the 1 to 31 days of hospitalization (mean, 9 days).

No learning curve was apparent in the United States study, and it is likely that the excellent results can be achieved at other centers. The second generation of extracorporeal lithotriptors uses ultrasonographic localization and a dry table; shock waves are delivered through a water bag.

▶ I had the opportunity to monitor this trial and was impressed with the efficacy and safety of the technique. It is important to recognize that the technology employed was the Dormier HMG3 kidney lithotriptor. Stones were targeted radiographically and were removed after fragmentation by transendoscopic extraction in the majority of patients. There was no randomizing curve because at each study site the stones were fragmented by urologists who were part of a bile duct stone team that included a surgeon and a gastroenterologist. The latter likely will become familiar with these techniques and, with the ultrasonographer and invasive radiologist, will be able to manage most bile duct stones without laparotomy.—F.G. Moody, M.D.

Selective ERCP and Preoperative Stone Removal in Bile Duct Surgery
Heinerman PM, Boeckl O, Pimpl W (Landeskrankenanstalten, Salzburg, Austria)
Ann Surg 209:267–272, March 1989   55–5

New diagnostic and therapeutic modalities have brought about many changes in biliary surgery during the last 15 years. For selected patients, preoperative endoscopic retrograde cholangiopancreatography and stone extraction (ERCP-ST EXTR) lowers morbidity and mortality. A series of 728 patients with primary (85.4%) or secondary (14.6%) biliary tract disease who were admitted to 1 institution in a 6-year period were prospectively evaluated.

When a pathologic condition of the bile duct system was suspected in patients scheduled for primary operations, preoperative ERCP was performed; all patients admitted for secondary operations underwent the procedure. Elective cholecystectomy was performed in all patients without excessive surgical risk.

Overall, the complication rate was 6%. Of 78 patients who underwent common duct stone removal, 21.8% had complications. The use of ERCP-ST EXTR reduced the incidence of complications to 2.1%, and retained stone rates were reduced from 2.2% to 0.5%. Patients with secondary stones who were treated only by ERCP-ST EXTR had a morbidity of 2%, a retained stone rate of 0%, and mortality of 0%.

With surgical exploration of the common bile duct, biliary and nonbiliary complications are at least doubled after cholecystectomy. Preoperative stone removal would presumably decrease the risk of complication. Results of this review indicate that endoscopic removal of common bile duct stones before elective cholecystectomy is indeed a means of reducing morbidity and mortality in patients undergoing biliary tract surgery.

▶ The results of this study are quite convincing: preoperative endoscopic clearance appears to lower the morbidity associated with removal of bile duct stones at the time of cholecystectomy. However, the trial was not randomized, and the biases expressed in the institution as to who received which approach are not known. It intuitively makes sense to take care of this complication of gallstones urgently and to remove the gallbladder, if at all, after a normal state of health has returned.—F.G. Moody, M.D.

Endoscopic Sphincterotomy for Bile Duct Stones in Patients With Intact Gallbladders
Hansell DT, Millar MA, Murray WR, Gray GR, Gillespie G (Victoria Infirmary; Western Infirmary, Glasgow, Scotland)

Br J Surg 76:856–858, August 1989   55–6

How often is cholecystectomy necessary after endoscopic sphincterotomy for bile duct stones? The procedure was carried out in 121 patients having intact gallbladders and bile duct stones. Seven patients needed a second endoscopic procedure to achieve adequate sphincterotomy. The patients' median age was 80 years. Where possible, endoscopic retrograde cholangiopancreatography and sphincterotomy were done with intravenous sedation and antibiotic coverage. Attempts were made to remove stones more than 1 cm in size using a Dormia basket or balloon catheter.

The first attempt at stone clearing succeeded in 57 patients. Ninety-three patients in all had their ducts cleared at the first admission. Three patients needed more than 2 endoscopic procedures. Retroperitoneal perforation occurred 3 times. One of 3 patients who sustained hemorrhage died after emergency surgery. Cholangitis developed in 3 patients after sphincterotomy, and in 5 patients, symptomatic pancreatitis occurred for the first time. Of 101 patients followed up for a median of 2 years after sphincterotomy, 76 had remained asymptomatic; 25 had sustained additional biliary tract symptoms. Of these 25 patients, 18, plus 1 asymptomatic patient needed cholecystectomy. Of 7 patients having recurring biliary symptoms, 2 required enlargement of the sphincterotomy. Three patients had recurring cholangitis that necessitated further stone retrieval.

Endoscopic sphincterotomy is an effective approach to treating bile duct stones in patients at high risk, but a significant number will need subsequent cholecystectomy.

▶ This sizable experience with retrograde transendoscopic removal of bile duct stones in the elderly provides a good idea of the limits of this approach. Three patients had hemorrhage, and 1 died. Three had a retroperitoneal perforation; 3, cholangitis; and 5, acute pancreatitis. The gallbladder subsequently was removed from 19. Only 1 death among 101 patients aged more than 80 years is a remarkable achievement.—F.G. Moody, M.D.

Endoscopic Cholangiography and Stone Removal Prior to Cholecystectomy: A More Cost-Effective Approach Than Operative Duct Exploration?
Van Stiegmann G, Pearlman N W, Goff JS, Sun JH, Norton LW (Univ of Colorado; Denver VA Hosps)
Arch Surg 124:787–790, July 1989   55–7

To determine whether it is cost-effective to perform endoscopic cholangiography and remove common bile duct stones before cholecystectomy in patients suspected of having common duct stones, the data were reviewed on 173 patients who had cholecystectomy, including 30 who also had exploration of the common bile duct. Another 31 patients had endoscopic cholangiography and endoscopic stone removal in the same period.

All common duct stones were successfully removed from 87% of the 31 patients who had endoscopy only. Cholecystectomy with common bile duct exploration cost $6,730 more per patient than cholecystectomy alone. If endoscopic cholangiography and stone removal had been done before operation in patients suspected of having choledocholithiasis, 21 of 30 common bile duct explorations could theoretically have been avoided. This would have saved $2,851 per patient who had common bile duct exploration.

Endoscopic cholangiography and stone removal is a cost-effective approach to patients who require cholecystectomy and are suspected of having choledocholithiasis. A prospective comparison will more definitively show how cost-effective this alternative is.

▶ I tend to agree with the authors' conclusion that preoperative endoscopic removal of stones from bile ducts should reduce primarily the cost of a surgical approach to the problem. Whether to remove the gallbladder at a later date is an unsolved problem in my own mind.—F.G. Moody, M.D.

Endoscopic Biliary Therapy Using the Combined Percutaneous and Endoscopic Technique

Dowsett JF, Vaira D, Hatfield ARW, Cairns SR, Polydorou A, Frost R, Croker J, Cotton PB, Russell RCG, Mason RR (Univ College; Middlesex Hosp Med School, London)
Gastroenterology 96:1180–1186, April 1989   55–8

A combined percutaneous transhepatic and endoscopic transpapillary approach was used in 74 patients in whom endoscopy procedures alone had failed but in whom there were contraindications to surgery. Sixty-six patients needed palliation of malignant biliary obstructions (41 common duct, 25 hilar); 6 patients had common bile duct stones and 2 had benign biliary stenosis (Fig 55–1).

Percutaneous transhepatic biliary drainage succeeded in all patients but 1. The bile duct was drained externally for 3.4 days on average before the combined procedure, which succeeded in 53 (80%) of 66 patients with malignant stricture and in 5 (83%) of 6 with common duct stones. Both patients with benign stricture did well.

Procedure-related mortality was 3% in patients with malignant disease and morbidity was 36% in this group. Four patients with hilar strictures needed intervention for probable sepsis in undrained segments. Seven patients had 16 episodes of late stent blockage, and in 3 of them a repeat combined procedure was necessary.

Percutaneous drainage should be done promptly if placement of an endoscopic stent fails, especially when sepsis is suspected. The combined procedure probably should be done in 1 stage, perhaps immediately after endoscopy fails. Central puncture should be avoided.

▶ The combined approach to the intubation of bile duct strictures from above and

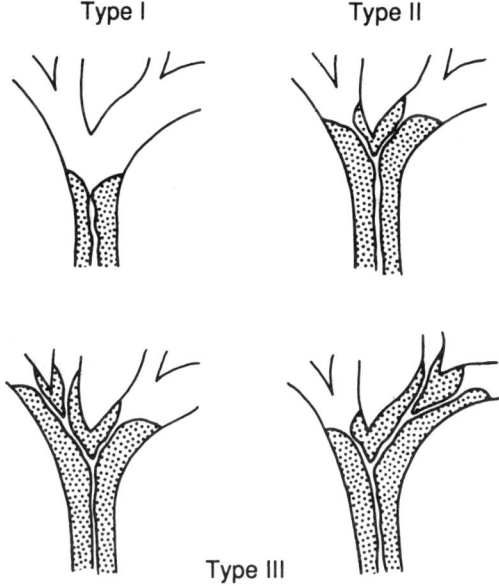

Fig 55-1.—Type I: obstruction of common hepatic duct below confluence; type II: obstruction of confluence so that right and left hepatic ducts do not communicate; type III: similar to type II, but stricture now extends into first-order branches of right or left hepatic ducts, or both. (Courtesy of Dowsett, JF, Vaira D, Hatfield ARW, et al: *Gastroenterology* 96:1180–1186, April 1989.)

below offers an opportunity to place larger stents and to evaluate more effectively the proximal biliary tree. The admonition to use this technique soon after the transpapillary approach fails is well taken.—F.G. Moody, M.D.

Sclerosing Cholangitis

Primary Sclerosing Cholangitis: Natural History, Prognostic Factors and Survival Analysis

Wiesner RH, Grambsch PM, Dickson ER, Ludwig J, MacCarty RL, Hunter EB, Fleming TR, Fisher LD, Beaver SJ, LaRusso NF (Mayo Clinic and Found, Rochester, Minn)
Hepatology 10:430–436, October 1989   55-9

The natural course of primary sclerosing cholangitis (PSC) was studied in 174 patients seen between 1970 and 1984; 137 had symptoms of underlying liver disease. The mean age at diagnosis was 40 years. Seventy-one percent of patients had associated inflammatory bowel disease, most often chronic ulcerative colitis. The mean follow-up was 6 years.

Biochemical findings at the outset were more abnormal in the patients with symptoms. Advanced septal fibrosis or cirrhosis was also significantly more common in these patients.

Fifty-nine patients (34%) died during follow-up. Fifty-one symptomatic patients and 3 without symptoms died of their underlying liver disease (Fig

55–2). Survival declined with increasing histologic stage at entry to the study (Fig 55–3).

During the study symptoms of hepatobiliary disease developed in 22 initially asymptomatic patients (59%). Eleven patients, all with symptoms, later had bile duct carcinoma. Independent predictors of high risk of mortality included age, serum level of bilirubin, blood concentration of hemoglobin, presence or absence of inflammatory bowel disease, and histologic stage of liver biopsy specimen.

Primary sclerosing cholangitis often is a progressive disease, even in patients who are asymptomatic at time of diagnosis. The rate of progression is, however, quite variable. The development of a multivariate statistical survival

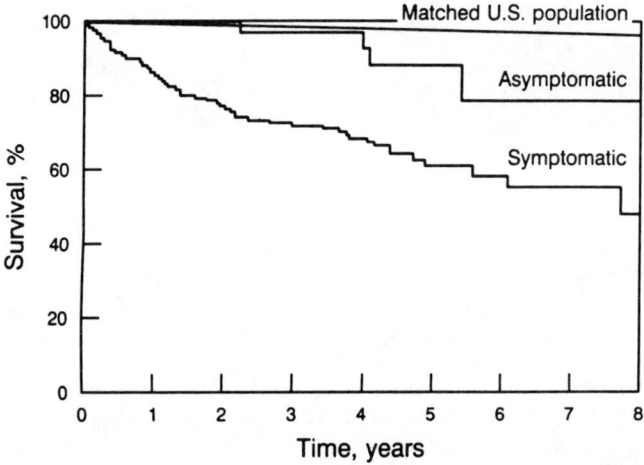

Fig 55–2.—Kaplan-Meier estimated survival curves of asymptomatic and symptomatic patients with PSC. For comparison, survival curve of United States population, matched for age, sex, and race to asymptomatic population, also is shown. For difference in survival: asymptomatic versus control, $P < .0001$; symptomatic versus asymptomatic, $P < .003$. (Courtesy of Weisner RH, Grambsch PM, Dickson ER, et al: *Hepatology* 10:430–436, October 1989.)

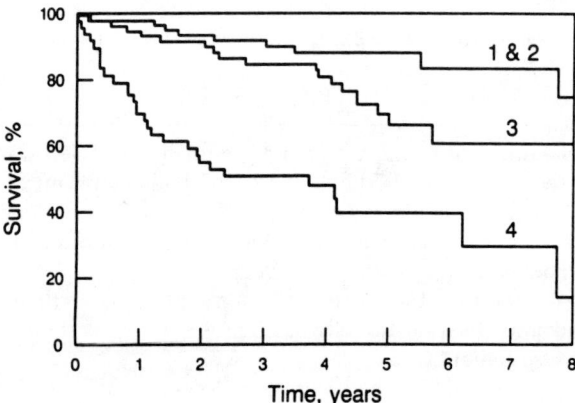

Fig 55–3.—Kaplan-Meier estimated survival by histologic stage on liver biopsy specimen at entry to study. (Courtesy of Weisner RH, Grambsch PM, Dickson ER, et al: *Hepatology* 10:430–436, October 1989.)

model is useful for stratifying patients in therapeutic trials and for planning liver transplantation.

▶ Little data exist as to the effect of inflammatory bowel disease on the presenting symptoms, radiologic features, response to liver transplantation, and potential risk of bile duct carcinoma in persons with primary sclerosing cholangitis. In an effort to answer these questions, Rabinowitz and colleagues (1) studied 66 patients with primary sclerosing cholangitis. The definitive diagnosis of primary sclerosing cholangitis in each was accomplished using cholangiography, which in each case demonstrated characteristic beading, ectasia, and stricturing of the intrahepatic and extrahepatic bile ducts.

Inflammatory bowel disease was present in 47 patients (71.2%). Thirty-nine (59.1%) had ulcerative colitis. In addition, 8 patients (12.1%) had Crohn's colitis, 19 patients (28.8%) had primary sclerosing cholangitis with no inflammatory bowel disease, and 72% of the patients without inflammatory bowel disease had jaundice, pruritus, or fatigue at presentation, compared with 41% of the patients with inflammatory bowel disease. In contrast, abnormal liver function tests were more common as the first manifestation of liver disease in the latter group (38% vs. 11%).

The intrahepatic and extrahepatic bile ducts together were involved more frequently in patients with inflammatory bowel disease than in those without inflammatory bowel disease (81.5% vs. 46.2%). In contrast, the extrahepatic bile ducts alone were involved more frequently in patients without inflammatory bowel disease (38.4% vs. 7.4%). Thirty-eight patients (58%) underwent orthotopic liver transplantation. Rates of 2-year survival after orthotopic liver transplantation for the groups with and without inflammatory bowel disease were 84% and 100%, respectively (NS).

Based on these observations, Rabinowitz and associates conclude that primary sclerosing cholangitis occurring in association with inflammatory bowel disease differs from primary sclerosing cholangitis occurring in the absence of inflammatory bowel disease in terms of its location and sex distribution.—N.J. Greenberger, M.D.

Reference

1. Rabinowitz M, Gavaler JS, Schade RR, et al: Does primary sclerosing cholangitis occurring in association with inflammatory bowel disease differ from that occurring in the absence of inflammatory bowel disease? A study of sixty-six subjects. *Hepatology* 11:7–11,1990

AIDS-Related Cholangiopathies

Radiological Features of AIDS Related Cholangitis
McCarty M, Choudhri AH, Helbert M, Crofton ME (St Mary's Hosp, London)
Clin Radiol 40:582–585, 1989   55–10

Patients with AIDS have been examined with acalculous cholecystitis, distal bile duct strictures, and proximal bile duct changes like those seen in sclerosing cholangitis. Five patients were seen since 1986 having AIDS-related biliary tract disease caused by cryptosporidial infestation. None of the patients had factors predisposing to biliary tract disease. All the patients had diarrhea, and all had right upper quadrant pain, nausea-vomiting, and biochemical evidence of cholestasis at the time of referral. The alkaline phosphatase was consistently increased. No patient was jaundiced at presentation.

All the patients had irregular intrahepatic bile ducts with areas of dilatation and focal strictures (Fig 55–4). Mildly dilated extrahepatic ducts also were a constant finding. Two patients had markedly irregular and thickened common duct walls (Fig 55–5). Two had hyperechoic areas in the periductal regions of the liver. Thickening of the gallbladder wall occurred in 4 cases, and a dilated pancreatic duct was seen in 2 patients (table).

Cryptosporidium produces a severe enteritis in the immunocompromised host, which is difficult to treat. The gallbladder may provide a reservoir for the organism, making it difficult to eradicate from the gut. Biliary tract changes can precede the onset of severe diarrhea in infected patients. Pancreatic duct dilatation might reflect pancreatic involvement instead of obstruction by a stricture. If the diagnosis is made ultrasonically, endoscopic cholangiopancreatography can be avoided.

▶ Cholangitis is increasing in importance in patients with AIDS. Most of the cases of cholangitis are related to cryptosporidial enteritis, although cytomegalovirus can produce similar features. The implications of this study are important not only for

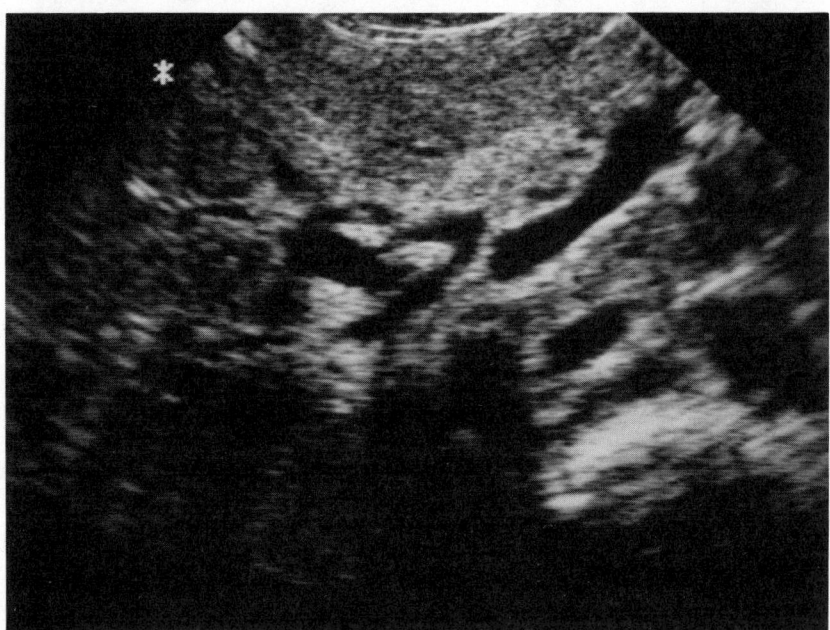

Fig 55–4.—An oblique scan showing the right lobe of the liver. The intrahepatic bile ducts are dilated and irregular with areas of tapering. There is also increased echogenicity in the periductal regions. A similar appearance was seen in the left lobe. (Courtesy of McCarthy M, Choudhri AH, Helbert M, et al: *Clin Radiol* 40:582–585, 1989.)

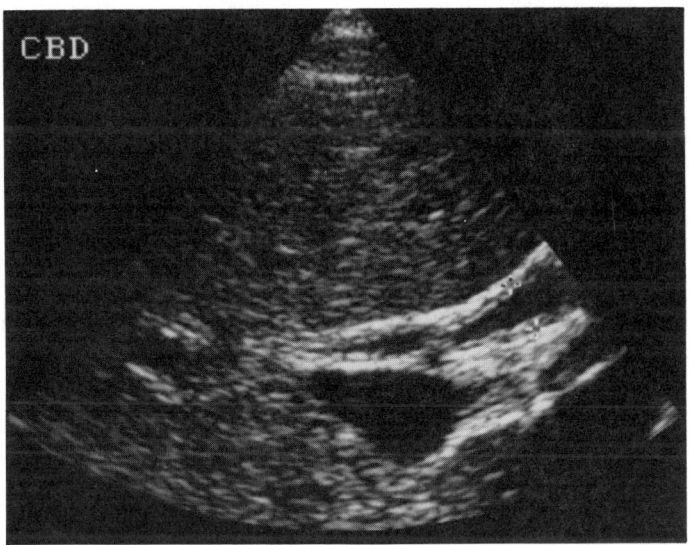

Fig 55–5.—An oblique scan through the common duct showing marked irregular thickening of its wall. The duct is slightly dilated (7.5 m). (Courtesy of McCarthy M, Choudhri AH, Helbert M, et al: *Clin Radiol* 40:582–585, 1989.)

Summary of Ultrasound Findings

Findings	No. of patients
Intrahepatic bile duct dilatation	5
Irregularity & focal strictures of intrahepatic ducts	5
Extrahepatic bile duct dilatation	5
Thickening of gall-bladder wall	4
Thickening and irregularity of common bile duct wall	2
Periductal hyperechoic areas	2
Pancreatic duct dilatation	2

(Courtesy of McCarthy M, Choudhri AH, Helbert M, et al: *Clin Radiol* 40:582–585, 1989.)

patients with AIDS in whom endoscopic retrograde cholangiopancreatography (ERCP) can be avoided, but also for patients in whom cholangitis may be diagnosed or suspected before ERCP: for example, patients with inflammatory bowel disease with suspected sclerosing cholangitis.—P.B. Miner, Jr., M.D.

Acquired Immunodeficiency Syndrome Cholangiopathy: Spectrum of Disease
Cello JP (San Francisco Gen Hosp)
Am J Med 86:539–546, May 1989   55–11

Nine previous patients with AIDS had features of papillary stenosis and sclerosing cholangitis, and another had primary bile duct lymphoma. Sixteen patients with AIDS seen subsequently had clinical and laboratory findings suggestive of biliary tract disease. All of these patients had retrograde cholangiopathy. Twenty-five patients were homosexual men, and 1 was a woman with a history of intravenous drug abuse who was HIV antibody positive.

Twenty patients (77%) had markedly abnormal findings on cholangiography. Sclerosing cholangitis and papillary stenosis occurred together in 10 patients. Eleven patients had an AIDS-associated pathogen or malignancy; cytomegalovirus was most frequent. Ductal dilation was seen on CT scanning or ultrasonography, or both, in 15 of 20 patients in whom abnormalities were found at cholangiography and in 1 of 6 patients in whom no abnormalities were seen at cholangiography. Three patients had long, irregular extrahepatic bile duct strictures.

Many HIV-infected patients may have marked biliary tract abnormalities. Early endoscopy with cholangiography maximizes the chances of detecting anatomical changes and instituting early treatment.

▶ This article is a reminder that profound biliary tract abnormalities may develop in a large number of HIV-infected patients. Although an earlier publication by Cello and his associates (1) reported a favorable response, both clinical and biochemical, to sphincterotomy, the short-term beneficial results were not sustained when the patients were followed for a longer period. Pain relief continued for the 12 patients who underwent sphincterotomy, but serum alkaline phosphatase levels rose. Cello suggests that progressive *intrahepatic* sclerosing cholangitis or diffuse parenchymal liver disease can account for the rising serum alkaline phosphatase levels in these patients.—N.J. Greenberger, M.D.

Reference

1. Schnerderman DJ, Cello JP, Laing FC: Papillary stenosis and sclerosing cholangitis in the acquired immunodeficiency syndrome. Ann Intern Med 106:546–549, 1987.

Bile Duct Strictures and Atresia

Benign Postoperative Biliary Strictures: Operate or Dilate?
Pitt HA, Kaufman SL, Coleman J, White RI, Cameron JL (Johns Hopkins Med Institutions)
Ann Surg 210:417–427, October 1989 55–12

Forty-two patients with benign postoperative biliary strictures had 45 procedures from 1979 through 1987. Three of them had both surgery and balloon dilatation. Twenty-five patients had a Roux–en-Y choledochojejunostomy or hepaticojejunostomy with postoperative transhepatic stenting for a mean of 14 months. Twenty patients had a mean of 4 balloon dilatations and transhepatic stents for a mean of 13 months. The mean follow-up was 57 months for surgery and 59 months for balloon dilatation.

A successful outcome was achieved in 88% of the surgically treated patients and in 55% of those who had balloon dilatation. Three surgically treated patients had recurrent strictures, as did 9 of the patients having balloon dilatation (45%). Significant hemobilia was more frequent after balloon dilatation. The total hospital stay and costs did not differ significantly between the 2 treatment groups. There were no deaths.

Surgical repair of benign postoperative biliary strictures results in fewer problems with cholangitis or jaundice that requires further treatment. Balloon dilatation is, however, an alternative for patients who are at high risk or who are not willing to have further surgery.

▶ The only situation whereby I have found balloon dilatation to be of lasting value in bile duct strictures is that which comprises a biliary-enteric anastomosis. Postoperative strictures should be repaired surgically when identified, except in those patients who pose a formidable operative risk. Delay or procrastination by balloon dilatation poses the risk of biliary cirrhosis and outcome that will lead to foreshortening of a patient's life.—F.G. Moody, M.D.

The Surgery of Biliary Atresia
Lilly JR, Karrer FM, Hall RJ, Stellin GP, Vasquez-Estevez JJ, Greenholz SK, Wanek EA, Schroter GPJ (Univ of Colorado)
Ann Surg 210:289–296, September 1989   55–13

The outcomes of surgery in 131 infants with biliary atresia, seen from 1973 to 1988, were reviewed. Six of the patients did not have biliary reconstruction because of advanced cirrhosis or preference for liver transplantation. The others had all nonpatent extrahepatic bile ducts excised. Biliary drainage was provided by a Roux-en-Y portoenterostomy in 111 infants and by a gallbladder-common duct conduit in 14. A conduit intussusception valve now is incorporated.

Immediate drainage was achieved in 82%. Reoperation restored bile flow in 14 of 18 infants in the first 6 postoperative weeks. Biliary obstruction remained relieved for longer than a year in 57% of patients. Morbidity was, however, substantial. Twenty-one infants with sustained bile flow had clinical signs of portal hypertension. Seventeen patients had antibiotic-resistant cholangitis. Fifty-seven patients were alive at last follow-up; 13 of them had undergone liver transplantation. Sixty-eight of the 125 patients having the Kasai operation died an average of 25 months after surgery. The survivors who have not had transplantation are not "cured," but many have nearly normal or normal liver function and they have grown normally and are active. The average follow-up is 86 months.

When possible the Kasai procedure should be the initial operative approach to biliary atresia. The best results have been reported in infants aged less than 3 months at operation.

▶ There is no doubt that the portoenterostomy biliary enteric anastomosis developed by Kasai for the treatment of biliary atresia was a major advance in therapy for this difficult neonatal disease. One must question, as have many of the transplant surgeons, whether a primary liver transplant at an appropriate age might not be the best therapy except for the unusual patients with accessible and dilated extrahepatic ducts. The authors recommend a Kasai procedure before 3 months of age as the initial approach in spite of a relatively high morbidity and only a 50% long-term survival. It is possible that further evaluation of their experience will offer clear indications for either a Kasai or a primary liver transplant.—F.G. Moody, M.D.

56 Carcinoma of the Gallbladder

Carcinoma of the Gallbladder: The Roswell Park Experience
Silk YN, Douglass HO Jr, Nava HR, Driscoll DL, Tartarian G (Roswell Park Meml Inst, Buffalo)
Ann Surg 210:751–757, December 1989   56–1

Gallbladder carcinoma is the fifth most common tumor of the gastrointestinal tract. The records of 71 patients seen between 1964 and 1986 with histologically proved carcinoma of the gallbladder were reviewed. The mean age of the 17 men and 54 women was 62 years. Four patients had squamous cell cancer rather than adenocarcinoma. Fifty-two patients had invasive or metastatic disease when first seen. In no case was the diagnosis made before surgery. Nine patients had, or had had, a second cancer.

Forty-seven patients initially had cholecystectomy. Most operations were palliative in intent. Forty-four patients (62%) received chemotherapy, and 17 patients received radiation therapy, which was often combined with 5-fluorouracil. Patients given chemotherapy lived somewhat longer than the others, but many variables were uncontrolled. The only factor that consistently influenced survival was stage of disease at diagnosis. Four patients were alive at last analysis.

Early diagnosis remains the key to managing gallbladder cancer. New treatments are needed urgently.

▶ It is fortunate that gallbladder carcinoma is a relatively uncommon disease considering the high incidence of 1 of its risk factors, gallstones. It is unfortunate that it is incurable when discovered during its symptomatic phase. The frequent use of ultrasonography seems not to influence the state of detection. More work on the pathogenesis of this neoplasm must be done because it may increase in its incidence as we leave more gallbladders in place after removal of stones from their lumina.—F.G. Moody, M.D.

The Pancreas

Chapter 57. Physiology and Pathophysiology
Chapter 58. Radiographic Considerations
Chapter 59. Cystic Fibrosis
Chapter 60. Acute Pancreatitis
        Gallstone Pancreatitis
        Severe Acute Pancreatitis and Complications
Chapter 61. Chronic Pancreatitis
        Pancreatitis Stone Protein
        Clinical Studies
        Surgical Therapy
Chapter 62. Pancreatic Neoplasms
        Evaluation of Ca19-9
        Clinical Studies
Chapter 63. Pancreatic Trauma
Chapter 64. Pancreas Transplantation

57 Physiology and Pathophysiology

Comparative Effects of CCK Receptor Antagonists on Rat Pancreatic Secretion In Vivo
Niederau M, Niederau C, Strohmeyer G, Grendell JH (Univ of Düsseldorf, West Germany; San Francisco Gen Hosp; Univ of San Francisco)
Am J Physiol 256:G150–G157, January 1989   57–1

Several new cholecystokinin (CCK) antagonists that are more potent in vitro than proglumide have been studied. The in vivo effects of peptide and nonpeptide antagonists and their relative potency in inhibiting the action of CCK on exocrine pancreatic secretion were studied in anesthetized rats with bile duct cannulation. Secretion was stimulated by intravenous caerulein or secretin, and the antagonists were administered 10 minutes before the agonists.

Increasing doses of 3 peptide and 2 nonpeptide antagonists lowered the caerulein-stimulated secretion of protein and enzymes (Fig 57–1). They did not, however, alter unstimulated or secretin-stimulated secretion, indicating their specificity for the CCK receptor. The order of potency of the antagonists in countering caerulein-stimulated secretion agreed with their potency in antagonizing caerulein-stimulated amylase secretion in vitro (table), and with their affinity to bind to peripheral CCK receptors.

The new CCK receptor antagonists specifically counter CCK-facilitated exocrine pancreatic secretion of protein and enzymes in vivo. The effect is specific for the CCK receptor. Both peptide and non peptide antagonists may have therapeutic value.

▶ Adler and associates (1) have evaluated the effect of atropine and of the cholecystokinin receptor antagonist loxiglumide on feedback regulation of basal pancreatic secretion in 6 healthy volunteers. The intraduodenal instillation of the protease inhibitor camostate reduced enzymatic activities of trypsin and chymotrypsin by 80%. This reduction was accompanied by a strong increase in output of amylase and lipase. The intravenous infusion of atropine completely abolished the stimulatory effect of camostate on enzyme output. The infusion of loxiglumide (10 mg/kg/hr) caused no changes in camostate-induced stimulation of enzyme output. Plasma levels of cholecystokinin were not altered after intraduodenal instillation of camostate whether atropine, loxiglumide, or saline were infused. Adler and colleagues suggest that the protease inhibitor camostate, by inhibition of the enzymatic activity of trypsin and chymotrypsin, interferes with feedback regulation of basal

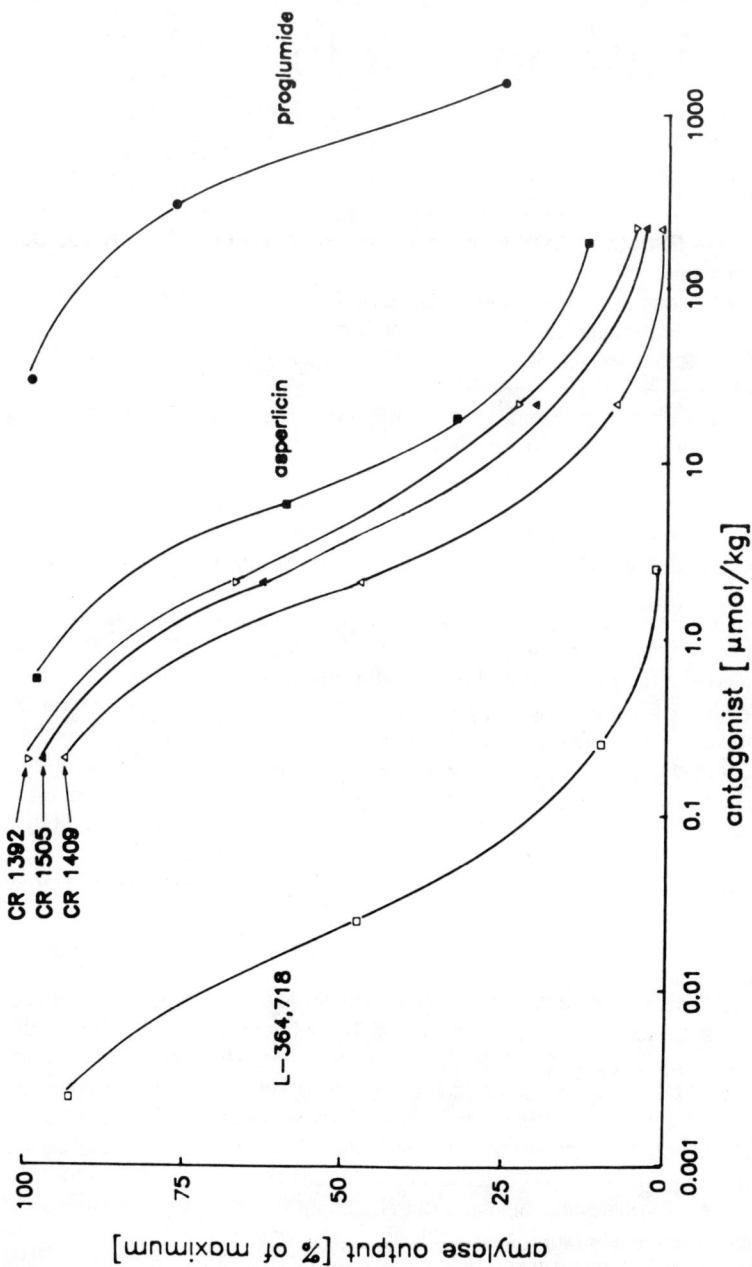

Fig 57-1.—Effects of various antagonists on mean integrated 1-hour response to .25 µg/kg of caerulein. Data are calculated as percentage of response to this caerulein dose in absence of antagonists and are given for amylase output in pancreaticobiliary secretions as mean values for the 4–8 independent experiments. Standard errors are omitted for illustrative reasons and were 1% to 5%. For CR 1409, CR 1505, and CR 1392, 2 µmol/kg or higher doses significantly inhibited mean integrated response to .25 µg/kg of caerulein ($P \leq .05$, analysis of variance) for proglumide only, a dose of 1.5 mmol/kg significantly inhibited mean integrated response ($P \leq .05$). For L364,718, .025 µmol/kg was already sufficient to significantly inhibit mean integrated response ($P \leq .05$): for asperlicin 5.5 µmol/kg or higher doses, significantly inhibited the mean integrated response ($P \leq .05$).

(Courtesy of Neiderau M, Neiderau C, Strohmeyer G, et al: *Am J Physiol* 256:G150–G157, January 1989.)

Potencies of Various CCK Antagonists in Relation to Proglumide

Antagonist	IC_{50}, $\mu mol/kg$	In Vivo Secretion	In Vitro Secretion	In Vitro Binding
Proglumide	740	1	1	1
Asperlicin	11	67	300	600*
CR 1392	9	82	800	1,000
CR 1505	6	123	900	1,000
CR 1409	3	250	2,500	4,000
L364,718	0.025	30,000	1,000,000	3,000,000*

IC_{50}, mean inhibitory concentration.
*In vitro binding data for asperlicin and L364,718 are derived from studies performed in another laboratory (Proc Natl Acad Sci USA 83:4923–4926, 1986) and are included for purpose of comparison.
(Courtesy of Niederau M, Niederau C, Strohmeyer G, et al: Am J Physiol 256:G150–G157, January 1989.)

pancreatic secretion in human beings and that this mechanism is mediated predominantly by the cholinergic system.—N.J. Greenberger, M.D.

Reference

1. Adler G, Reinshagen M, Koop L, et al: Differential effects of atropine and a cholecystokinin receptor antagonist on pancreatic secretion. *Gastroenterology* 96:1158–1164, 1989.

Effect of Alcohol and Alcoholic Beverages on Meal-Stimulated Pancreatic Secretion in Humans

Hajnal F, Flores MC, Radley S, Valenzuela JE (Los Angeles County–Univ of Southern California Med Ctr)
Gastroenterology 98:191–196, January 1990

The effects of an alcohol solution, beer, wine, and gin secretion of pancreatic enzyme after stimulation by a meal were examined and compared with the effects of a glucose solution. Six healthy men participated in the study. The meal-stimulated release of gastrin, cholecystokinin, and trypsin also was studied.

The alcohol solution and all the alcoholic beverages produced similar elevations in blood level of alcohol. Secretion of pancreatic enzyme was significantly less than when glucose solution was administered. Plasma levels of trypsin were unchanged. Wine and beer promoted a higher release of gastrin than glucose solution did. Beer also released significantly more cholecystokinin than when glucose accompanied the meal.

Ingestion of alcohol inhibits secretion of postprandial pancreatic enzyme in normal human beings. A better understanding of what happens in the pancreas under these conditions might shed light on the pathogenic mechanisms of alcoholic pancreatitis.

▶ I would like to recapitulate the major findings in this study:

1. A liquid meal plus a glucose solution resulted in significant stimulation of pancreatic secretion.
2. By contrast, when an alcoholic solution or alcoholic beverages were added to the meal, the pancreatic enzyme secretory response was inhibited.
3. Plasma cholecystokinin (CCK) was increased to similar levels after the meal on all study days except for the study with beer, which caused a higher peak and postprandial CCK response.
4. Significant increments in plasma gastrin were observed on each study day with similar releases after glucose, alcohol, and gin solutions were added and even higher levels after beer or wine was added to the meal.

These studies indicate that *inhibition* of pancreatic enzyme secretion stimulated by a meal eaten by nonalcoholic persons is a common effect of alcohol and alcoholic beverages despite appropriate but variable increases in the release of gastrointestinal peptides such as CCK and gastrin.—N.J. Greenberger, M.D.

Fecal Triglyceride Excretion Is Not Excessive in Pancreatic Insufficiency
Khouri MR, Ng S-N, Huang G, Shiau Y-F (VA Med Ctr, Philadelphia; Univ of Pennsylvania)
Gastroenterology 96:848–852, March 1989

The validity of the neutral fat and split fat stains, the 2-step Sudan stain, in differentiating between disorders of maldigestion and malabsorption is contingent on the premise that patients with maldigestive disorders excrete an excessive amount of fecal triglyceride, whereas patients with disorders of malabsorption excrete an excess amount of fecal fatty acid. The validity of the 2-step Sudan stain in differentiating between maldigestion and malabsorption was assessed in 6 patients with pancreatic insufficiency and 6 normal controls. Fecal triglyceride and fatty acid were measured after extraction and thin-layer chromatographic separation and compared with the 2-step Sudan stain (Fig 57–2).

The fecal triglyceride contents in patients with pancreatic insufficiency did not differ from those in the normal controls. In contrast, the fecal fatty acid content of patients with pancreatic insufficiency was increased fivefold to sixfold over that of controls.

As patients with maldigestion do not excrete an excess of fecal triglycerides, it is not possible to differentiate disorders of maldigestion from malabsorption by quantifying fecal triglyceride and fatty acid. The Sudan stain for split fat alone, however, is sufficient for the detection of fat malabsorption.

▶ The Sudan stain of fecal fat, which involves tests for neutral fat (triglycerides) and split fats (fatty acids), is widely used as a screening test to document the presence of steatorrhea. It also has been used to differentiate between primary *malabsorptive* disorders such as celiac sprue and *maldigestive* disorders such as pancreatic exocrine insufficiency. The study of Khouri clearly demonstrates that patients with maldigestion do not excrete an excess of undigested triglyceride; therefore it is not feasible to differentiate between malabsorption and maldigestion by either qualita-

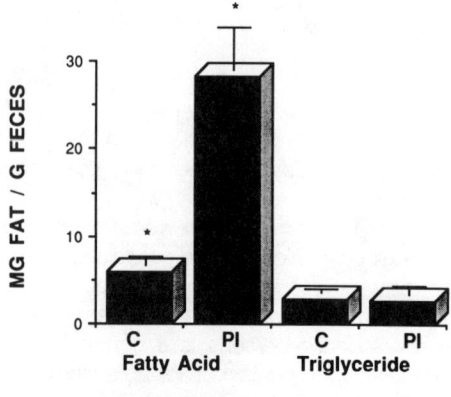

Fig 57-2.—Chemical quantitation of fecal triglyceride and fatty acid in healthy persons, controls (C), and patients with pancreatic insufficiency (PI). The measurement was performed on freshly collected spot fecal samples. There were 6 persons in each group. (Courtesy of Khouri MR, Ng S-N, Huang G, et al: *Gastroenterology* 96:848–852, March 1989.)

tive or quantitative examination of stool specimens for triglycerides or fatty acids. The practical implication is that doing the stains for split fat alone is sufficient as a screening test for steatorrhea.—N.J. Greenberger, M.D.

58 Radiographic Considerations

Prediction of Pancreatic Necrosis by Dynamic Pancreatography
Bradley EL III, Murphy F, Ferguson C (Emory Univ)
Ann Surg 210:495–503, October 1989   58–1

The overall mortality from acute pancreatitis is still 10% to 12%. Eighty percent of the deaths can be attributed to infectious complications occurring late in the disease course. A link recently has been established between the severity of clinical presentation and histologic changes in the pancreas, particularly pancreatic necrosis. The results of a noninvasive technique for measuring the integrity of the pancreatic microcirculation with parenchymal contrast enhancement were reported.

Thirty-seven patients with acute pancreatitis and 5 healthy controls were studied prospectively with intravenous bolus, contrast-enhanced CT, also known as dynamic pancreatography. When there was no pancreatic necrosis, no significant differences in parenchymal enhancement were found among the controls, patients with uncomplicated pancreatitis, patients with pancreatic abscess, or patients with peripancreatic necrosis (Fig 58–1). However, pancreatic parenchymal enhancement was decreased significantly in or absent from all 6 patients with segmental or diffuse pancreatic necrosis. Postcontrast

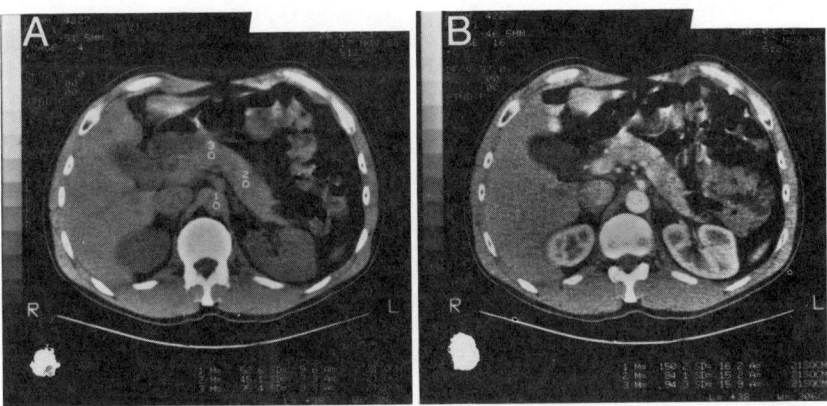

Fig 58–1.—Dynamic pancreatogram in a control patient. **A,** precontrast density is 52.6 Hounsfield units (HU) in the aorta (1M), 45.1 HU in the tail of the pancreas (2M), and 35.4 HU in the body of the pancreas (3M). **B,** rise in corresponding aortic and pancreatic densities and overall enhancement of the pancreatic parenchyma during the dynamic phase (pancreas:aorta ratio, 60%). (Courtesy of Bradley EL III, Murphy F, Ferguson C: *Ann Surg* 210:495–503, October 1989.)

enhancement of pancreatic parenchyma was inversely correlated with the number of Ranson signs.

Pancreatic necrosis is the primary risk factor in the incidence of infectious complications in acute pancreatitis. Necrosis is a principal determinant of outcome. Dynamic pancreatography is a safe, reliable method for distinguishing patients with parenchymal necrosis from those with uncomplicated acute pancreatitis.

► There is no doubt that bolus contrast vascular-enhanced CT imaging of the pancreas provides useful information about acute pancreatitis. Whether such imaging is sufficiently sensitive to detect true pancreatic necrosis will require a larger series than reported here. Furthermore, whether infection precedes or causes pancreatic necrosis must be resolved. It is becoming clear that most of the retroperitoneal debris is not necrotic pancreas but exudate and saponified fat. Computed tomography-guided aspiration cultures have emerged among the most useful diagnostic maneuvers for ascertaining the presence or absence of pancreatic or peripancreatic colonization. Recovery of organisms has become the major indication for surgical intervention.—F.G. Moody, M.D.

Grey Turner's Sign and Cullen's Sign in Acute Pancreatitis
Meyers MA, Feldberg MAM, Oliphant M (State Univ of New York, Stony Brook; Univ of Utrecht, the Netherlands; Crouse-Irving Mem Hosp, Syracuse, NY)
Gastrointest Radiol 14:31–37, 1989   58–2

Cullen's sign of periumbilical staining and Grey Turner's sign of flank discoloration are long recognized as indicating severe acute pancreatitis. Computed tomographic studies were done for 4 patients with acute pancreatitis and cutaneous discoloration of the abdomen. Grey Turner's sign reflects spread from the anterior pararenal space to between the leaves of the posterior renal fascia, and subsequently to the lateral edge of the quadratus lumborum muscle (Fig 58–2). Cullen's sign (Fig 58–3) is secondary to the tracking of freed pancreatic enzymes to the anterior abdominal wall.

Discoloration may be seen 3–7 days after the onset of symptoms. Typically a blue-black color is present at first and fades through greenish and yellowish tints before disappearing. Most affected patients have severe disease and major complications. Flank discoloration is rarely a result of subcutaneous fat necrosis. Cullen's sign has been confused in the literature by attempts to establish a route common to cases of ruptured ectopic pregnancy and acute pancreatitis. Cullen's sign in acute pancreatitis is dependent on dissemination along the falciform ligament.

► This paper illustrates the anatomical path of fluid dissection in the evolution of Cullen's sign with the tracking of pancreatic enzymes to the anterior abdominal wall from the inflamed gastrohepatic ligament and across the falciform ligament. Grey Turner's sign represents fluid spread from the anterior pararenal space to the posterior renal fascia, and subsequently to the lateral edge of the quadrus lumborum

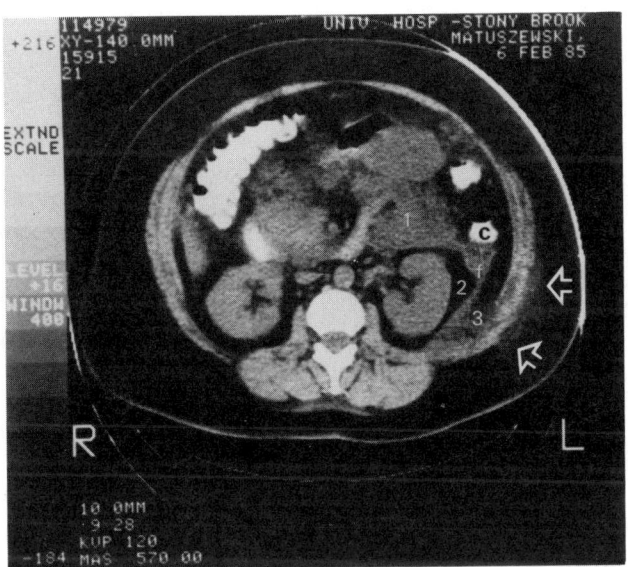

Fig 58–2.—Grey Turner's sign secondary to pancreatitis. Extravasated pancreatic fluid in the left anterior pararenal space (1) dissects between the leaves of the posterior renal fascia with a loculated fluid collection (f) near the descending colon (c). The perirenal space (2) is maintained. Inflammatory changes have reached an adjacent portion of the posterior pararenal space (3) and the subcutaneous tissues in the left flank (arrows) at the clinical site of discoloration. (Courtesy of Meyers MA, Feldberg MAM, Oliphant M: Gastrointest Radiol 14:31–37, 1989.)

muscle. The description of the anatomical pathway illustrated with the CT scan is too complex to explain in a short synopsis, but readers interested in the origin of these 2 physical findings will find a careful review of this paper rewarding.—P.B. Miner, M.D.

The Interpretation of Retrograde Pancreatography in the Elderly
Jones SN, McNeil NI, Lees WR (Middlesex Hosp, London)
Clin Radiol 40:393–396, 1989
58–3

Although endoscopic retrograde pancreatography is considered the most specific means of diagnosing chronic pancreatitis, its relevance for elderly patients is uncertain. Interpreting pancreatograms of the elderly is difficult because of pancreatic atrophy and calcification. Dilation of the main pancreatic duct and formation of cysts also may be incidental findings with elderly persons. Thus the pancreatograms of 101 patients aged 75 years and older who were examined because of suspected biliary or pancreatic disease were studied.

Differences in diameters of the main pancreatic ducts between different pathologic groups were not significant (Fig 58–4). Dilatation of the entire main pancreatic duct was uncommon, with no substantial group differences (Fig 58–5). The side branches were usually normal (Fig 58–6). Only 1 patient with definite chronic pancreatitis had a stone. None of the 4 with acinar

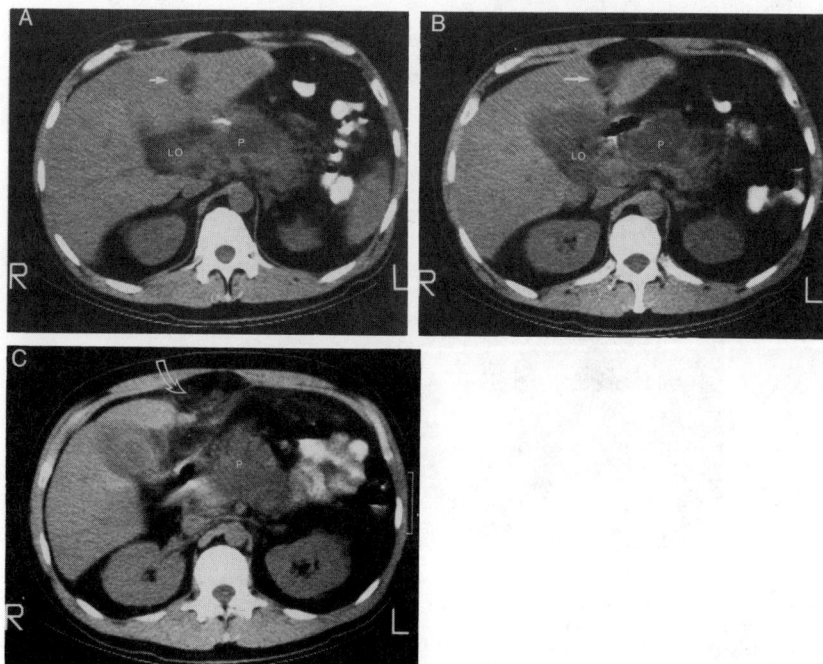

Fig 58-3.—Cullen's sign secondary to spread of pancreatitis along falciform ligament. A-C, inflammatory process of pancreas (P) has extended into the lesser omentum (LO) toward the liver and porta hepatis. There is extension of disease to the ligamentum teres as shown by increased density of fat in region (*white arrow*). Inflammatory densities extend throughout the falciform ligament and involve the properitoneal fat of anterior abdominal wall (*open arrow*) immediately deep to the site of clinical periumbilical discoloration. Inflammatory changes consequent to the pancreatitis also involve the greater omentum lateral to the falciform ligament. Incidentally noted is mural thickening of the gallbladder. (From Meyers MA, Feldberg MAM, Oliphant M: *Gastrointest Radiol* 14:31–37, 1989. Parts A and C Courtesy of Meyers MA, Oliphant M, Berne AS, et al: *Radiology* 163:593–604, 1987.)

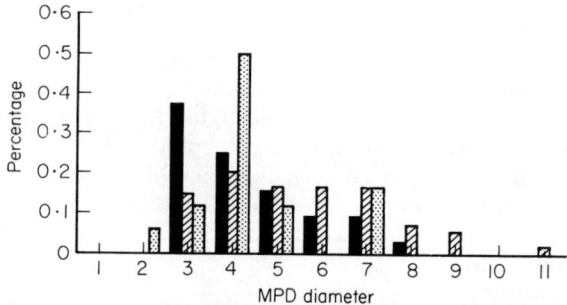

Fig 58-4.—Distribution of main pancreatic duct diameters in the 3 groups. CHD disease = biliary pathology remote from the pancreas. CBD stones = common bile duct stones. Pain ? pancreatic = pain suggestive of a pancreatic cause. *Black column,* CHD disease; *diagonal column,* CBD stones; *dotted column,* pain, ? pancreatic. (Courtesy of Jones SN, McNeil NI, Lees WR: *Clin Radiol* 40: 393–396, 1989.)

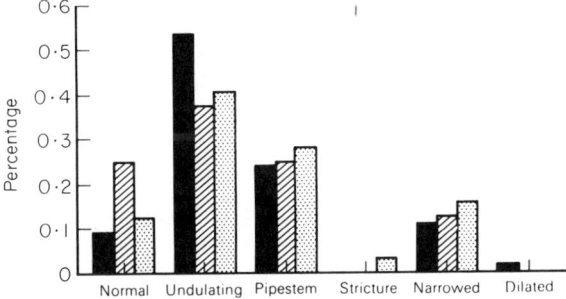

Fig 58-5.—Distribution of main pancreatic duct contour in the 3 groups. CBD stones = common bile duct stones. CHD disease = biliary pathology remote from the pancreas. Pain ? pancreatic = pain suggestive of a pancreatic cause. *Black column,* CBD stones; *diagonal column,* pain; ? pancreatic; *dotted column,* CHD disease. (Courtesy of Jones SN, McNeil NI, Lees WR: *Clin Radiol* 40: 393–396, 1989.)

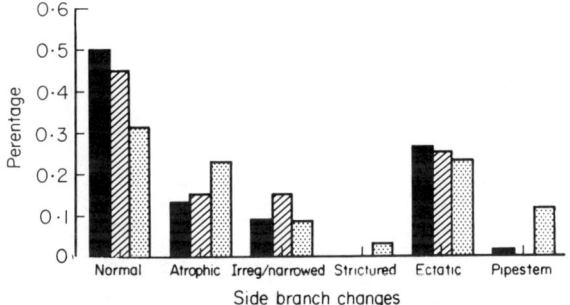

Fig 58-6.—Distribution of side branch changes in the 3 groups. CBD stones = common bile duct stones. Pain ? pancreatic = pain suggestive of a pancreatic cause. CHD disease = biliary pathology remote from the pancreas. *Black column,* CBD stones; *diagonal column,* pain; ? pancreatic; *dotted column,* CHD disease. (Courtesy of Jones SN, McNeil NI, Lees WR: *Clin Radiol* 40: 393–396, 1989.)

calcification had chronic pancreatitis. Two of 13 patients with cavity formation had definite chronic pancreatitis.

Most of the changes in these patients are normal age-related findings. Definite criteria for chronic pancreatitis in elderly persons include duct obstruction by stricture, a grossly irregular main pancreatic duct, and cavities greater than 5 mm.

▶ An age-related decrease in pancreatic weight and enlargement of the main pancreatic duct have been recognized since the 1920s. The authors demonstrate that many of the usual radiographic changes associated with chronic pancreatitis (atrophy, calcification, cavity formations) were absent. The authors found evidence of chronic pancreatitis in only 4 of the 101 cases evaluated. It is unfortunate that the specific tests of pancreatic function were not delineated in this paper, nor is it certain that pancreatic function was normal in the remaining 97. The anatomical changes seen with aging and the association of pancreatic insufficiency with pancreatic atrophy (Abstract 58-4) illustrate the need to correlate pancreatic function with abnormalities on endoscopic retrograde cholangiopancreatography in a formal way.—P.B. Miner, M.D.

CT Demonstration of Pancreatic Atrophy Following Acute Pancreatitis
Magnuson JE, Stephens DH (Mayo Clinic, Rochester, Minn)
J Comp Assist Tomogr 12:1050–1053, Nov–Dec 1988   58-4

Single episodes of uncomplicated acute pancreatitis usually resolve without functional sequelae. Four patients were studied who had pancreatic atrophy after acute pancreatitis, documented with serial CT. Three of the patients ultimately had pancreatic insufficiency. The course of pancreatic atrophy during 6 months of observation is documented in Figure 58-7.

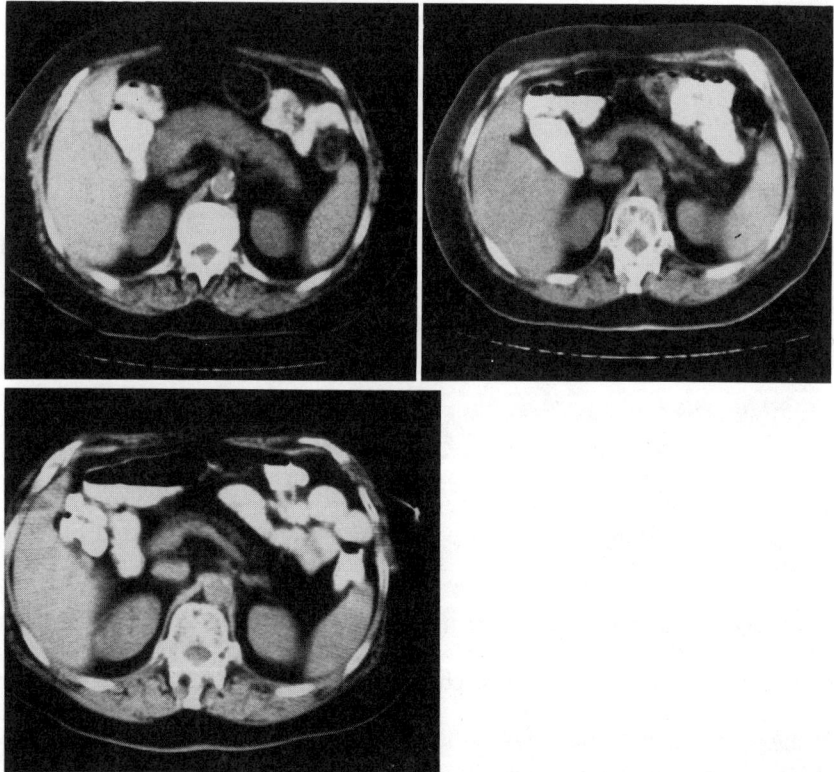

Fig 58-7.—Top left, a 68-year-old woman with elevated urinary amylase and abdominal pain. The pancreas is moderately enlarged. Top right, two months later, marked reduction in the size of the pancreas. Bottom left, 4 months later (6 months after top left photo), further atrophy of the organ. (Courtesy of Magnuson JE, Stephens DH: J Comp Assist Tomogr 12:1050–1053, November–December 1988.)

Progressive glandular destruction and functional insufficiency had been considered hallmarks of chronic, not acute, pancreatitis. Acute pancreatitis complicated by formation of abscesses or pseudocysts can cause permanent anatomical change. None of the 4 patients had an indication of chronic pancreatitis, and 2 patients had causes that do not often produce chronic disease (e.g., biliary stone and penetrating peptic ulcer). In 3 patients CT failed to show peripancreatic fluid during the acute event. Pancreatic integrity usually is maintained when significant extrapancreatic fluid accumulates early in the course of acute pancreatitis.

Acute pancreatitis must be added to the differential diagnosis of pancreatic atrophy, which includes chronic pancreatitis, pancreatic tumor, pancreatic duct stone or stricture, mucoviscidosis, and old age.

➤ It is important to recognize that pancreatic atrophy can follow acute pancreatitis. The pancreatic insufficiency that developed in 3 cases was easily treated with enzyme supplementation.—P.B. Miner, M.D.

59 Cystic Fibrosis

Identification of the Cystic Fibrosis Gene: Genetic Analysis
Kerem B, Rommens JM, Buchanan JA, Markiewicz D, Cox TK, Chakravarti A, Buchwald M, Tsui L-C (Hosp for Sick Children, Toronto; Univ of Pittsburgh)
Science 245:1073–1080, September 8, 1989   59-1

Linkage analysis produces evidence of a single cystic fibrosis (CF) locus on human chromosome 7 (region q31). The number of mutations in CF is probably small, and in Northern European populations, a single mutational event may account for most CF mutations. The clinical subgroups of CF patients—those with and those without pancreatic insufficiency—can be accounted for by different mutations.

About 70% of mutations in patients with CF correspond to a specific deletion of 3 base pairs leading to loss of a phenylalanine residue at amino acid position 508 of the putative gene product. With the polymerase chain reaction technique, 68% of CF chromosomes in a general patient population were found to have the ΔF_{508} mutation. Haplotype data based on DNA markers closely linked to the disease gene locus suggest that the rest of the mutant gene pool consists of multiple, different mutations. About 8% of those mutant alleles may confer residual pancreatic exocrine function.

The available data are most consistent with CF and pancreatic insufficiency being caused by the presence of 2 severe alleles, whereas patients who do not have pancreatic insufficiency carry either a single severe allele or 2 mild alleles. A complete molecular account of all CF mutations could well lead to more effective treatment of the disease.

▶ The successful identification of the CF gene is a dramatic and major breakthrough that will have important clinical implications. The reader is referred to 3 back-to-back articles in Science (1,2) that report the successful isolation and cloning of the defective gene that causes CF. This work should facilitate the development of definitive screening tests for the most common form of the gene, estimated to be carried by approximately 12 million Americans. Further, it offers the ultimate prospect of gene therapy to cure the disease.—N.J. Greenberger, M.D.

References

1. Rommens JM, Iannuzzi MC, Kerem B, et al: Identification of the cystic fibrosis gene: Chromosome walking and jumping. Science 245:1059–1065, Sept 8, 1989.
2. Riorden JR, Rommens JM, Kerem B, et al: Identification of the cystic fibrosis gene: Cloning and characterization of complementary DNA. Science 245:1066–1072, Sept 8, 1989

60 Acute Pancreatitis

Gallstone Pancreatitis

Management of Gallstone Pancreatitis During Pregnancy and the Postpartum Period
Block P, Kelly TR (Northeastern Ohio Univ, Akron)
Surg Gynecol Obstet 168:426–428, May 1989   60–1

Eleven women were pregnant at the time gallstone pancreatitis was diagnosed in 1965 through 1987. Ten others had gallstone pancreatitis within 6 weeks after delivery. During the last 15 years of the study gray-scale ultrasonography was used in diagnosing cholelithiasis in 14 patients.

Management did not differ from that of nonpregnant patients except that conventional roentgenography was avoided. Nineteen patients had elective surgery, but 2 had to be operated on during their episodes of pancreatitis because of worsening symptoms. No patient had recurrent pancreatitis during follow-up for 3 to 5 years.

None of the patients operated on during pregnancy had operative cholangiography. There were no maternal or fetal deaths. All 4 patients in whom pancreatitis developed in the second trimester were operated on uneventfully shortly after symptoms subsided. Four of 5 third-trimester patients did well with conservative management and had surgery in the early postpartum period.

Patients who have gallstone pancreatitis in the first trimester of pregnancy should have conservative management and operations during the second trimester. Those presenting in midpregnancy are operated on when symptoms subside. Third-trimester patients are best operated on early during the postpartum period. Worsening symptoms, however, call for prompt exploration.

▶ Surgeons and their obstetrical colleagues will welcome this report, which supports their current practice. Defer cholecystectomy to the second trimester when confronted with gallstone pancreatitis during pregnancy. Delay cholecystectomy in the third trimester until after parturition unless one's hand is forced. Do not use ionizing radiation (cholangiogram or CT) for imaging. Ultrasound provides all the information you need.—F.G. Moody, M.D.

Severe Acute Pancreatitis and Complications

Surgical Intervention in Severe Acute Pancreatitis: 476 Cases in 20 Years
Kune GA, Brough W (Univ of Melbourne; Repatriation Gen Hosp, Heidelberg, Australia)
Ann R Coll Surg Engl 71:23–27, January 1989   60–2

Physicians continue to disagree about the indications for and correct timing of surgical intervention for severe acute pancreatitis. A large series of patients with acute pancreatitis in the care of 1 surgeon from 1967 to 1986 was reviewed.

In the 20-year period, 476 patients with severe acute pancreatitis had treatment, and 173 underwent surgery. Seventy-seven of the procedures were laparotomies for diagnosis, 7 were for the excision of necrotic pancreatic tissue, and 89 were for complications of pancreatitis. Pancreatic complications included 18 pseudocysts, 53 pancreatic abscesses, 1 large-bowel perforation, 17 cases of persistent obstructive jaundice, and 1 acute hemorrhage into a cyst, causing obstructive jaundice. Fifty patients (11%) died: 38 early in the course of the disease, 2 after total pancreatectomy, and 10 as a result of pancreatic abscess.

▶ Kune and Brough review Kune's experience with severe acute pancreatitis in 476 patients over 2 decades. The 11% mortality attests to the quality of care these patients received. It is possible that in the early years of the study, some patients had exploration because of uncertainty of diagnosis. Modern imaging techniques have almost eliminated this practice, which lends to contamination of the retroperitoneum. The authors report on all of the complications associated with severe pancreatitis except one: pancreatic ascites. The diagnosis of severe pancreatitis, however, is a subjective call, and I would suggest that possibly at least half of the patients had only moderately severe disease if judged with Ranson's or Imnie's signs.—F.G. Moody, M.D.

Automated Selection of High-Risk Patients With Acute Pancreatitis
de Bernardinis M, Violi V, Roncoroni L, Montanari M, Peracchia A (Univ of Parma, Italy)
Crit Care Med 17:318–322, April 1989   60–3

Therapeutic decision making in cases of acute pancreatitis can be difficult, partly because of the lack of criteria available to assess disease severity. Computer-aided management of acute pancreatitis was investigated, and the value of automatic processing of clinical and laboratory features in providing an accurate prediction of severity was determined.

Forty-four patients were studied retrospectively. One hundred six early features were collected and stored in a data base programmed on a microcomputer. On the basis of intraoperative or autopsy findings or clinical course, 16 patients had severe pancreatitis and 28, mild pancreatitis. The frequency of 88 early features was analyzed, and 20 significant differences were identified. Assuming their independence, those variables were used to program a Bayesian prediction of severity.

An additional 47 patients were studied prospectively. All 91 patients were assessed with the early predictive Ranson's signs, and the results were compared with those produced by the computer. In the prospective assessment, the computer was 89.4% accurate, 100% sensitive, and 84.8% specific. Physicians were 65.9% accurate, 71.4% sensitive, and 63.6% specific.

Decisions regarding treatment of patients with acute pancreatitis are difficult because of the many variables involved in clinical judgment. Computer-aided processing of data may provide better guidelines than an unaided clinical estimate.

▶ De Bernardinis and associates use quasi-artificial intelligence to demonstrate that a well-programmed computer can outperform tired and worried physicians in assessing the severity of a complex disease. I found the study to be consistent with our previous experience with the early warning systems that were developed more than a decade ago by the computer group at the LDS Hospital in Salt Lake City. More work of this type and sharing of software are needed. The computer was 100% sensitive (it identified the severity of the illness precisely) and 85% specific (it overdiagnosed 15% of the time). Sounds good to me.—F.G. Moody, M.D.

Direct Retroperitoneal Approach to Necrosis in Severe Acute Pancreatitis
Fagniez P-L, Rotman N, Kracht M (Hôpital Henri Mondor, Créteil, France)
Br J Surg 76:264–267, March 1989   60–4

The appropriate extent of surgery in patients with necrotizing pancreatitis has been widely debated. Some propose extensive pancreatectomy, but others advocate limited débridement of necrosis. Data were reviewed on surgical treatment of 40 patients with a direct retroperitoneal approach in 1981 to 1987. Eighteen patients had had previous surgery through another incision. Ranson's bioclinical and CT scan scoring systems were used to assess the severity of disease.

The retroperitoneal approach involved a left lateral incision just anterior to the 12th rib, permitting direct access to the pancreas and a complete manual exploration of the gland and peripancreatic spaces. All patients but 1 were operated on for infected necrosis. The overall mortality was 33%, but the rate among patients operated on primarily through a direct retroperitoneal approach was 18.2%. Fifty percent of patients had hemorrhage, colon fistula, or necrosis.

The surgical treatment of severe acute pancreatitis through a direct retroperitoneal approach is a relatively safe, simple way to remove necrosis and infected fluid collections. This approach allows the removal of necrosis and several reoperations without the risk of large wound dehiscence. It also does not preclude the extension of the incision to a subcostal incision when needed.

▶ The retroperitoneal approach to the infected, necrotic pancreas has some pluses and some negatives. As pointed out by the authors, it is possible to explore the necrotic retroperitoneum through the lesser sac in this way but with a high morbidity, as was reported. The approach is best reserved for drainage of collections that occur in the left subdiaphragmatic space and paracolic gutter. The same approach can be used for the right. The retroperitoneal approach is best reserved for drainage in the later phases of pancreatitis when the acute inflammation has subsided. Otherwise, a bilateral subcostal incision offers the best approach to the lesser sac. The direct approach offers a safe way to obtain bilateral frank drainage.—F.G. Moody, M.D.

Delayed Débridement and External Drainage of Massive Pancreatic or Peripancreatic Necrosis
Howard JM (Med College of Ohio, Toledo)
Surg Gynecol Obstet 168:25–29, January 1989   60–5

Thirty-six consecutively seen patients aged 27 to 81 years with massive tissue necrosis caused by acute pancreatitis first had treatment without operation. In each case a mass of necrotic tissue bathed in fluid became evident. Unless a life-threatening complication occurred, laparotomy was delayed. In no instance did the "cavitary necrosis" disappear before laparotomy. Laparotomy was avoided in 5 cases in which chronic pseudocysts evolved.

When 31 patients underwent laparotomy, usually after 1 or 2 months, the necrotic tissue was found to be retroperitoneal in every case and clearly demarcated from viable tissue. In most patients the necrotic area was primarily retroperitoneal adipose tissue. In these cases the anatomical definition of the pancreas was impractical.

Diagnosing secondary infection of the necrotic tissue before or during surgery, which consisted of débridement and external drainage, was often difficult. The amount of necrotic tissue often exceeded 1 kg. Secondary explorations and débridement sometimes were needed when initial débridement was incomplete. In only a few cases did necrosis and débridement appear to result in the loss of an appreciable amount of pancreatic tissue. One of the 36 patients died.

Delaying surgical treatment of severe necrotizing pancreatitis allows the recognition of vast amounts of necrotic tissue bathed in fluid. After 1 or 2 months the process essentially is restricted to the retroperitoneum. Dead tissue may be tolerated fairly well for a long time. After a month nonviable tissue usually is demarcated clearly. Complete débridement combined with external pancreatic drainage results in significantly lower mortality than early pancreatic resection.

▶ John Howard again has made a definitive statement about how best to treat necrotizing pancreatitis. Let the process demarcate, and you are left with necrotic fat, a relatively normal pancreas, and a live patient. But it takes time (1–2 months) and patience. The volume of necrotic tissude is impressive. This report should bring forward a strong challenge to early surgical débridement.—F.G. Moody, M.D.

Débridement and Closed Cavity Irrigation for the Treatment of Pancreatic Necrosis

Larvin M, Chalmers AG, Robinson PJ, McMahon MJ (St James's Univ Hosp, Leeds, England)
Br J Surg 76:465–471, May 1989   60–6

The overall mortality from acute pancreatitis in the United Kingdom is still about 10%, although most attacks have a benign course and result in uncomplicated recovery. Serious complications often result from necrosis of parts of the gland or adjacent tissues. Recurrent necrosis and sepsis are a problem in many patients after necrotic tissue initially is removed, and traditional methods of drainage appear to be inadequate to prevent it.

Fourteen patients aged 17 to 77 years had pancreatic and peripancreatic débridement combined with a closed cavity system of drainage (Fig 60–1). Intravenous contrast-enhanced CT or incremental dynamic CT angiography was used to accurately detect and localize necrotic tissue.

In 9 patients a retrocolic route of access was used. Purpose-made silicone elastomer tubes with an outside diameter of 20 mm were placed so that drainage was assisted by gravity when patients were supine. Cavities were irrigated with saline, initially 2 L daily. In the last 7 patients Trasylol was included in the irrigation fluid for the first week after surgery. The drainage tubes were removed when contrast studies showed cavities to be small and superficial. Drainage lasted a median of 28 days.

Sinograms showed fistulas between the cavity and small bowel in 4 patients

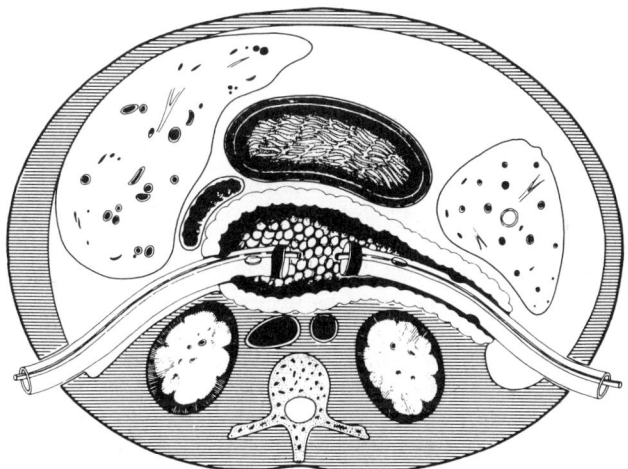

Fig 60–1.—Transverse section of drains in situ. Side holes were fashioned as shown if cavity was extensive. (Courtesy of Larvin M, Chalmers AG, Robinson PJ, et al: *Br J Surg* 76:465–471, May 1989.)

and small bowel and colon in 2, but there were no clinical problems and all closed spontaneously. Two patients had planned reoperations. Three elderly patients died, but all those aged less than 68 years survived.

Closed drainage may be as effective as methods of marsupialization and obviates the need for frequent relaparotomy. Although mortality in this series was 21%, all 3 patients who died were aged more than 65 years, and the youngest was chonically ill with multiorgan failure.

▶ Closed drainage with irrigation of the retroperitoneum after surgical débridement of pancreatic necrosis makes sense. However, the mortality (21%) was high in this series, suggesting that the technique is not as good as the authors surmise. I do not see how antiproteolytic agents in the perfusate can help. It is possible they made the physicians treating the patient feel better. A large number of patients would be required for a trial to show efficacy of such therapy.—F.G. Moody, M.D.

Percutaneous Drainage of Infected and Noninfected Pancreatic Pseudocysts: Experience in 101 Cases

van Sonnenberg E, Wittich GR, Casola G, Brannigan TC, Karnel F, Stabile BE, Varney RR, Christensen RR (Univ of California, San Diego; Univ of Vienna)
Radiology 170:757–761, March 1989   60-7

Percutaneous drainage of pancreatic pseudocysts remains controversial. Of 101 pseudocysts in 77 patients that were drained, most were drained because of fever and sepsis or pain. Those cysts suspected of being infected were drained on an emerency basis. In most cases, drainage was done under CT guidance; ultrasound guidance was used in a few cases. Most often a fine-needle localization, tandem trocar catheter-insertion technique was used.

Drainage was successful in treating 91 of the 101 pseudocysts; surgery was avoided in these cases. Forty-eight of 51 infected lesions were successfully drained. In 2 instances, drainage was protracted; the mean duration was 20 days. In 7 patients, there was spontaneous fistulization of the pseudocyst to the gastrointestinal tract, most often the stomach. Ten patients (13%) had complications, and 4 had major complications, most often bacterial superinfection of a previously uninfected pseudocyst.

Percutaneous catheter drainage is an effective approach to treating pancreatic pseudocysts. Infected pseudocysts are cured as often as abscesses at other abdominal sites. Drainage will likely become the preferred procedure for most pancreatic pseudocysts. Success is independent of the access route used. In some cases, multiple catheters may be necessary.

▶ Diagnostic percutaneous aspiration of pancreatic pseudocysts is useful in distinguishing between the infected and noninfective pseudocysts. This paper defines a role for percutaneous drainage as treatment of pseudocysts. Prior failure of percutaneous pseudocyst drainage was caused by insufficient duration of catheter placement. The average duration of drainage in these patients was 19.6 days. Catheters were left in place until the drainage ceased and fistulas had disappeared.

Grosso and colleagues (1) had success with internal transgastric drainage. These 2 studies emphasize that pseudocyst drainage should be prolonged and can be done with either percutaneous or internal drainage placed via radiographic means.—P.B. Miner, M.D.

Reference

1. Grosso M et al: *Radiology* 173:493, 1989.

61 Chronic Pancreatitis

Pancreatitis Stone Protein

Secretory Pancreatic Stone Protein Messenger RNA: Nucleotide Sequence and Expression in Chronic Calcifying Pancreatitis
Giorgi D, Bernard J-P, Rouquier S, Iovanna J, Sarles H, Dagorn J-C (Inst Natl de la Santé et de la Recherche Médicale, Marseille, France)
J Clin Invest 84:100–106, July 1989

Secretory pancreatic stone protein (PSP-S) is a glycoprotein secreted by the pancreas that is immunologically identical to the major protein component of calculi from patients with chronic calcifying pancreatitis (CCP). Secretory pancreatic stone protein comprises 10% to 14% of normal pancreatic juice and may function to inhibit crystallization of $CaCO_3$, in which normal pancreatic secretion is supersaturated. To better understand the function of this protein, an attempt was made to clone and sequence the messenger RNA (mRNA) for PSP-S and to investigate its expression in patients with CCP. Cadaver kidney transplant donors or patients with obstructive pancreatitis without calcifications served as controls.

A complementary DNA library from human pancreas was probed with a mixed oligonucleotide whose sequence was derived from the partial amino acid sequence of PSP. A clone that encodes a preprotein of 166 amino acids was selected and sequenced. Homology between the nucleotide sequence of PSP-S mRNA was found to several serine proteases, including trypsinogen, bovine chymotrypsinogen, and plasmatic kallikrein. Dot blot hybridizations were performed on total RNA extracted from pancreatic tissue from 5 patients with CCP and 7 controls. Significantly less PSP-S mRNA (388 ± 70 OD_{492} units per µg total RNA) was found in persons with CCP than in controls ($1{,}167 \pm 187$ OD_{492} units per µg total RNA), although no significant differences between the groups were found in the levels of expression of trypsinogen, chymotrypsinogen, or colipase mRNAs (Fig 61–1).

This work achieved the cloning and sequencing of mRNA for PSP-S mRNA. This mRNA was found much reduced in concentration in patients with CCP. This is consistent with a previous report that CCP juice contains decreased levels of PSP-S. Although these findings do not establish whether reduced expression of PSP-S is primary or secondary to CCP, they suggest that altered expression confers predisposition to the disease.

▶ Human pancreatic juice contains approximately 20 major protein components, most of which have been well characterized. For example, secretory proteins include zymogens such as trypsinogen and chymotrypsinogen, enzymes such as

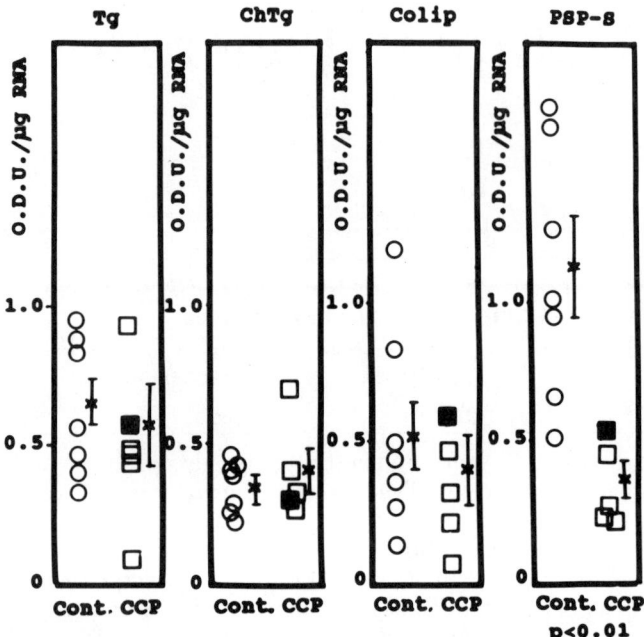

Fig 61-1.—Messenger RNA concentrations of trypsinogen, chymotrypsinogen, colipase, and PSP-S in the pancreases of CCP patients and in controls. Messenger RNA concentrations were measured by dot-blot hybridization of equal amounts of RNA from control (*Cont.*) or CCP tissues (*CCP*) to ^{32}P-labeled cDNA probes. They were expressed as arbitrary OD$_{492}$ units per µg of RNA obtained after scanning the autoradiograms of the blots. *Circles,* individual data controls; *open squares,* individual data CCP patients, respectively; ×, mean values (±SE) for each group. *Shaded squares* in the CCP groups, the patient presenting with a mild form of the disease. The significance of the difference in PSP-S mRNA concentration between controls and CCP patients was estimated by Wilcoxon test. (Courtesy of Giorgi D, Bernard J-P, Rouquier S, et al: *J Clin Invest* 84:100–106, July 1989.)

lipase and amylase, enzyme cofactors such as colipase, and inhibitors such as trypsin inhibitor, all of which are directly involved in the digestive process. Recently, Montalto Giorgi, Caro Sarles, and their associates reported the presence in human pancreas of a polymorphic glycoprotein, that is, PSP-S, without any recognized enzymatic activity. Evidence that PSP-S plays a role in the exocrine function of the pancreas is being accumulated. Normal pancreatic juice is supersaturated with $CaCO_3$ (1), and PSP-S has been shown to inhibit $CaCO_3$ crystal growth. Further, it has been shown that the concentration of PSP-S in pancreatic juice is decreased in patients with chronic calcific pancreatitis (3). These observations have led to the hypotheses that the physiologic role of PSP-S is to prevent the formation of stones and proteinaceous plugs in pancreatic juice and that a deficiency of PSP-S facilitates the development of pancreatic calculi.

This elegant study by Giorgi and co-workers provides further support for their concept that altered PSP-S gene expression predisposes to the development of chronic calcific pancreatitis. However, whether decreased PSP-S gene expression is *primary* or *secondary* to chronic pancreatic disease remains uncertain and awaits further study.—N.J. Greenberger, M.D.

References

1. Moore EW, Vérine HJ: Pathogenesis of pancreatic and biliary $CaCO_3$ lithiasis: The solubility product K¢sp) of calcite determined with the Ca++ electrode. *J Lab Clin Med* 106:611–618, December 1985.
2. Multigner LH, De Caro A: Pancreatic stone protein: Kinetic studies on calcium carbonate crystal growth inhibition by human pancreatic stone protein. *Digestion* 38:43–44, 1985.
3. Multigner LH, Sarles H, Lombardo D, et al: Pancreatic stone protein: II. Implication in stone formation during the cause of chronic calcifying pancreatitis. *Gastroenterology* 89:387–391, August 1985.

Clinical Studies

Mortality Factors Associated With Chronic Pancreatitis: Unidimensional and Multidimensional Analysis of a Medical-Surgical Series of 240 Patients
Levy P, Milan C, Pignon JP, Baetz A, Bernades P (Hôpital Beaujon, Clichy; Faculté de Medecine, Dijon; Hôpital Antoine Béclère, Clamart, France)
Gastroenterology 96:1165–1172, April 1989   61-2

Only 1 study, with a small number of patients and limited follow-up, has compared the mortality of patients with chronic pancreatitis with that of a matched reference population. The frequency and cause of death in a large series of patients with chronic pancreatitis, the cumulative survival rates of those patients corrected by comparing them with a matched population, and the factors associated with mortality were investigated using unidimensional and multidimensional analyses.

Two hundred forty patients were followed up for a mean 8.7 years. Of 32 women and 208 men, 210 were alcoholic and 30 were nonalcoholic. Chronic pancreatitis had begun at a mean age of 41.5 years. Fifty-seven patients died at a mean age of 52.3 years. "Overmortality" after 20 years was 35.8% compared with the matched reference population. Chronic pancreatitis directly caused the deaths of only 19.3% of the patients. The main causes of death were alcoholic hepatopathy, cancer, and postoperative complications.

Variables associated with mortality were male sex, surgery, hepatopathy, diabetes mellitus, and absence of attack of acute pancreatitis, according to unidimensional analysis. Multidimensional analysis showed that surgery, hepatopathy, no attack of acute pancreatitis, and male sex were associated with mortality in the overall patient population; when patients with cirrhosis were excluded, surgery, male sex, and diabetes mellitus were associated with mortality. However, surgery did not appear to interfere with long-term death rates. The lower death rate among patients with attacks of acute pancreatitis suggests a favorable influence for alcohol abstinence.

▶ Chronic pancreatitis shortens life expectancy as a consequence of liver disease and diabetes. Surgery and cancer each played a significant role in the overmortality in comparison with a reference control. The mean age of onset of chronic pancreatitis (42 years) seems greater than what would be experienced in the United States.

It is of interest that only 19% of deaths were attributed directly to the disease in contradistinction to acute necrotizing pancreatitis.—F.G. Moody, M.D.

Pseudocysts in Chronic Pancreatitis: Surgical Results in 102 Consecutive Patients
Kiviluoto T, Kivisaari L, Kivilaakso E, Lempinen M (Helsinki Univ Central Hosp)
Arch Surg 124:240–243, February 1989   61–3

Data for 102 consecutively seen patients with pancreatic pseudocysts were reviewed to analyze preoperative symptoms, diagnoses, and postoperative outcomes. The mean age of the 81 men and 21 women was 39 years.

The most common preoperative symptoms were upper epigastric pain, loss of weight, obstructive jaundice, and sudden arterial bleeding from the pseudocyst. The most useful diagnostic tools in evaluating the presence, size, location, and possible pancreatic ductal communications of the pseudocyst were ultrasonography, CT, and endoscopic retrograde cholangiopancreatography.

In patients with a single thick-walled pseudocyst, internal drainage produced the best long-term results. Pancreatic resection was used in patients who already had diabetes or multiple pseudocysts or if a pseudocyst was not amenable to internal drainage. The most serious preoperative complication was sudden arterial bleeding from a pseudocyst. Hemostasis with transcystic arterial ligation and external drainage of the pseudocyst produced the best results in these cases.

Hospital mortality was 7%. Fourteen (19%) of 75 reexamined patients were unable to work because of symptoms attributable to chronic pancreatitis.

Factors to be considered when suitable surgical treatment for pancreatic pseudocysts in chronic pancreatitis is being determined include the patient's general condition; the pancreatic endocrine and exocrine functional capacity; and the site, number, and possible complications of the pseudocysts.

▶ The surgeons at the Helsinki University Central Hospital provide an overview of their experience with pseudocysts in chronic pancreatitis. I agree with their general tenet: resect if the cysts are multiple or not amenable to internal drainage.—F.G. Moody, M.D.

Biliary Tract Dilatation in Chronic Pancreatitis: CT and Sonographic Findings
Huntington DK, Hill MC, Steinberg W (George Washington Univ Med Ctr, Washington, DC)
Radiology 172:47–50, July 1989   61–4

The features of chronic pancreatitis associated with biliary tract dilatation were examined in 30 male and 14 female patients with an average age of 47 years, who were seen between 1983 and 1988. All but 3 patients had histories of alcohol abuse. Twenty-three patients had follow-up CT or sonography, the average time to the last study averaging 16 months.

Twenty-four patients had biliary tract dilatation. Of these, 88% had pancreatic calcifications and 75% had a focal mass in the pancreatic head. Twelve of 16 patients who were followed up had no change in the degree of biliary tract dilatation or the appearance of the pancreas. There was no consistent relationship between serum alkaline phosphatase and bilirubin levels and the radiologic findings at follow-up.

About half of the patients with chronic pancreatitis may have biliary tract dilatation that persists. If the disease is moderate or severe in degree, liver biopsy should be considered. A biliary-enteric bypass procedure may be helpful if the biopsy specimen shows cholestasis or biliary cirrhosis.

▶ Compression of the intrapancreatic portion of the common bile duct by pancreatic inflammation is well recognized. This study was not only an evaluation of the frequency of biliary tract dilatation in chronic pancreatitis, but an attempt to assess the natural history as well. As may be expected, a patient with a mass in the pancreatic head (generally calcified) and dilatation of the pancreatic duct was more likely to have bile duct dilatation. The continued dilatation of the bile duct in 75% of patients in conjunction with abnormal liver tests emphasizes the importance of recognizing common bile duct obstruction to monitor liver injury and decide whether bypass surgery may be needed.—P.B. Miner, M.D.

Surgical Therapy

Treatment of Chronic Alcoholic Pancreatitis by Pancreatic Resection
Keith RG, Saibil FG, Sheppard RH (Univ of Toronto)
Am J Surg 157:156–162, January 1989   61–5

Although pancreatic duct decompression is a widely accepted treatment for painful chronic pancreatitis when the ducts are diffusely dilated, the appropriate surgical management of painful chronic pancreatitis in patients with stenotic pancreatic ducts is still controversial. The long-term results of resective procedures for selected patients with chronic pancreatitis caused by alcoholism in whom pancreatography demonstrated stenotic pancreatic duct abnormalities precluding decompressive procedures were reviewed.

Forty-one patients underwent resective surgery. Five had Whipple resections, 32 had 80% resections, and 7 had total pancreatectomies. Mortality was 10%, with 1 perioperative and 3 late deaths. On long-term follow-up, complete freedom from pain was reported by all of the patients who had total pancreatectomy, half of those who had 80% resection, and only 1 of 5 patients who had Whipple resection. Diabetes occurred in 1 patient who had Whipple resection, almost half of those who underwent 80% pancreatectomy, and in all those who had total resection. In the last group, diabetes frequently was complicated by recurrent alcoholism. Jaundice was a rare complication of disease progression; none of the patients had cholestasis preoperatively.

Recurrent alcoholism was reported in 32% and contributed to 2 deaths.

Recurrent alcoholism is a serious risk in this population, with devastating effects on treatment outcome.

▶ There appears to be no ideal operation for the pain of chronic pancreatitis, especially when the main pancreatic duct is small and not suitable for a pancreaticojejunostomy. Resection unfortunately is associated with a high incidence of diabetes, which in association with alcoholism leads to a high mortality in late follow-up. I favor a procedure that preserves as much pancreas as possible and leaves the duodenum in place, a so-called ventral-dorsal pancreatic disconnection with denervation. Because no procedure guarantees a pain-free state (except total pancreatectomy in this report), one should preserve as much islet cell function as possible; it is the combination of insulin-requiring diabetes and alcoholism that kills those operated on and not the pain that was the indication.—F.G. Moody, M.D.

Severe Chronic Cephalic Pancreatitis: Use of Partial Duodenopancreatectomy With Occlusion of the Pancreatic Duct in 289 Patients
Gall FP, Gebhardt C, Meister R, Zirngibl H, Schneider MU (Friedrich-Alexander-Univ of Erlangen-Nuremberg, Erlangen, West Germany)
World J Surg 13:809–817, November–December 1989   61–6

Over a 9-year period partial duodenopancreatectomy and occlusion of the remaining ductal system by Ethibloc to induce rapid exocrine atrophy were used in treating severe chronic cephalic pancreatitis in 268 male and 21 female patients with an average age of 41.6 years. Ethibloc is a slowly hardening injectable solution of prolamin that is readily absorbed in the ductal system and followed by recanalization of the efferent ducts.

Twelve percent of the 289 patients had postoperative morbidity, and there were 5 pancreatic and 3 biliary fistulas. One percent of the patients died after surgery. Relapses of pancreatitis occurred in 2.2% because of incomplete filling of ducts with Ethibloc. Eight-eight percent of the patients were pain free and asymptomatic after treatment. Eleven percent had minor complaints, and 85.9% gained an average of 7.8 kg after the surgery.

Ethibloc occlusion is an effective technique for inducing complete exocrine atrophy, abolishing the inflammatory process, preventing relapses of chronic pancreatitis, and preserving the endocrine function from further damage. Partial duodenopancreatectomy combined with Ethibloc occlusion of the pancreatic duct is the procedure of choice in the surgical management of patients with severe chronic cephalic pancreatitis.

▶ This unique approach to the pain of chronic pancreatitis was associated with a high success rate (88% pain free). Time and the experience of others with the technique will reveal its true value. It is interesting that the patients gained weight in spite of acinar ablation. The authors should perform and report on the results of glucose blood tests to demonstrate that islet function was not disturbed by Ethibloc occlusion.—F.G. Moody, M.D.

Duodenum-Preserving Resection of the Head of the Pancreas in Severe Chronic Pancreatitis: Early and Late Results
Beger HG, Büchler M, Bittner RR, Oettinger W, Roscher R (Univ of Ulm, West Germany)
Ann Surg 209:273–278, March 1989   61-7

Surgical treatment is needed for patients with severe chronic pancreatitis when the patients also have medically intractable pain, stenosis of the common bile duct, severe obstruction of the duodenum, or compression of the portal vein producing portal hypertension. A stomach-, duodenum-, and biliary-tree-preserving resection of the head of the pancreas has been introduced to minimize the high morbidity and mortality associated with the use of major pancreatic resection, such as the Whipple procedure. Duodenum-preserving resection of the head of the pancreas was performed in 128 patients with severe chronic pancreatitis, and early and late results were presented.

The median length of hospitalization after surgery was 15.5 days. Reoperation was needed in 5.5%. One patient died in the early postoperative phase, yielding a hospital mortality of 0.8%. At a median follow-up of 3.6 years, 6 patients were dead, for a late mortality of 4.7%. Seventy-seven percent of the patients were totally free of pain, and 67% returned to their former work. Late in the follow-up, glucose metabolism was not changed in 80.7% of the patients, had deteriorated in 13.7%, and had improved permanently in 5.5%. Eighty percent of the patients had a marked increase in weight, averaging 8.7 kg.

In comparison with the Whipple technique, duodenum-preserving resection of the head of the pancreas spares patients with chronic pancreatitis a gastrectomy, duodenectomy, and resection of the extrahepatic biliary ducts. The limited surgical intervention at the head of the pancreas and the preservation of the duodenum account for the low early and late rates of postoperative complications and death.

▶ Beger and his colleagues from Ulm, West Germany, provide an excellent report on the treatment of chronic pancreatitis by a duodenal-preserving resection of the head of the pancreas. The low morbidity and high success rate makes this approach one to be recommended for those who specialize in pancreatic surgery. The mortality was low (< 1%), but the reoperation rate was relatively high (> 5%), suggesting that perioperative complications were common.—F.G. Moody, M.D.

62 Pancreatic Neoplasms

Evaluation of Ca19-9

Evaluation of a Serologic Marker, CA19-9, in the Diagnosis of Pancreatic Cancer

Pleskow DK, Berger HJ, Gyves J, Allen E, McLean A, Podolsky DK (New England Deaconess Hosp, Boston; Harvard Med School; Massachusetts Gen Hosp, Boston; Centocor, Inc, Malvern, Pa)
Ann Intern Med 110:704–709, May 1, 1989

The diagnosis of pancreatic cancer is difficult because various diagnostic imaging tools are limited by their specificity, sensitivity, safety, or cost. Efforts have been made to develop useful serologic markers for this disease, and 1 candidate marker is the epitope reactive with monoclonal antibody Ca19-9. This study blindly evaluated frozen serum for Ca19-9 antibody reactivity using samples from 261 patients collected between 1978 and 1980. The results were compared with the final diagnosis, based in part on retrospective review after an 8-year follow-up.

In 54 patients with pancreatic cancer, the median level of Ca19-9 was 349 units per mL, with values ranging from 7.3 to 2,859,964 units per mL. In patients without pancreatic cancer, the median level of Ca 19-9 was 15 units per mL, with values ranging from 7.3 to 35,914 units per mL. In this population, which included 20% with pancreatic cancer, a cutoff value of 70 units per mL had a sensitivity of 70% and a specificity of 87% (table). The positive predictive value of this test was 59% and the negative predictive value, 92%.

Comparison of CA19-9 and Carcinoembryonic Antigen Test Parameters in Identification of Patients with Pancreatic Carcinoma

Test Parameter	CA19-9 (%)	Carcinoembryonic Antigen (%)	P Value
Sensitivity	38/54*(70)	20/61*(33)	<0.0001
Specificity	181/207†(87)	190/209†(91)	0.0966
Positive Predictive Value	38/64 (59)	20/39 (49)	0.1281
Negative Predictive Value	181/197 (92)	190/231 (83)	0.0033
Accuracy	219/261 (84)	210/270 (77)	

*Number of positive test/total with pancreatic cancer.
†Number negative test/all persons without pancreatic cancer.
(Courtesy of Pleskow DK, Berger HJ, Gyves J, et al: Ann Intern Med 110:704–709, May 1, 1989.)

Among patients with pancreatic cancer, no significant linear relationship was found between tumor stage and median Ca19-9 values.

The Ca19-9 antibody could be useful for evaluating patients with suspected pancreatic disease. The marker is highly specific but limited in sensitivity. A positive test with Ca19-9 might be used to indicate the need for further evaluation in patients with a moderate to low probability of pancreatic cancer, whereas in patients with strong clinical findings of pancreatic cancer the marker is of little use. Although determinations of Ca19-9 combined with a single imaging modality are highly accurate in diagnosing pancreatic cancer, it is cautioned that Ca19-9 should not be used as a screening tool in an asymptomatic population.

▶ This investigation as well as other recent studies, indicates that Ca19-9 is an accurate tool that can be useful for evaluating patients with suspected pancreatic disease. Although its sensitivity is limited, the high specificity of the marker in conditions that are often difficult to diagnose underscores its potential value. Illustrative examples include patients with suspected chronic pancreatitis and unrelenting pain, chronic pancreatitis with cholestasis, and acute pancreatitis with persistent pain (2% of patients with pancreatic carcinoma have acute pancreatitis).

Heptner and co-workers (1) have reported that Ca19-9 is clearly superior to 2 other tumor-associated markers, CEA and Ca72-4, in the serodiagnosis of pancreatic cancer. Using a cutoff level of 37 units per mL (a cutoff value of 70 units per mL was used by Pleskow and associates), 56 (82%) of 68 patients with pancreatic cancer had a positive test. Obviously, the sensitivity will vary depending on the cutoff value.

Finally, I would underscore the cautionary note by Pleskow and colleagues that the Ca19-9 test not be used as a screening test for asymptomatic patients.—N.J. Greenberger, M.D.

Reference

1. Heptner G, Domschke S, Domschke W: Comparison of Ca72-4 with Ca19-9 and carcinoembryonic antigen in the serodiagnostics of gastrointestinal malignancies. *Scand J Gastroenterol* 24:745–750, 1989.

The Clinical Utility of the Ca19-9 Radioimmunoassay for the Diagnosis of Pancreatic Cancer Presenting as Pain or Weight Loss: A Cost-Effectiveness Analysis
Richter JM, Christensen MR, Rustgi AK, Silverstein MD (Massachusetts Gen Hosp, Boston; Harvard Med School; Mayo Clinic, Rochester, Minn)
Arch Intern Med 149:2292–2297, October 1989

The Ca19-9 radioimmunoassay (RIA) is a relatively new serologic test for the detection of gastrointestinal carcinoma, particularly pancreatic carcinoma. Although previous studies have shown that the Ca19-9 RIA is substantially more sensitive and specific than carcinoembryonic antigen testing and more practical than other diagnostic tests currently in development, its clinical role and cost-effectiveness have not yet been determined. Clinical decision analysis was used to model and analyze diagnostic strategies for patients with pancreatic cancer whose initial symptoms were pain or weight loss.

Six strategies were developed and analyzed. Each was modeled as a decision tree consisting of a combination of tests. These 6 comprehensive diagnostic strategies were developed based on current and projected patterns of clinical practice, using the Ca19-9 RIA either to yield biopsy-proven pancreatic cancer or exclude its presence with certainty. The comparison was made between ultrasonography first and Ca19-9 RIA first.

The Ca19-9 RIA proved most valuable as an initial office-based diagnostic test for use by the primary care physician when the possibility of pancreatic carcinoma initially is considered for a patient with pain or weight loss. In the context of a comprehensive diagnostic strategy, the Ca19-9 RIA test did not particularly improve the overall diagnostic accuracy of the strategy. However, the use of the Ca19-9 RIA test did decrease the need for noninvasive and invasive diagnostic tests at a savings in direct health care cost of 24% to 28% per patient tested when compared with the ultrasound-first strategy (table).

The results of this decision analysis indicate that Ca19-9 RIA is a cost-effective, useful *initial* test for the examination of patients with suspected pancreatic cancer, but does not contribute to the overall diagnostic accuracy of a comprehensive diagnostic strategy.

▶ The diagnosis of cancer of the pancreas is often difficult and frequently requires invasive and expensive diagnostic tests. An accurate serologic marker for this disease would simplify diagnosis. As the authors point out, earlier assays such as carcinoembryonic antigen, galactosyltransferase II, leukocyte adherence assay, pancreatic oncofetal antigen, and serum ribonuclease have not proved to be reliable or practical. The carcinoembryonic antigen assay currently is commercially available, but is insufficiently sensitive to be of clinical utility except in the exceptional case. The Ca19-9 RIA appears to be promising, with a substantially better sensitivity and specificity than carcinoembryonic antigen. In this study, the role of Ca19-9 RIA was evaluated and proved most valuable as an initial, office-based diagnostic study to be used by the primary care physician when the possibility of pancreatic carcinoma in patients with pain or weight loss initially was considered.—N.J. Greenberger, M.D.

Clinical Studies

Distal Pancreatectomy With and Without Splenectomy: A Comparative Study
Richardson DQ, Scott-Conner CEH (Univ of Mississippi)
Am Surg 55:21–25, January 1989

Ten of 21 patients who had distal pancreatectomy from January 1980 through April 1987 had splenectomy, and in 11 cases the spleen was preserved. Mean age and the extent of pancreatic resection were comparable between the 2 groups. Operating time averaged 3.7 hours with splenectomy and 2.9 hours without, unless the patient needed additional major surgery.

Performance of Strategies

	Predictive Value		No. of Tests/100 Patients					Cost/
Prevalence	Positive	Negative	Noninvasive Tests	EGD	ERCP	Needle Biopsy	Laparotomy	Patient, $
			CA19-9 First					
0.02	0.999	0.996	130	10	2	3	0	848
0.05	0.999	0.991	132	10	2	5	1	908
0.10	0.999	0.981	135	10	2	9	1	1009
0.15	0.999	0.969	139	9	3	13	2	1120
0.20	0.999	0.958	142	9	3	17	2	1211
0.30	0.999	0.930	149	9	4	25	3	1413
			Ultrasonography First					
0.02	0.992	0.998	193	8	8	5	1	1186
0.05	0.997	0.994	192	8	8	8	1	1257
0.10	0.999	0.988	192	7	8	12	2	1375
0.15	0.999	0.978	192	7	8	17	3	1515
0.20	0.999	0.974	191	7	9	20	3	1612
0.30	0.999	0.955	190	7	9	29	4	1848

Abbreviations: EGD, esophagogastroduodenoscopy; *ERCP*, endoscopic retrograde cholangiopancreatography.
(Courtesy of Richter JM, Christensen MR, Rustgi AK, et al: *Arch Intern Med* 149:2292–2297, October 1989.)

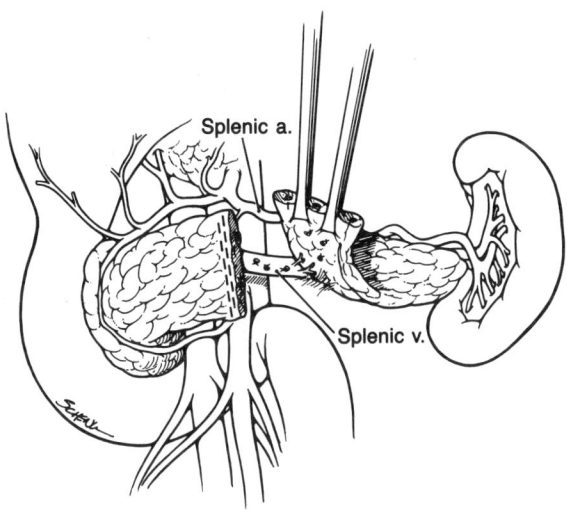

Fig 62–1.—Distal pancreatectomy with splenic preservation. Retrograde dissection of distal pancreas after early transection. (Courtesy of Richardson DQ, Scott-Conner CEH: Am Surg 55:21–25, January 1989.)

No deaths occurred in either group; however, there were complications in 36% to 40% of cases. There were no new cases of insulin-dependent diabetes after surgery. The splenic vein was ligated in 1 case without adverse sequelae. A second patient, in whom both the splenic artery and vein were ligated, needed splenectomy; this was the only patient for whom splenic preservation failed. The postoperative hospital stay was similar in the 2 surgical groups.

The spleen may be preserved in selected patients who undergo distal pancreatectomy (Fig 62–1). An alternative to retrograde dissection of the distal pancreas is to begin dissection at the splenic hilum (Fig 62–2). In both instances multiple small feeding vessels must be ligated individually. Management of a large benign cyst is shown in Figure 62–3. In cases of chronic pancreatitis Roux-en-Y drainage of the pancreatic stump may be preferable to simple closure.

▶ Splenic preservation should be attempted when the pancreas is being resected for benign disease. Preservation can be accomplished in most cases, but does require a more tedious dissection.—F.G. Moody, M.D.

An Analysis of the Reduced Morbidity and Mortality Rates After Pancreaticoduodenectomy
Pellegrini CA, Heck CF, Raper S, Way LW (VA Med Ctr; Univ of California, San Francisco)
Arch Surg 124:778–781, July 1989   62–4

Traditionally, Whipple's pancreaticoduodenectomy for carcinoma of the ampulla of Vater has been associated with mortality of more than 20% and

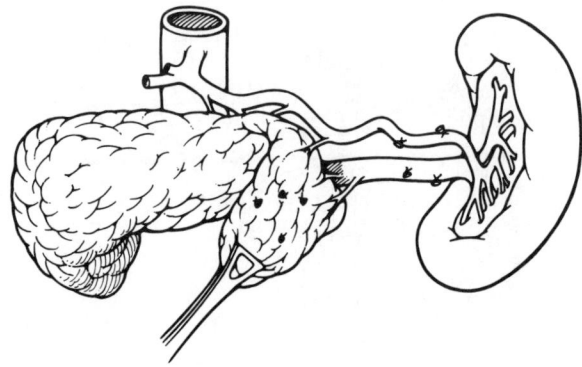

Fig 62-2.—Alternate technique for distal pancreatectomy with splenic salvage. Dissection begins at hilum of spleen and progresses toward body of pancreas. (Courtesy of Richardson DQ, Scott-Conner CEH: *Am Surg* 55:21–25, January 1989.)

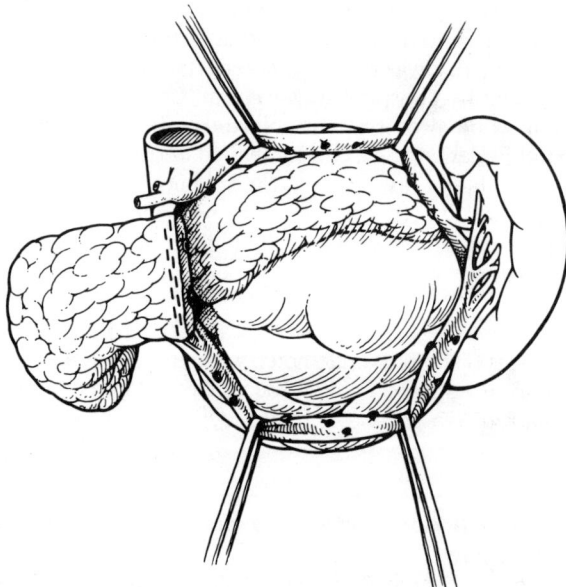

Fig 62-3.—Early mobilization of splenic vessels from large benign cyst. (Courtesy of Richardson DQ, Scott-Conner CEH: *Am Surg* 55:21–25, January 1989.)

morbidity of more than 50%. Some, however, have reported much better results.

Data were reviewed on 51 consecutively seen patients who had pancreaticoduodenectomy in 1979 through 1987. Thirty percent of patients had a traditional procedure and 70% had a pylorus-preserving procedure. The 2 groups were similar in amount of blood lost during surgery, resumption of oral intake, and time to discharge.

One patient died of surgical complications. Fourteen (27%) had nonfatal intra-abdominal complications. Two patients needed reoperation. Seventy-four percent of patients who had pancreaticoduodenectomy for cancer survived 1 year, 47% survived 3 years, and 33% survived 5 or more years.

In a center where a large number of pancreaticoduodenectomies are performed, mortality is substantially lower than in the past because of the greater experience of those who perform the operation and the availability of CT and skilled interventional radiologists. These allow for better control of postoperative infection and pancreatic fistulas. Although this procedure is only palliative in most patients with cancer, it provides the best palliation and the only chance of cure.

▶ These results are encouraging for the treatment of pancreatic cancer with pancreaticoduodenectomy. Not only is the mortality acceptable, but survival appears to be improved. The authors' point is well taken; the Whipple procedure is best employed by those who perform it frequently.—F.G. Moody, M.D.

Experience With 647 Consecutive Tumors of the Duodenum, Ampulla, Head of the Pancreas, and Distal Common Bile Duct
Michelassi F, Erroi F, Dawson PJ, Pietrabissa A, Noda S, Handcock M, Block GE (Univ of Chicago)
Ann Surg 210:544–556, October 1989   62–5

Between 1946 and 1987, 647 patients with periampullary tumors were treated at a university medical center. Included were 549 tumors in the head of the pancreas, 40 in the distal common bile duct, 29 in the duodenum, and 29 at the ampulla of Vater. Ninety-eight percent of all tumors were adenocarcinomas. Operability ranged from 81% to 97%. A combined laparotomy, biopsy, and bypass procedure (nonresection) was done in 433 patients, and only 1 survived for 5 years, for a 5-year survival rate of 0.2%.

The resectability rate ranged from 89.3% for ampullary lesions to 16.5% for pancreatic adenocarcinoma. The 133 resections included 80 pancreaticoduodenectomies, 29 total pancreatectomies, 7 duodenectomies, 2 gastroectomies, 8 common bile duct resections, and 7 local excisions.

Mortality in the immediate postoperative period among patients undergoing radical resection was 19%; however, this rate has dropped to 5% since 1981. Overall mortality was 20% after standard pancreaticoduodenectomy and 24.1% after total pancreatectomy.

The 5-year actuarial survival rates for pancreatic, duodenal, and ampullary adenocarcinoma were 8.8%, 20%, and 32%, respectively. Half the patients with sarcoma and two thirds of those with carcinoid of the duodenum were alive at 5 years. All patients with distal common bile duct adenocarcinoma were dead at 5 years.

Intent of surgery, tumor site, and histologic type appear to determine the outcome of patients with periampullary tumors. Although a curative resection provides the best chance for long-term survival, these findings stress the limitation of staging and selection. Multicentricity rarely occurs, and total pancreatectomy does not result in a lower perioperative mortality or better survival rate than standard pancreaticoduodenectomy, indicating that the latter is the resection of choice, unless multicentricity is obvious at exploration.

▶ This large series provides a panoramic view of the results to be expected in the management of periampullary carcinomas. It is of interest that total pancreatectomy did not improve the relatively poor 5-year survival rate when performed for pancreatic cancer. Bile duct cancers also fared poorly in this series.—F.G. Moody, M.D.

Total Pancreatectomy for Ductal Cell Carcinoma of the Pancreas: An Update

Brooks JR, Brooks DC, Levine JD (Harvard Med School; Brigham and Women's Hosp, Boston)
Ann Surg 209:405–410, April 1989   62–6

Some surgeons have suggested abandoning the Whipple procedure for ductal cell carcinoma of the head of the pancreas because of its operative mortality and lack of long-term survivors. The results of a 2.5- to 16-year follow-up of 48 patients with ductal cell carcinoma of the pancreas who were treated with total pancreatectomy were reported.

From 1970 to 1976, 4 patients died, a mortality of 18%. However, no hospital deaths occurred after the last 28 operations, performed from 1977 to 1986. Seventeen percent of the patients had intraoperative complications involving mesenteric vessels, and 27% of the patients suffered postoperative complications. Twenty-five percent were discharged from the hospital within 2 weeks of the surgery; 50%, within 4 weeks; and 25%, after 4 weeks. Thirty-five percent of the patients returned to preoperative work. An additional 35% were able to lead active lives but did not return to their regular work. The remaining 30% were incapacitated to some degree by the surgery and disease. The 4-year survival rate was 21% and the 5-year survival rate, 14%.

In the past 10 years, the postoperative mortality and 5-year survival rates for patients with ductal cell carcinoma of the pancreas treated by total pancreatectomy have improved significantly. Some of the patients in this series also received radiotherapy, chemotherapy, or both, but their use was not consistent enough to be assessed properly.

▶ Brooks and his associates provide an update of their experience with total pancreatectomy for pancreatic ductal cancer. They have performed 28 such procedures without a death and report a 14% 5-year survival. Unfortunately, only 35% of patients who survived were able to return to work, and a third were incapacitated by the operation or recurrence of their disease. The Whipple procedure appears to be associated with significantly less long-term morbidity.—F.G. Moody, M.D.

63 Pancreatic Trauma

Conservative Management of Combined Pancreatoduodenal Injuries
Mansour MA, Moore JB, Moore EE, Moore FA (Denver Gen Hosp; St Anthony Central Hosp; Univ of Colorado, Denver)
Am J Surg 158:531–535, December 1989   63–1

Combined injury to the pancreas and duodenum can be difficult to manage. A unified approach to the treatment of patients with such injury based on an anatomical classification of injury was described.

Sixty-two patients with combined injury to the pancreas and duodenum were treated in 12 years. Sixty percent of the injuries resulted from penetrating wounds, and 40%, from blunt trauma. Grades of I through V were assigned to classify the severity of injury. Sixteen percent of the injuries were grade I, and 23% were grade II. Those injuries were treated with simple repair and drainage. Nineteen percent of the injuries were grade III, and 32% were grade IV. Those injuries were treated primarily with pyloric exclusion. Grade V injuries, occurring in 10% of the patients, were managed with pancreatoduodenectomy. Pancreatic and duodenal complications occurred in 35% and 2% of the patients, respectively. Nineteen percent of the patients died, 83% of them within the first 24 hours as a result of exsanguination or severe head injury.

Although no one procedure is uniformly applicable to combined pancreatoduodenal injuries, the mainstay treatment principles are active sump drainage of the pancreas, pyloric exclusion of the duodenum, and early nutritional support through needle catheter jejunostomy.

▶ The authors provide a useful grading system for determining the choice of procedure for combined duodenopancreatic injuries. I agree in general with their proposed management plan and would emphasize the importance of the use of needle catheter jejunostomy as a site for enteral feeding.—F.G. Moody, M.D.

64 Pancreas Transplantation

A 10-Year Experience With 290 Pancreas Transplants at a Single Institution
Sutherland DER, Dunn DL, Goetz FC, Kennedy W, Ramsay RC, Steffes MW, Mauer SM, Gruessner R, Moudry-Munns KC, Morel P, Viste A, Robertson RP, Najarian JS
(Univ of Minnesota Hosp)
Ann Surg 210:274–288, September 1989   64-1

Pancreas transplants are being performed more often for patients with diabetes mellitus and its complications.

Two hundred ninety transplants were performed in a 10-year period at 1 institution. Duct management methods included free intraperitoneal drainage in 44 cases, duct occlusion in 44, enteric drainage in 89, and bladder drainage in 128. Overall, the 1-year patient and graft survival rates were 91% and 42%, respectively. Patient and graft survital rates progressively improved. Bladder drainage appeared to be better than enteric drainage.

The best results were achieved in patients receiving primary simultaneous pancreas and kidney bladder-drained transplants, with a 1-year pancreas graft survival rate of 75%, kidney graft survival rate of 80%, and patient survival rate of 95%. Significant predictors of success were technique, with bladder drainage better than enteric drainage and enteric drainage better than duct injection; category, with simultaneous pancreas and kidney transplants better than a pancreas transplant after a kidney transplant (PAK) from the same donor, which was better than PAK from a different donor, which was better than pancreas transplants alone; and donor HLA DR mismatch, with 0 antigens better than 1, and 1 better than 2.

Pancreas transplantation has been increasingly successful in patients with diabetes with and without uremia. Transplantation may also ameliorate secondary complications of diabetes. Pancreas transplants should be done in most uremic diabetic recipients of kidney transplants and may be considered for selected patients without uremia who have other complications of diabetes.

▶ Sutherland reports on the Minnesota experience with pancreatic transplantation. Progress clearly has been significant in the last decade. A survival rate of 75% for grafts performed simultaneously with a renal transplant bodes well for long-term success as more effective and less toxic agents become available.—F.G. Moody, M.D.

Capsules and Comments

Esophagus and Stomach

C–1 Ingestion of Corrosive Acids: Spectrum of Injury to Upper Gastrointestinal Tract and Natural History
C–2 Refractory Duodenal Ulcers (Nonhealing Duodenal Ulcers With Standard Doses of Antisecretory Medication)
C–3 Postbulbar Duodenal Ulcer in a Patient With Pentagastrin-Fast Achlorhydria

Small Bowel and Colon

C–4 Enteroclysis in the Evaluation of Suspected Small Intestinal Bleeding
C–5 Cholera in Louisiana: Widening Spectrum of Seafood Vehicles
C–6 Healing of Severe Perineal and Cutaneous Crohn's Disease With Hyperbaric Oxygen
C–7 Inadequate Barium Enemas in Hospitalized Elderly Patients: Incidence and Risk Factors
C–8 Bacteriotherapy for Chronic Relapsing *Clostridium difficile* Diarrhea in Six Patients
C–9 Clinical Features of Abdominal Tuberculosis
C–10 5-Aminosalicylic Acid Suppositories in the Management of Ulcerative Colitis
C–11 Protein-Losing Enteropathy Associated With *Clostridium difficile* Infection
C–12 Primary Malignant Lymphoma of the Large Intestine Complicating Chronic Inflammatory Bowel Disease

Liver

C–13 Extrahepatic Malignancy Following Long-Term Immunosuppressive Therapy of Severe Hepatitis B Surface Antigen-Negative Chronic Active Hepatitis
C–14 Autonomic Neuropathy and Chronic Liver Disease
C–15 Prognosis of Corticosteriod-Treated Hepatitis B Surface Antigen-Negative Chronic Active Hepatitis in Postmenopausal Women: A Retrospective Analysis
C–16 Polymorphonuclear Cell Count Response and Duration of Antibiotic Therapy in Spontaneous Bacterial Peritonitis
C–17 Fulminant Hepatitis A in Intravenous Drug Users Wtih Chronic Liver Disease
C–18 Sexual Behavior in Women With Nonalcoholic Liver Disease
C–19 Delta Hepatitis in Homosexual Men in the United States
C–20 Development of Large Spleno-Adreno-Renal Shunt After Endoscopic Sclerotherapy

C-21 Treatment of Chronic Hepatitis Delta Virus (HDV) Infection With Human Lymphoblastoid Alpha Interferon
C-22 Evidence for Disease Recurrence After Liver Transplantation for Primary Biliary Cirrhosis: Clinical and Histologic Follow-Up Studies
C-23 Prospective Evaluation of Esophageal Varices in Primary Biliary Cirrhosis: Development, Natural History, and Influence on Survival
C-24 Correlation of IgM Anti-Hepatitis D Virus (HDV) to HDV RNA in Sera of Chronic HDV

Gallbladder and Biliary Tract

C-25 Abdominal Symptoms and Gallstone Disease: An Epidemiological Investigation
C-26 Prospective Randomized Comparison of Mezlocillin Therapy Alone With Combined Ampicillin and Gentamicin Therapy for Patients With Cholangitis
C-27 Cholecystokinin Prevents Parenteral Nutrition Induced Biliary Sludge in Humans

Pancreas

C-28 Acute Pancreatitis and Normoamylasemia: Not an Uncommon Combination
C-29 The Spectrum and Natural History of Common Bile Duct Stenosis in Chronic Alcohol-Induced Pancreatitis

Esophagus and Stomach

Ingestion of Corrosive Acids: Spectrum of Injury to Upper Gastrointestinal Tract and Natural History
Zargar SA, Kochhar R, Nagi B, et al.
Gastroenterology 97:702–707, September 1989   C-1

▶ These investigators prospectively have evaluated 41 patients who ingested acid for location, extent, severity, and outcome of the injury to the upper gastrointestinal tract. The injuries were assessed within 36 hours of acid intake by endoscopy or surgery, or at autopsy. Symptoms and signs were unreliable in predicting the extent and severity of injury. The degree of burns was classified as follows: grade 0 in 2 patients, grade 1 in 3, grade 2 in 16, and grade 3 in 20. Esophageal injury was seen in 87.8% of the patients; gastric injury, in 85.4%; and duodenal injury, in 34.1%. All patients with grade 0, 1, or 2a injury recovered without sequelae. Acute complications occurred in 39.1% of patients, and death, in 12.2%. It is significant that all such patients had grade 3 burns. Five of the 8 patients with grade 2b injury and all survivors of grade 3 injury had esophageal or gastric cicatrization, or both, which subsequently needed endoscopic or surgical treatment. The authors find that endoscopy is not only the tool of choice for diagnosis in such cases, but also aids in deciding on treatment and prognosis. The authors conclude that acid injury of the upper gastrointestinal tract is a serious condition that affects the esophagus and stomach equally and results in high morbidity and mortality.—N.J. Greenberger, M.D.

Refractory Duodenal Ulcers (Nonhealing Duodenal Ulcers with Standard Doses of Antisecretory Medication)
Collen MJ, Stanczak VJ, Ciarleglio CA
Dig Dis Sci 34:233–237, February 1989   C–2

▶ To evaluate possible differences between patients with refractory duodenal ulcers and those with duodenal ulcers that respond to standard doses of antisecretory medications, Collen and colleagues determined basal acid outputs by nasogastric suction and daily smoking histories for 75 patients with endoscopically documented active duodenal ulcers. Patients had treatment for at least 8 weeks with standard doses of antisecretory medications; endoscopic healing or nonhealing was documented. Fifty-five patients who had complete healing of their duodenal ulcers had a mean basal acid output of 6.6 ± 5.3 mEq/hr, and 18 of 55 had histories of daily cigarette smoking, whereas 20 patients who had nonhealing duodenal ulcers had a mean basal acid output of 20.0 ± 9.6 mEq/hr, and 8 of 20 had histories of daily cigarette smoking. Differences between the 2 groups were not significant with regard to age, duodenal ulcer size, or cigarette smoking history. However, differences in male-female ratio and in mean basal acid output were significant, and all patients with nonhealing duodenal ulcers had basal acid outputs greater than 10.0 mEq/hr. Patients with nonhealing duodenal ulcers were given increased doses of ranitidine (mean, 675 mg/day; range, 600–1,200 mg/day), and all had endoscopically documented complete healing. These results indicate that patients with nonhealing duodenal ulcers who are given standard doses of antisecretory medications have increased basal acid outputs of more than 10.0 mEq/hr, and the duodenal ulcers heal with increased doses of antisecretory medication.—N.J. Greenberger, M.D.

Postbulbar Duodenal Ulcer in a Patient With Pentagastrin-Fast Achlorhydria
Goldschmiedt M, Peterson WL, Vuitch F, et al.
Gastroenterology 97:771–774, September 1989   C–3

▶ This report describes the clinicopathologic features of a 55-year-old man found to have a bleeding, postbulbar duodenal ulcer and fasting hypergastrinemia. Gastric analysis revealed pentagastrin-fast achlorhydria. Healing of the ulcer was documented 8 weeks after vagotomy, antrectomy, gastrojejunostomy, and a course of sucralfate therapy. The etiology of the postbulbar ulcer was uncertain. This is the first documented case of a duodenal ulcer with pentagastrin-fast achlorhydria.—N.J. Greenberger, M.D.

Small Bowel and Colon

Enteroclysis in the Evaluation of Suspected Small Intestinal Bleeding
Deuglar KR, Lappas JC, Maglinte DDT, et al.
Gastroenterology 97:58–60, 1989   C–4

▶ One hundred twenty-five consecutive enteroclysis studies performed for the indication of gastrointestinal bleeding were reviewed. The overall yield of positive studies was low (10%), but important lesions were found. Patients with unequivocally normal evaluations of the upper gastrointestinal tract and colon had the highest yield of positive enteroclysis studies (20%). The specific type of bleeding, the presence or absence of abdominal symptoms or physical examination findings, and the results of laboratory tests were not associated with a positive or negative enteroclysis study.—N.J. Greenberger, M.D.

Cholera in Louisiana: Widening Spectrum of Seafood Vehicles
Lowry PW, Pavia AT, McFarland LM, et al.
Arch Intern Med 149:2079–2084, 1989   C–5

▶ The largest cholera outbreak in the United States in more than a century occurred in Louisiana from August through October 1986. Eighteen persons in 12 family clusters had stool cultures or serologic evidence of infection with toxigenic Vibrio cholerae 0-group 1. Thirteen of these persons had severe diarrhea, and 4 needed treatment in an intensive care unit. Although all 18 survived, 1 96-year-old woman with suspected cholera died shortly after hospital admission. A case-control study showed that case-patients were more likely than neighborhood controls to have eaten cooked crabs or cooked or raw shrimp during the week before illness. Case-patients who ate crabs were more likely than controls who ate crabs to have undercooked and mishandled the crabs after cooking. A third vehicle from the Gulf waters, raw oysters, caused V. cholerae 01 infection in 2 persons residing in Florida and Georgia. All 3 seafood vehicles came from multiple sources. Stool isolates from the Louisiana case-patients were genetically identical to other North American strains isolated since 1973, but different from African and Asian isolates. Crabs are the most important vehicle for V. cholerae 01 infection in the United States, but shrimp and oysters from the Gulf coast also can be vehicles of transmission. A persisting reservoir of V. cholerae 01 along the Gulf coast may continue to cause sporadic cases and outbreaks of cholera in Gulf states and in states importing Gulf seafood.—N.J. Greenberger, M.D.

Healing of Severe Perineal and Cutaneous Crohn's Disease With Hyperbaric Oxygen
Brady CE, Cooley BJ, Davis JC
Gastroenterology 97:756–760, 1989   C–6

▶ Recurrent perineal Crohn's disease can be an extremely debilitating complication that may be difficult to treat. Brady and associates report a patient with progressively worsening perineal and biopsy-proven cutaneous Crohn's disease that had been refractory to surgery and medical treatment (sulfasalazine, steroids, 6-mercaptopurine, metronidazole, antibiotics). As the lesions were reminiscent of problem wounds occurring in other situations, hyperbaric oxygen treatment was instituted while the patient was continued on metronidazole. Response was dramatic with almost immediate relief of symptoms and regression within 2.5 months of wounds that had defied therapy for 8 years. Clinical remission has not been sustained as 4 subsequent courses of hyperbaric oxygen have been given for 11 months. Nevertheless, the patient has been essentially asymptomatic since her initial course, and the extent of her cutaneous disease has been minimal compared with that before hyperbaric oxygen. Hyperbaric oxygen treatment is costly and should not be used routinely for every patient with perineal Crohn's disease. However, this case report may herald an advance in the understanding of the pathogenesis of this complication and ultimately its therapy.—N.J. Greenberger, M.D.

Inadequate Barium Enemas in Hospitalized Elderly Patients: Incidence and Risk Factors
Tinetti ME, Stone DL, Cooney L, et al.
Arch Intern Med 149:2014–2016, 1989   C-7

▶ The likelihood of obtaining interpretable results is as important as sensitivity and specificity in selecting diagnostic tests. The authors reviewed medical and radiologic records of 140 consecutively seen inpatients aged more than 65 years who underwent nonemergent barium enemas. For 43 (31%) of these patients, examinations were incomplete or the results were uninterpretable. Thirteen patients could not retain the barium, and 27 patients had too much stool. Characteristics significantly associated with an inadequate barium enema included confusion, fever, and cachexia. Characteristics more common among persons unable to retain barium than among persons with too much stool were diarrhea (38% vs. 18%) and fecal incontinence (31% vs. 0%). The high frequency of inadequate results suggests that clinicians should consider whether a barium enema is an appropriate test for elderly patients with these characteristics and, if so, what interventions may increase the chance for success.—N.J. Greenberger, M.D.

Bacteriotherapy for Chronic Relapsing *Clostridium difficile* Diarrhea in Six Patients
Tvede M, Rask-Madsen J
Lancet 1:1156–1160, 1989   C-8

▶ Six patients with chronic relapsing diarrhea caused by *Clostridium difficile* were treated with rectal instillation of homologous feces (1 patient) or a mixture of 10 different facultatively aerobic and anaerobic bacteria diluted in sterile saline (5 patients). The mixture led to a prompt loss of *Cl. difficile* and its toxin from the stools and to bowel colonization by *Bacteroides* sp., which had not been present in pretreatment stool samples. Strains of *Escherichia coli, Cl. bifermentans,* and *Peptostreptococcus productus* in the mixture inhibited the in vitro growth of *Cl. difficile,* which in turn inhibited the growth of *Bacteroides ovatus, B. vulgatus,* and *B. thetaiotaomicron.* The findings that *Bacteroides* sp. had been absent during the patients' illness but was present after recovery suggests that the absence of *Bacteroides* sp. may result in chronic relapsing *Cl. difficile* diarrhea, and that its presence may prevent colonization by *Cl. difficile.*—N.J. Greenberger, M.D.

Clinical Features of Abdominal Tuberculosis
Jakubowski A, Elwood RK, Enarson DA
J Infect Dis 158:687–692, 1989   C–9

▶ The clinical features of 81 cases of abdominal tuberculosis (TB) diagnosed in British Columbia are presented. The peritoneum was involved in 41 patients; the ileocecal area, in 17; the anorectal area, in 16; and mesenteric glands, in 8. One case each involved the liver and sigmoid colon. Most patients were young women. The tuberculin reaction was clearly positive in 83% of patients tested, and 54% had evidence of TB elsewhere. Tuberculous peritonitis was more common in native North Americans and presented as an acute abdomen, abdominal tumor, or cirrhosis. Most ileocecal and mesenteric lymph node disease developed in Asians, who frequently had diagnoses of Crohn's disease, appendicitis, or cancer. Anorectal cases were apparent as fistulas or abscesses and usually had concomitant pulmonary TB. The disease was fatal in 5 patients (6%), 4 of whom had diagnoses only after death. One noncompliant patient had a relapse. All other patients had cures after receiving treatment.—N.J. Greenberger, M.D.

5-Aminosalicylic Acid Suppositories in the Management of Ulcerative Colitis
Campieri M, Gionchetti P, Belluzzi A, et al.
Dis Colon Rectum 33:398–399, 1989   C–10

▶ 5-Aminosalicylic acid (5-ASA) suppositories have been used in the authors' outpatient clinic in Bologna for the treatment of distal ulcerative colitis (UC). Mild or moderate attacks of UC in 156 patients were treated with different protocols for controlling active disease. Improvement was observed in 88.5% of the therapeutic cycles after 1 month. A small preliminary maintenance study using only 400-mg suppositories of 5-ASA twice a day for 6 to 12 months showed a remission percentage similar to that for salicylazosulfapyridine (SASP).—N.J. Greenberger, M.D.

Protein-Losing Enteropathy Associated With *Clostridium difficile* Infection
Rybolt AH, Laughon BE, Greenough WB, et al.
Lancet 1:1583–1585, 1989 C–11

➤ A commercially available radial immunodiffusion assay was used to measure serum alpha$_1$-antitrypsin levels in stool samples from patients aged more than 60 years as a marker of protein-losing enteropathy. Alpha$_1$-antitrypsin was found in all of 12 patients with colonoscopy-confirmed pseudomembranous colitis, 6 (43%) of 14 patients with *Clostridium difficile* diarrhea without pseudomembranes, 6 (50%) of 12 nursing-home patients with cultures positive for *Cl. difficile* but negative for its cytotoxin, and none of 15 healthy controls. It is concluded that serum protein loss into the gastrointestinal tract can occur as a result of *Cl. difficile* infection, that its presence is correlated with the severity of disease, and that it may occur even in the absence of diarrhea. The diagnosis of protein-losing enteropathy should be considered for all patients with *Cl. difficile* infection, particularly elderly nursing home patients, for whom the risk of *Cl. difficile* disease and the frequency of severe malnutrition are high.—N.J. Greenberger, M.D.

Primary Malignant Lymphoma of the Large Intestine Complicating Chronic Inflammatory Bowel Disease
Shepherd NA, Hall PA, Williams GT, et al.
Histopathology 15:325–337, 1989 C–12

➤ Ten cases of malignant lymphoma of the colon and rectum complicating chronic inflammatory bowel disease are presented. Seven patients had chronic ulcerative colitis with a history varying from 6 to 20 years. Six of these patients had extensive colitis, and 1 had left-sided colitis. All seven lymphomas had the pathologic and immunohistologic features of primary B cell tumors of the gastrointestinal tract with a predominance of high-grade tumors. Three patients had Crohn's disease of the large intestine complicated by malignant lymphoma of the sigmoid colon or rectum. The history of Crohn's disease varied from 30 months to 20 years, and each patient has fissuring and fistulas. Two patients had extensive anal involvement. The 3 lymphomas were histologically heterogeneous: 1 was of "granulomatous" T cell type and the other 2 were markedly polymorphic and of equivocal phenotype. They also were characterized by numerous multinucleate tumor giant cells. Primary colorectal malignant lymphoma should be regarded as a rare, but significant, complication of ulcerative colitis. Immunosuppression may be an additional factor in the genesis of intestinal lymphoma in Crohn's disease. The prognosis appears to be dependent on factors already known to be prognostically significant in primary gut lymphomas: a predominance of high-grade tumors suggests that the outlook is generally worse than that for idiopathic primary large intestinal lymphoma.—N.J. Greenberger, M.D.

Liver

Extrahepatic Malignancy Following Long-Term Immunosuppressive Therapy of Severe Hepatitis B Surface Antigen-Negative Chronic Active Hepatitis
Wang KK, Czaja AJ, Beaver SJ
Hepatology 10:39–43, 1989

▶ To determine the frequency, predisposing factors, and consequences of extrahepatic malignancy after long-term immunosuppressive therapy of severe hepatitis B surface antigen-negative chronic active hepatitis, 149 patients who had received prednisone, 20 mg daily, or prednisone, 10 mg daily, in combination with azathioprine, 50 mg daily, for at least 6 months were evaluated systematically for an average of 109 months (range, 7–223 months). Seven neoplasms involving cervix (2), lymphatic tissue (1), breast (1), bladder (1), soft tissue (1) and unknown site (1) developed in 7 patients after 116 ± 23 months (range, 18–164 months). The incidence of extrahepatic neoplasm was 1 per 194 patient-years of surveillance, and the probability of tumor occurrence was 3% after 10 years. Tumor frequency was similar among men and women, and the risk was 1.4-fold greater than that in an age- and sex-matched healthy population. Patients with extrahepatic malignancy were not distinguished by age, sex, treatment regimen, cumulative duration of treatment, or individual features of the liver disease. Five of the 7 patients survived during 48 ± 25 months of follow-up, including 2 patients who have lived for at least 5 years after the diagnosis of malignancy. Wang and co-workers conclude that extrahepatic malignancy develops infrequently during long-term immunosuppressive therapy. Its occurrence is not related to the type or duration of treatment, and long-term survival after tumor detection is possible. The low but probably increased risk of extrahepatic neoplasm does not militate against the use of immunosuppressive therapy in these patients.—N.J. Greenberger, M.D.

Autonomic Neuropathy and Chronic Liver Disease
Thuluvath PJ, Triger DR
Q J Med 72:737–747, 1989

▶ Autonomic neuropathy has been associated with alcoholic cirrhosis, but no information exists on its occurrence with nonalcoholic liver disease. The authors have examined autonomic function in 64 patients with biopsy-proven liver disease (22 with alcoholic liver disease and 42 with nonalcoholic liver disease) and in 29 age-matched controls. Forty-five percent of patients with alcoholic liver disease and 43% with nonalcoholic liver disease had evidence of parasympathetic damage; 11% of patients with alcoholic liver disease and 12% with nonalcoholic liver disease had sympathetic damage. Forty-five percent of patients with alcoholic liver disease and 22% with nonalcoholic liver disease had peripheral neuropathy on clinical examination. Sixty-eight percent of those with peripheral neuropathy also had autonomic neuropathy. This study confirms that autonomic neuropathy is common in alcoholic patients, but its being found with comparable frequency in nonalcoholic liver disease suggests that the neurologic defect may be secondary to the disturbed liver function.—N.J. Greenberger, M.D.

Prognosis of Corticosteroid-Treated Hepatitis B Surface Antigen-Negative Chronic Active Hepatitis in Postmenopausal Women: A Retrospective Analysis
Wang KK, Czaja AJ
Gastroenterology 97:1288–1293, 1989   C-15

➤ To determine the consequences of corticosteroid treatment in postmenopausal patients with severe chronic active hepatitis negative for hepatitis B surface antigen, the findings for 43 such patients (mean age, 59 years) were compared retrospectively with those for 46 premenopausal counterparts (mean age, 31 years) after similar durations of therapy. Postmenopausal patients entered remission as frequently as premenopausal women during initial treatment (81% vs. 83%), deteriorated as often (7% vs. 7%), and had drug-related complications as frequently (49% vs. 33%). Postmenopausal women, however, had a higher cumulative frequency of complications (77% vs. 48%) and a greater occurrence of multiple complications (44% vs. 13%) than premenopausal counterparts during follow-up. Vertebral compression occurred more frequently (23% vs. 7%), and lumbar spine densities were below the spontaneous fracture threshold more often (85% vs. 22%). Longer initial and cumulative durations of therapy were associated with the development of complications. Wang and associates conclude that initial corticosteroid treatment is as safe and effective for postmenopausal women as for their premenopausal counterparts. Postmenopausal women, however, have a higher cumulative frequency of complications over the long term and a lower net ratio of benefit to risk than premenopausal women given comparable treatment.—N.J. Greenberger, M.D.

Polymorphonuclear Cell Count Response and Duration of Antibiotic Therapy in Spontaneous Bacterial Peritonitis
Fong TL, Akriviadis EA, Runyon BA, et al.
Hepatology 9:423–426, 1989   C-16

➤ The purposes of this study were (1) to measure serially ascitic fluid polymorphonuclear cell response in treated spontaneous bacterial peritonitis and (2) to determine whether an ascitic fluid polymorphonuclear cell count of less than $250/mm^3$ on serial paracenteses was a satisfactory end point for antibiotic therapy. Thirty of 33 patients had exponential falls in counts of polymorphonuclear cells in ascitic fluid after 48 hours of antibiotic therapy; the magnitude of decrease was correlated with survival. Among the patients whose antibiotic therapy was discontinued when the ascitic fluid polymorphonuclear cell count reached $250/mm^3$ or less, the duration of therapy was considerably shorter than for the patients who received "conventional" therapy. Recurrence of spontaneous bacterial peritonitis was similar in the 2 groups.

Mortality was correlated with the severity of underlying liver disease, but not with duration of antibiotic therapy.—N.J. Greenberger, M.D.

Fulminant Hepatitis A in Intravenous Drug Users With Chronic Liver Disease
Akriviadis EA, Redeker AG
Ann Intern Med 110:838–839, 1989   C–17

➤ During the last 2 years, 16 of 113 patients with hepatitis A seen at the liver unit of the University of Southern California needed hospitalization. Among those hospitalized, 6 eventually had fulminant hepatitis and 4 patients died (those whose cases are reported here). The 2 patients who survived neither used intravenous drugs nor had evidence of chronic liver disease.

In all 4 patients who died, heroin was self-injected, creating a distinctly identifiable risk factor. Recent reports show a striking increase in hepatitis A infection among intravenous drug users, and injection or ingestion of contaminated drugs has been suggested in the common-source spread of the virus. In the 4 cases reported here, percutaneous transmission may have occurred, although fecal-oral transmission through close contact also is possible. The short period of hepatitis A viremia makes needle-mediated transmission unlikely, although not impossible.

Intravenous drug users are at high risk for chronic liver disease, which, superimposed on hepatitis A infection, may cause unusually severe hepatic injury. Regardless of the mode of transmission, a recent Centers for Disease Control report of hepatitis A outbreaks involving intravenous drug users suggests that hepatitis A infection may be a real threat for these patients.—N.J. Greenberger, M.D.

Sexual Behavior in Women With Nonalcoholic Liver Disease
Bach N, Schaffner F, Kapelman B
Hepatology 9:698–703, 1989   C–18

➤ Sexual behavior among women with liver disease was examined with 150 women to determine whether liver disease influenced sexual desire, frequency, or performance. The average age of women studied was 53 years (range, 26–76 years), and a wide variety of liver diseases was represented. Sexual desire was reduced in 33%. Difficulty in becoming sexually aroused was noted by 18%. Orgasm during intercourse was not experienced by 25%. The frequency of sexual intercourse was decreased since onset of disease in 27%. Dyspareunia was reported by 21% and most often was attributed to decreased vaginal lubrication. Liver disease was considered by 17% to be significant in interfering with sexual function. No statistical difference was found between sexual desire or function in this study and that in other large studies of sexual behavior of women. Each category was subdivided by the presence or absence of cirrhosis, premenopausal or postmenopausal state, laboratory values, and duration of disease. Except for a greater number of postmenopausal women with complaints of painful intercourse, no statistical differences or trends were found. Nonalcoholic liver disease does not affect sexual desire, function, or performance. Variables other than liver disease influence sexuality. Women with liver disease thus can be reassured that they can maintain normal sexual relations.—N.J. Greenberger, M.D.

Delta Hepatitis in Homosexual Men in the United States
Weisfuse IB, Hadler SC, Fields HA, et al.
Hepatology 9:872–874, 1989   C–19

➤ To assess the incidence and prevalence of delta hepatitis in homosexual men, the authors tested serum specimens for delta markers in participants of 2 previous studies: a hepatitis B vaccine trial among homosexual men conducted in the early 1980s and the Centers for Disease Control sentinel counties hepatitis study for 1983–1984. In the vaccine trial, men found to be positive for hepatitis B surface antigen (HBsAg) at the time of enrollment and those men who had serologic evidence of new hepatitis B virus infection during follow-up were tested. In the sentinel counties' determination of risk factors for viral hepatitis in reported cases, all homosexual men with acute and chronic hepatits B virus infections were tested for delta markers. Specimens were tested for delta antigen and immunoglobulin M and total delta antibody. In 7 different cities, among 321 men found to be positive for HBsAg at the time of screening, only 8 (2%) were positive for any delta marker. Among 290 men with new hepatitis B virus infections during follow-up, 3 (2 coinfections, 1 superinfection) had serologic evidence of delta hepatitis. In the sentinel counties study, none of 63 acute hepatitis B virus infections in homosexual men were associated with delta hepatitis. This study indicates that the delta agent is an infrequent cause of viral hepatitis in homosexual men in the United States.— N.J. Greenberger, M.D.

Development of Large Spleno-Adreno-Renal Shunt After Endoscopic Sclerotherapy
Dilawari JB, Raju GS, Chawla YK
Gastroenterology 97:421–426, 1989   C–20

➤ Endoscopic sclerotherapy is now well established as a treatment for bleeding esophageal varices. However, the effect that obliteration of varices has on the development of natural portosystemic shunts is not known. These investigators have studied 15 patients wtih bleeding from esophageal varices caused by extra-hepatic portal venous obstruction with splenoportovenography, before and after endoscopic obliteration of varices. A splenorenal (natural) shunt was defined when the contrast, injected into the spleen, immediately revealed the inferior vena cava. Such shunts were seen in 6 (40%) of 15 patients after the obliteration of esophageal varices and a mean interval between the 2 sessions of splenoportovenography of

23.5 months. In contrast, none of the 13 patients with bleeding caused by extrahepatic portal venous obstruction had splenorenal shunts in the absence of treatment over a mean period of 40.8 months. After obliteration, only patients without the development of shunts had reappearance of esophageal varices requiring sclerotherapy. Because natural splenorenal shunts occurred frequently in a group of patients with extrahepatic portal venous obstruction who were observed for 23.5 months and who also underwent sclerotherapy, it appears that splenorenal shunts result from sclerotherapy and protect patients from rebleeding and recurrence of varices.—N.J. Greenberger, M.D.

Treatment of Chronic Hepatitis Delta Virus (HDV) Infection With Human Lymphoblastoid Alpha Interferon
Farci P, Karayiannis P, Brook MG, et al.
QT J Med 73:1045–1054, 1989   C–21

▶ Ten patients with evidence of continuing HDV replication were given lymphoblastoid α-interferon and 8 more were followed up as a nonrandomized control group. In 4 of 8 patients who completed 1 year of follow-up, HDV-RNA had cleared from the serum, but in none of the control group did it clear. In these 4 responding patients transaminase levels were increased transiently during treatment, and in 2, the increases were followed by improvement. In 1 patient HBV also cleared and seroconverted to anti-HBs (antibody to hepatitis B surface antigen). In 1 patient with sustained loss of HDV, recurrence of HDV infection was detected 18 months after completion of treatment.

These data suggest that α-interferon can inhibit HDV replication in the short term, but relapse may occur after 1 to 2 years. Inhibition of HDV-RNA is associated with improvement in inflammatory liver disease; now larger studies must be done to determine whether it influences survival.—N.J. Greenberger, M.D.

Evidence for Disease Recurrence After Liver Transplantation for Primary Biliary Cirrhosis: Clinical and Histologic Follow-Up Studies
Polson RJ, Portmann B, Neuberger J, et al.
Gastroenterology 97:715–725, 1989   C–22

▶ Twenty-three patients with primary biliary cirrhosis who survived more than 1 year after liver transplantation were studied. All reported marked symptomatic improvement and had significant falls in serum bilirubin, alkaline phosphatase, immunoglobulin M, and antimitochondrial antibody levels. Beyond 1 year, liver biopsies showed features compatible with disease recurrence in 9 of 10 patients, and another 4 patients had pruritus or associated abnormalities. Levels of immunoglobulin M were raised in 80%, and antimitochondrial antibody titers were elevated in all those tested. Cyclosporine treatment for some patients initially given prednisone and azathioprine was followed by regression of histologic abnormalities.

Of 102 patients with nonprimary biliary cirrhosis who were followed similarly, 50 underwent biopsy, and although 12 had features of bile duct damage, all had additional histologic and clinical changes supporting alternative diagnoses. These findings are consistent with previous reports that primary biliary cirrhosis can recur after transplantation, possibly modified by the use of cyclosporine.—N.J. Greenberger, M.D.

Prospective Evaluation of Esophageal Varices in Primary Biliary Cirrhosis: Development, Natural History, and Influence on Survival
Gores GJ, Wiesner RH, Dickson ER, et al.
Gastroenterology 96:1552–1559, 1989   C-23

▶ The aims of this study were to determine the development and natural history of esophageal varices and variceal bleeding in patients with primary biliary cirrhosis. As part of a controlled clinical study, 265 patients with primary biliary cirrhosis who did not have esophageal varices at entry were followed for a median of 5.6 years. Their mean age was 49 years, 89% were women, and 69% had advanced histologic stage disease (stages 3–4) on liver biopsy at study entry. All patients underwent annual screening for esophageal varices by barium esophagogram, endoscopy, or both; endoscopy was used to diagnose all episodes of esophageal variceal bleeding. Esophageal varices developed in 83 patients (31%), and 40 (48%) of those with esophageal varices had 1 or more episodes of esophageal variceal bleeding. Cox regression analysis indicated that only serum bilirubin and histologic stage were associated independently with time to development of esophageal varices. Among patients with esophageal varices, 33% and 41% had esophageal variceal bleeding at 1 and 3 years, respectively. After development of esophageal varices, 1- and 3- year survival estimates were 83% and 59%, respectively. After the initial variceal bleeding episode, survival estimates were 65% and 46% at 1 and 3 years and were dependent on Child's classification. These findings are important in considering indications for prophylactic therapy for esophageal varices in primary biliary cirrhosis and may influence timing of liver transplantation.—N.J. Greenberger, M.D.

Correlation of IgM Anti-Hepatitis D Virus (HDV) to HDV RNA in Sera of Chronic HDV
Govindarajan S, Gupta S, Valinluck B, et al.
Hepatology 10:34–35, 1989   C-24

▶ One hundred forty-four serum samples from 52 patients with chronic hepatitis D virus infection were analyzed for hepatitis D virus RNA by dot-blot hybridization using hepatitis D virus complementary DNA probe labeled with ^{32}P. The results were correlated with the presence of serum immunoglobulin M (IgM) anti-hepatitis D virus and hepatitis D antigen in liver biopsy specimens when available. Although there was a trend of positive correlation between serum hepatitis D virus RNA and IgM anti-hepatitis D virus, no stastistical significance could be found. In the serum samples with hepatitis D virus RNA, 32% were found to be negative for IgM anti-hepatitis D virus. Therefore, in chronic hepatitis D virus, absence of IgM anti-hepatitis D virus does not rule out active viral infection, as suggested by previous studies. Serum hepatitis D virus RNA and hepatic hepatitis D virus antigen were strongly correlated. These data indicate that detection of hepatitis D virus RNA in serum samples is a reliable noninvasive marker of active viral infection.—N.J. Greenberger, M.D.

Gallbladder and Biliary Tract

Abdominal Symptoms and Gallstone Disease: An Epidemiological Investigation
Jorgensen T
Hepatology 9:856–860, 1989   C–25

▶ Which symptoms are caused specifically by stones in the gallbladder never has been established. To examine this issue, the relationship between occurrence of gallstone disease diagnosed with ultrasonography and complaints about abdominal pain and discomfort was assessed with a random sample comprising 4,581 males and females, of whom 3,608 (79%) took part in the investigation. Regarding the presence of gallstones, the predictive values of various complaints about pain and discomfort were very low, ranging from 0% to 25%, whereas for the absence of gallstones, the predictive value of no complaints about pain or discomfort was very high, ranging from 93.2% to 94.2%. In persons with gallstones, the prevalence of upper right quadrant pain during the last 12 months was equal to that in persons with normal gallbladders, whereas in cholecystectomized persons, the prevalence of pain was significantly higher. Pain was not associated with size, number, or motility of the stones. Jorgensen concludes that in a random population it is difficult to define the symptoms specific for gallstones and thereby to distinguish between symptomatic and asymptomatic gallstones.—N.J. Greenberger, M.D.

Prospective Randomized Comparison of Mezlocillin Therapy Alone With Combined Ampicillin and Gentamicin Therapy for Patients With Cholangitis
Gerecht WB, Henry NK, Hoffman WW, et al.
Arch Intern Med 149:1279–1284, 1989   C–26

▶ Forty-six patients with cholangitis were randomized to receive therapy with mezlocillin sodium (24 patients) or a combination of ampicillin sodium and gentamicin sulfate (22 patients). The biliary concentration of mezlocillin was 112 times greater than that of ampicillin and 778 times greater than that of gentamicin. The ratio of the concentration in serum or bile over the minimum inhibitory concentration against aerobic gram-negative bacilli (therapeutic index) was higher for mezlocillin than for either ampicillin or gentamicin. *Twenty (83%) of 24 patients were cured after mezlocillin therapy compared with 9 (41%) of 22 patients after ampicillin-gentamicin therapy.* The 3 patients with superinfection were in the ampicillin-gentamicin arm of the study. Fewer toxic or adverse effects occurred in association with mezlocillin treatment than with ampicillin-gentamicin treatment. Mezlocillin therapy was more effective, less toxic, and less expensive than treatment with ampicillin and gentamicin for patients with cholangitis.—N.J. Greenberger, M.D.

Cholecystokinin Prevents Parenteral Nutrition Induced Biliary Sludge in Humans
Sitzmann JV, Pitt HA, Steinborn PA, et al.
Surg Gynecol Obstet 170:25–31, 1990   C-27

▶ Long-term total parenteral nutrition (TPN) induces biliary sludge and formation of gallstones. A randomized, double-blind controlled study was designed to test the hypothesis that daily administration of cholecystokinin-octapeptide (CCK-OP) prevents the formation of biliary sludge in persons receiving long-term TPN. Adult patients receiving TPN for more than 21 consecutive days were studied. After randomization of 15 patients, the study was concluded because statistical significance was achieved. Eight patients received saline solution (placebo) intravenously, and 7 received CCK-OP (50 ng/kg) intravenously over a 10-minute period daily. The groups were similar with respect to age, sex, diagnosis, liver function tests, amylase levels, total TPN time, and time of study. All the patients underwent weekly ultrasound studies. Volume and emptying studies of the gallbladder in response to the study drug were performed after 1 week. None of the patients receiving CCK-OP had sludge, whereas 5 of 8 of the patients receiving placebo had sludge ($P < .02$). The results of emptying studies indicated significant contraction of the gallbladder in the CCK-OP group but not in the placebo group. These data suggest that CCK-OP given intravenously daily prevents TPN-induced stasis and sludge of the gallbladder. The authors conclude that CCK-OP should be used as routine prophylaxis against biliary sludge and formation of gallstones in patients receiving long-term TPN.—N.J. Greenberger, M.D.

Pancreas

Acute Pancreatitis and Normoamylasemia: Not an Uncommon Combination
Alain Clavien P, Robert J, Meyer P, et al.
Ann Surg 210:613–620, 1989   C-28

▶ A series of 352 consecutive attacks of acute pancreatitis (AP) in 318 patients was studied prospectively. The disease was ascertained with contrast-enhanced CT scan in all but 4 cases, in which diagnosis was made at operation or autopsy.

In 67 of these cases serum amylase levels were normal on admission (i.e., less than 160 IU/L, a limit that includes 99% of control values), a figure considerably higher than generally admitted. When compared with AP with elevated serum amylase, normoamylasemic pancreatitis was characterized by the following: (1) the prevalence of alcoholic etiology (58% vs. 33%, respectively); (2) a greater number of previous attacks in alcoholic pancreatitis (0.7 vs. 0.4); and (3) a longer duration of symptoms before admission (2.4 vs. 1.5 days, $P < .005$). In contrast AP did not appear to differ significantly in terms of CT findings, Ranson's score, and clinical course, when comparing normoamylasemic and hyperamylasemic patients, although normoamylasemic patients tended to have milder courses.

Serum lipase was measured in 65 of these normoamylasemic cases and was found to be elevated in 44 (68%), thus increasing diagnostic sensitivity from 81% when amylase alone is used to 94% for both enzymes. A peritoneal tap was obtained in 44 cases: amylase concentration in the first liter of dialysate was greater than 160 IU/L in 24 cases (55%), and lipase was greater than 250 U/L in 31 cases (70%). Twelve of these 44 cases had low peritoneal fluid and plasma concentration for both enzymes. Thus little gain in diagnostic sensitivity was obtained when adding peritoneal values (96%) to serum determinations. Acute pancreatitis is not associated invariably with elevated serum amylase. Multiple factors may contribute to the absence of hyperamylasemia on admission, including a return to normal enzyme levels before hospitalization or the inability of inflamed pancreases to produce amylase. Approximately two thirds of cases with normal amylasemia were properly identified by serum lipase determinations. Acute pancreatitis does not appear to behave differently when serum amylase is normal or elevated, and therefore should be submitted to similar therapeutic regimens in both conditions.—N.J. Greenberger, M.D.

The Spectrum and Natural History of Common Bile Duct Stenosis in Chronic Alcohol-Induced Pancreatitis
Kalvaria I, Bornman PC, Marks IN, et al.
Ann Surg 210:607–613, 1989   C-29

▶ Sixty patients wtih chronic alcohol-induced pancreatitis and evidence of common bile duct stenosis on endoscopic retrograde cholangiopancreatography (ERCP) were studied to determine the clinical spectrum and natural history of this complication, as well as the indications for biliary bypass. In 17% of patients, common bile duct stenosis (CBDS) was an incidental finding at ERCP, whereas in the remaining patients pain and jaundice were the predominant symptoms in 35% and 48%, respectively. Biliary drainage was done in 38% of patients for persistent or recurrent jaundice, for cholangitis, and while undergoing drainage of pancreatic ducts or cysts to alleviate pain. The benign nature of CBDS in chronic alcohol-induced pancreatitis (CAIP) in patients without persistent jaundice is emphasized. In particular, no histologically proved cases of secondary biliary cirrhosis were noted. Most cases of CBDS caused by CAIP may be managed safely without biliary bypass, but require close follow-up.—N.J. Greenberger, M.D.

Visual Vignettes

V–1   Esophageal Carcinoma Multiplex With Gastric Metastasis
V–2   Mycobacterial Esophagitis in AIDS
V–3   Heterotopic Gastric Mucosa of the Duodenum Mimicking a Duodenal Cancer
V–4   Gastrointestinal Sarcoidosis: Radiographic Findings
V–5   Lymphomatous Polyposis of the Colon
V–6   Colonic Aphthous Ulcers in Pseudomembranous Colitis
V–7   Magnetic Resonance Imaging in Hemochromatosis: Extrahepatic Iron Deposition
V–8   The Stilette Sign: The Appearance of Dilated Bile Ducts in the Fatty Liver

---

Esophageal Carcinoma Multiplex With Gastric Metastasis
Davis M, Gogel H, et al.
Gastrointest Radiol 14:6–8, 1989   V–1

➤ Multiple discrete squamous cancers of the esophagus are rare. In this case report a 50-year-old man who used ethanol and tobacco heavily was found to have 5 discrete foci of esophageal squamous carcinoma with a large metastasis to the stomach. The authors propose 3 possible explanations for the simultaneous appearance of these cancers: lymphatic metastasis, simultaneous primary tumors, and hematogenous metastasis. Of these possibilities, lymphatic spread of tumor appears to be most likely.—P.B. Miner, Jr., M.D.

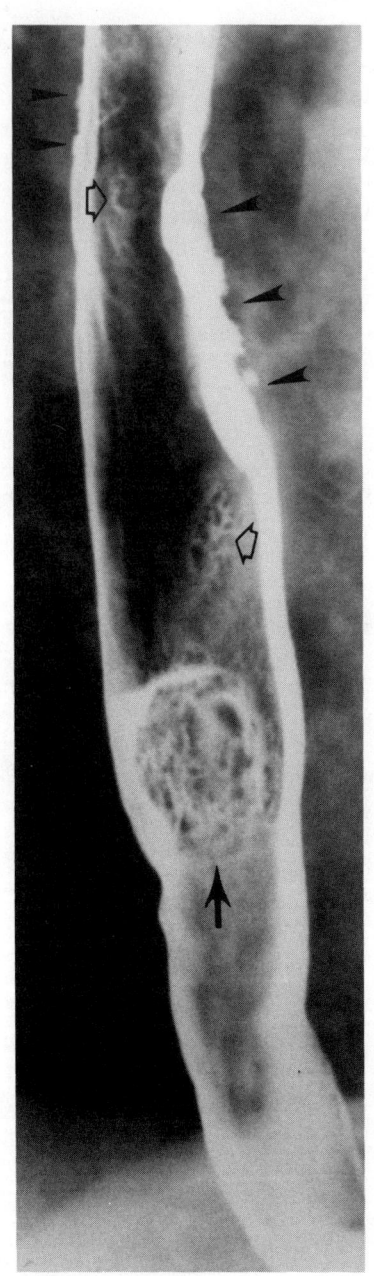

Double-contrast esophagogram shows 5 distinct lesions: 2 separate areas of ulcerations (*arrowheads*), 2 separate colonies of mucosal irregularity (*open arrows*), and 1 large tumor plaque with an irregular surface (*large arrows*). (Courtesy of Davis M, Gogel H, et al: *Gastrointest Radiol* 14:6–8, 1989.)

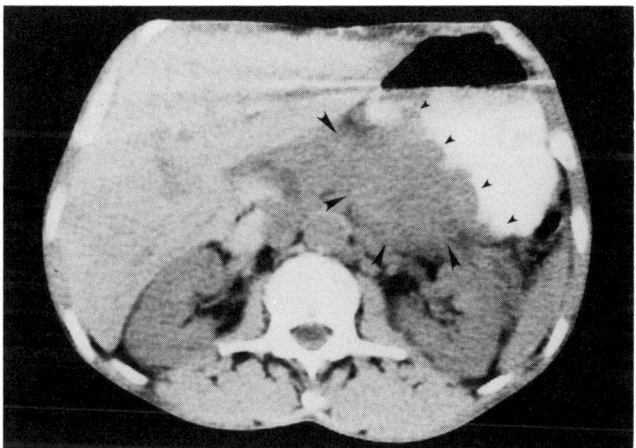

The CT examination of the abdomen at level of stomach shows a metastatic gastric tumor mass (*small arrowheads*) and retrogastric adenopathy (*large arrowheads*). (Courtesy of Davis M, Gogel H, et al: *Gastrointest Radiol* 14:6–8, 1989.)

Mycobacterial Esophagitis in AIDS
Goodman P, Pinero SS, et al.
Gastrointest Radiol 14:103–105, 1989   V-2

➤ Unusual infections with very severe manifestations occur in patients with acquired immune deficiency. In this case report *Mycobacterium tuberculosis* was cultured from a pleural effusion in a patient with severe esophagitis. Esophagitis was characterized by sinus tracts and deep ulcerations into the mediastinum. The presence of sinus tracts into the mediastinum should suggest an atypical manifestation of infection because this has not been reported with fungal or viral esophagitis in patients with AIDS.—P.B. Miner, Jr., M.D.

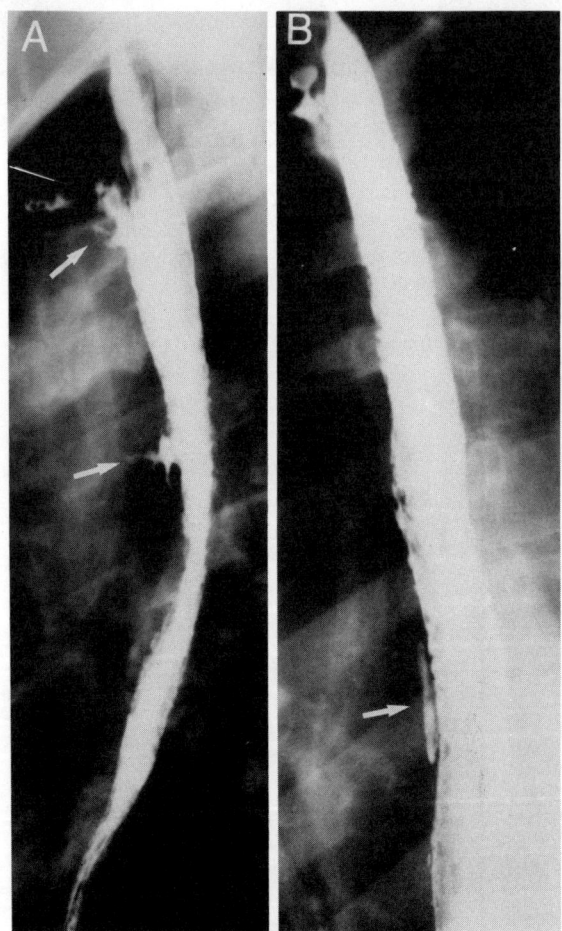

A, esophagogram shows sinus tracts extending anteriorly from the thoracic esophagus into the mediastinum (*arrows*). Diffuse mucosal irregularity of the esophagus is also present. **B,** a long, shallow ulceration is seen in the midportion of the esophagus (*arrows*). (Courtesy of Goodman P, Pinero SS, et al: *Gastrointest Radiol* 14:103–105, 1989.)

Heterotopic Gastric Mucosa of the Duodenum Mimicking a Duodenal Cancer
Yoshimitsu K, Yoshida M, et al.
Gastrointest Radiol 14:115–117, 1989

➤ Advanced diagnostic techniques indicate heterotopic gastric mucosa of the duodenum is far more common than previously suspected. Recently, Agha et al. (AJR 150:291–294, February 1988) described radiographic findings for 25 patients with heterotopic gastric mucosa. In most of the patients mucosal plaques were 1 to 3 mm and were raised above a flat, featureless mucosa of the duodenal bulb. A different appearance was coarse nodular mucosa in the duodenum with superficial erosions or ulcer craters. Patients occasionally can have solitary polyps in the duodenal bulb. This illustration presents a solitary lesion with a central depression that mimics an ulcerating cancer. The mucosa has a pattern similar to that of enhanced area gastrica seen in gastritis and was compressible during the examination. The importance of heterotopic gastric mucosa is unknown.—P.B. Miner, Jr., M.D.

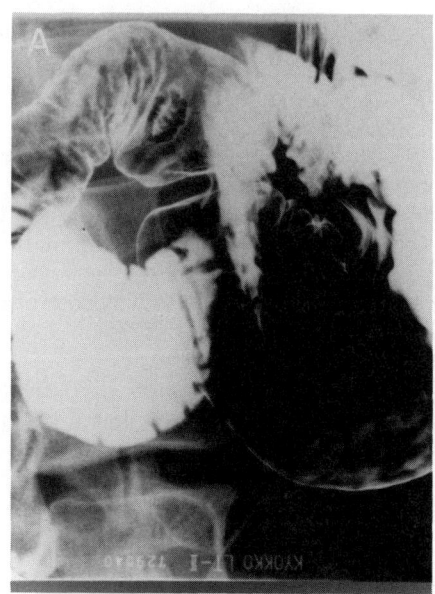

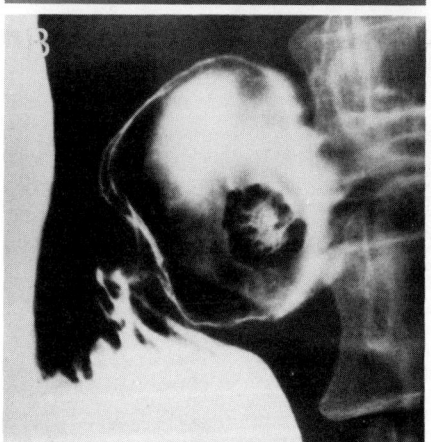

Radiography revealed a solitary polypoid lesion on the anterior wall of the duodenal bulb. **A,** double-contrast image, supine position, right anterior oblique view. **B,** compression image, prone position, left posterior oblique view. (Courtesy of Yoshimitsu K, Yoshida M, et al: *Gastrointest Radiol* 14:115–117, 1989.)

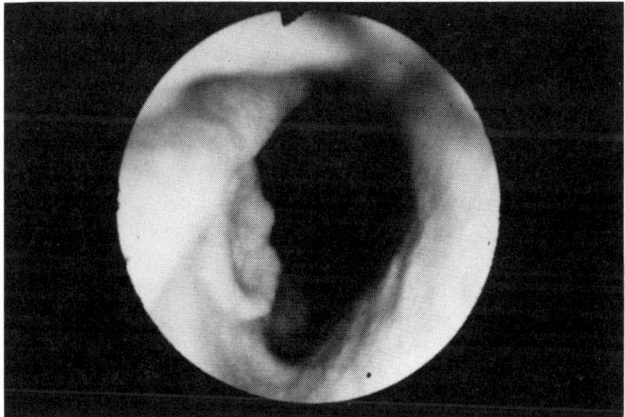

Endoscopy revealed the lesion's color to be indistinguishable from that of the normal duodenal mucosa surrounding it. (Courtesy of Yoshimitsu K, Yoshida M, et al: *Gastrointest Radiol* 14:115–117, 1989.)

Gastrointestinal Sarcoidosis: Radiographic Findings
Levine MS, Ekberg O, et al.
AJR 153:293–295, August 1989   V–4

➤ Although gastrointestinal involvement with sarcoidosis is considered unusual, E. D. Palmer reported noncaseating granulomas in mucosal biopsies of 10% of patients with known sarcoidosis (1). The findings in the figures in this case demonstrate nodularity in the gastric mucosa associated with sarcoidosis. The differential diagnosis of nodular gastric mucosa includes numerous diseases such as caustic ingestion, radiation, tuberculosis, fungal disease, syphilis, chronic gastritis, and Crohn's disease. Gastric polyps and tumors also can mimic this appearance, although they usually have a more prominent luminal definition. The authors mentioned a cecal stricture caused by sarcoid.—P.B. Miner, Jr., M.D.

Reference

1. Palmer ED: *J Lab Clin Med* 52:231, 1958.

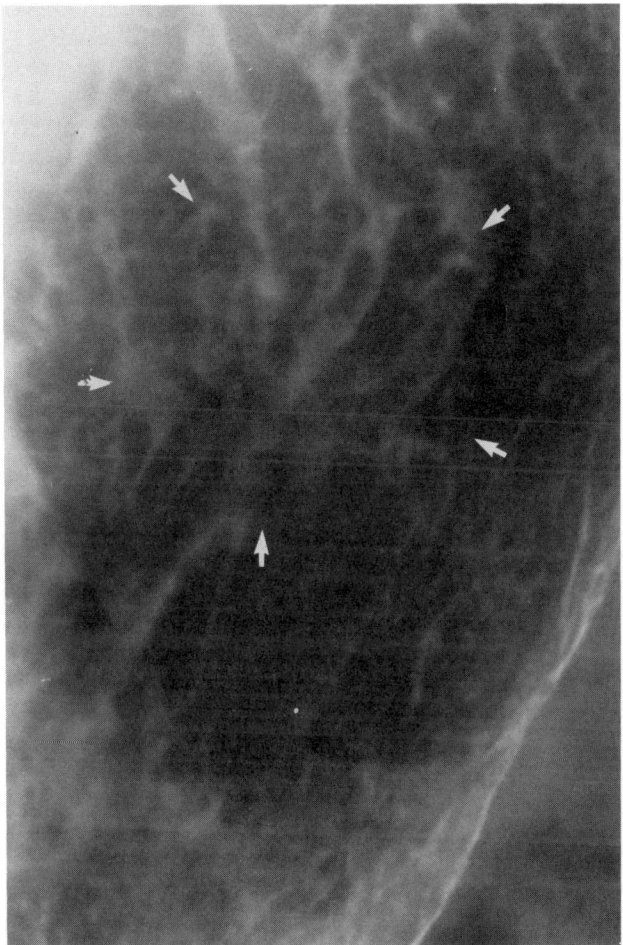

Man, 70, with known pulmonary sarcoidosis and epigastric pain. Double-contrast radiograph of stomach shows localized area of mucosal nodularity and thickened, irregular folds in the proximal stomach (*arrows*). Mucosal biopsies from this region revealed noncaseating granulomas. (Courtesy of Levine MS, Ekberg O, et al: *AJR* 153:293–295, August 1989.)

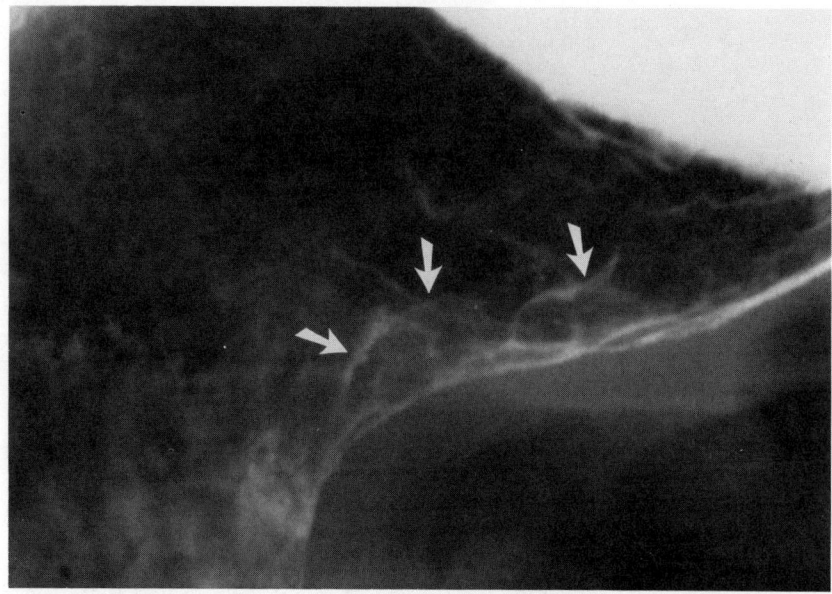

Double-contrast radiograph of stomach of man aged 72 years with pulmonary sarcoidosis, dysphagia, and epigastric pain shows focal area of mucosal nodularity on greater curvature of gastric body (*arrows*). Although endoscopic biopsies failed to reveal granulomas, the patient had a dramatic clinical response to steroid therapy with resolution of lesions on repeat endoscopy 6 weeks later. (Courtesy of Levine MS, Ekberg O, et al: *AJR* 153:293–295, August 1989.)

Lymphomatous Polyposis of the Colon
Davis M, Maxwell G, et al.
Gastrointest Radiol 14:70–72, 1989   V–5

➤ Lymphoma commonly involves the gastrointestinal tract. Diffuse lymphomatous polyposis is unusual, occurring in approximately 3% of patients with lymphoma involving the colon. The radiographic patterns include multiple intraluminal masses, intraluminal infiltration, multiple small umbilicated nodules of various size and distribution, and an ileocecal mass.—P.B. Miner, Jr., M.D.

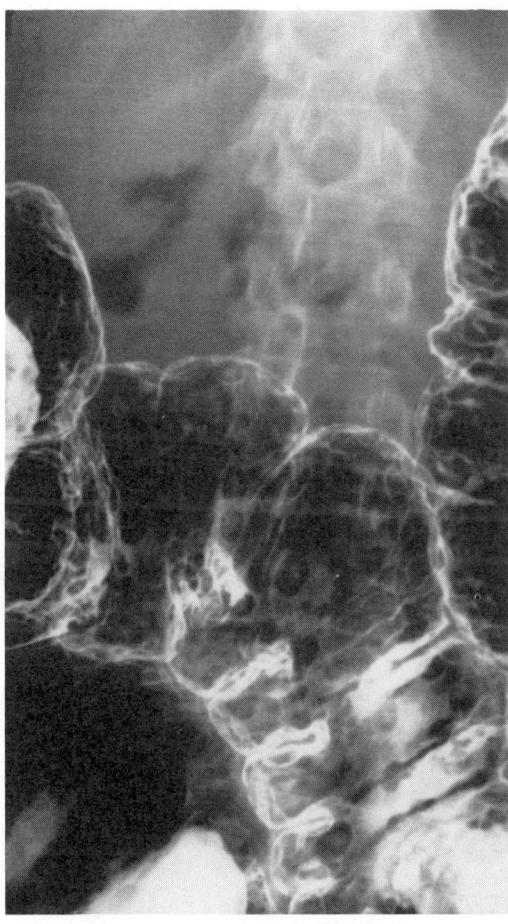

Magnified view of double-contrast enema of transverse colon shows innumerable umbilicated lymphomatous nodules. (Courtesy of Davis M, Maxwell G, et al: *Gastrointest Radiol* 14:70–72, 1989.)

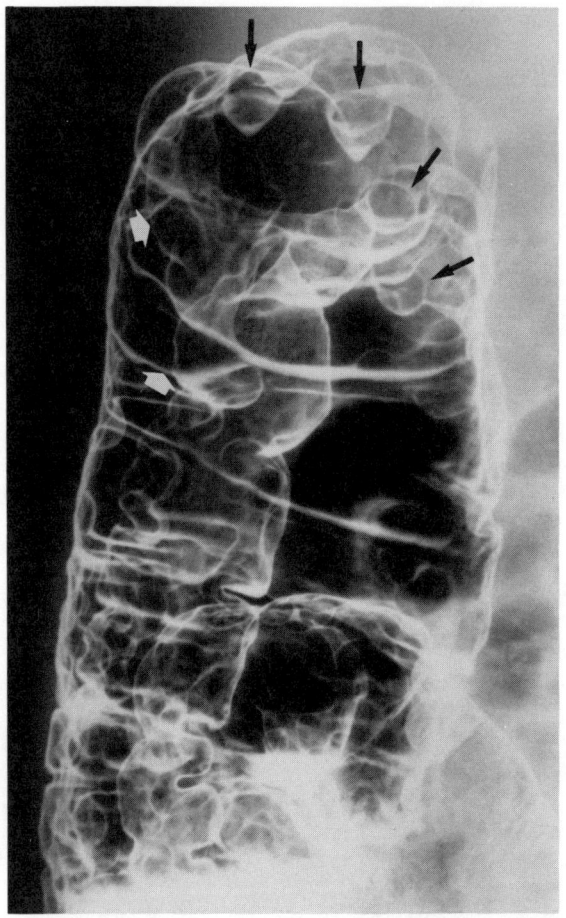

Double-contrast enema of hepatic flexure shows numerous lymphomatous polyps (*arrows*), appearing elongated or filiform *(arrowheads)*. (Courtesy of Davis M, Maxwell G, et al: *Gastrointest Radiol* 14:70–72, 1989.)

Colonic Aphthous Ulcers in Pseudomembranous Colitis
Millward S, Salonen D, Joanes F
J Can Assoc Radiol 40:53–54, February 1989   V–6

➤ An edematous colonic wall with multiple aphthous ulcers caused by *Clostridium difficile* broadens the differential of aphthous ulceration in the colon. The thickened mucosa narrows the differential diagnosis to the more inflammatory lesions of colon, which include Crohn's disease, Behçet's disease, *Yersinia enterocolitica,* shigellosis, *Campylobacter jejuni,* ischemia colitis, diversion colitis, *Entamoeba histolytica,* herpes, tuberculosis, cytomegalovirus, candida, and histoplasmosis. Many patients with resolving pseudomembranous colitis have nodular areas with plaque-like lesions. This radiographic picture fits nicely between resolving, active pseudomembranes and nodularity associated with resolution.—P.B. Miner, Jr., M.D.

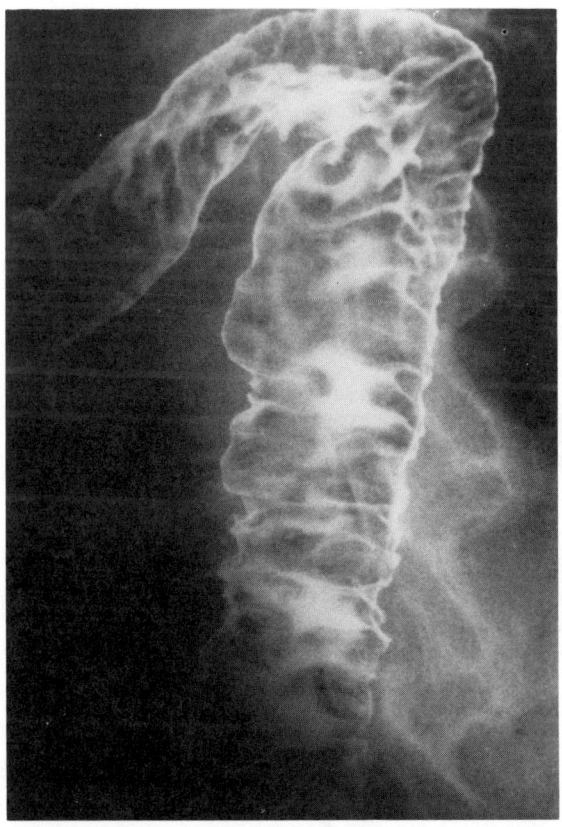

Spot film of the descending colon reveals numerous aphthous ulcers. (Courtesy of Millward S, Salonen D, Joanes F: *J Can Assoc. Radiol* 40:53–54, February 1989.)

Magnetic Resonance Imaging in Hemochromatosis: Extrahepatic Iron Deposition
Housman JF, Chezmar JL, Nelson RC
Gastrointest Radiol 14:59–60, 1989   V-7

▶ Computed tomography has been used to identify hemochromatosis by the increase in alternation of a variety of organs including liver, spleen, pancreas and lymph nodes containing increased iron. In this case magnetic resonance imaging (MRI) indicates extrahepatic iron deposition as well as deposition of iron in the liver suggested by striking decrease in signal intensity. These findings suggest MRI is sensitive to changes in tissue iron, which may allow its use for indicating extrahepatic iron overload.—P.B. Miner, Jr., M.D.

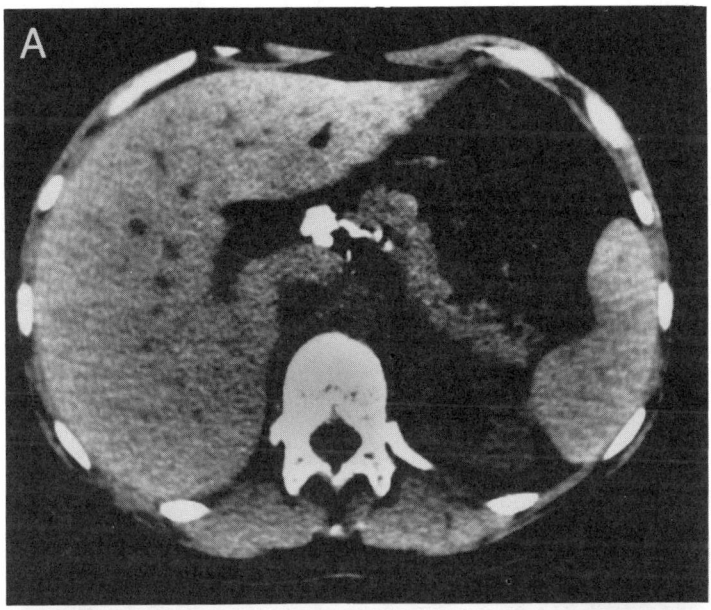
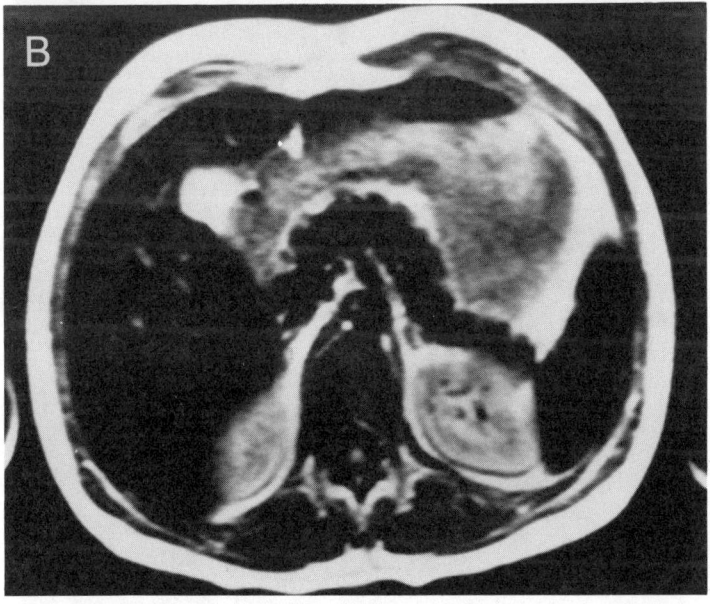

A, noncontrast CT image demonstrates increased attenuation of liver and spleen. The pancreas is also of slightly increased density. The porta hepatis lymph nodes are strikingly dense secondary to iron deposition. **B,** magnetic resonance image (spin echo, 30/1,000) at a slightly different level demonstrates marked decrease in signal intensity of liver, spleen, and pancreas. Low-signal peripancreatic nodes could not be distinguished from pancreatic tissue of similar low intensity. (Courtesy of Housman JF, Chezmar JL, Nelson RC: *Gastrointest Radiol* 14:59–60, 1989.)

The Stilette Sign: The Appearance of Dilated Bile Ducts in the Fatty Liver
Ingram C, Joseph AEA
Clin Radiol 40:257–258, 1989   V–8

➤ Fatty changes in the liver decrease the ultrasound characteristics of the portal vein and bile duct. The usual double-barreled shotgun sign seen in the presence of dilated ducts in a normal liver is lost with fatty liver because of these changes in the ultrasound resolution. Loss of the walls of the tubular structure results in an apparent fluid-filled tube with a central echogenic line indicating the adjacent portal vein and bile duct.—P.B. Miner, Jr., M.D.

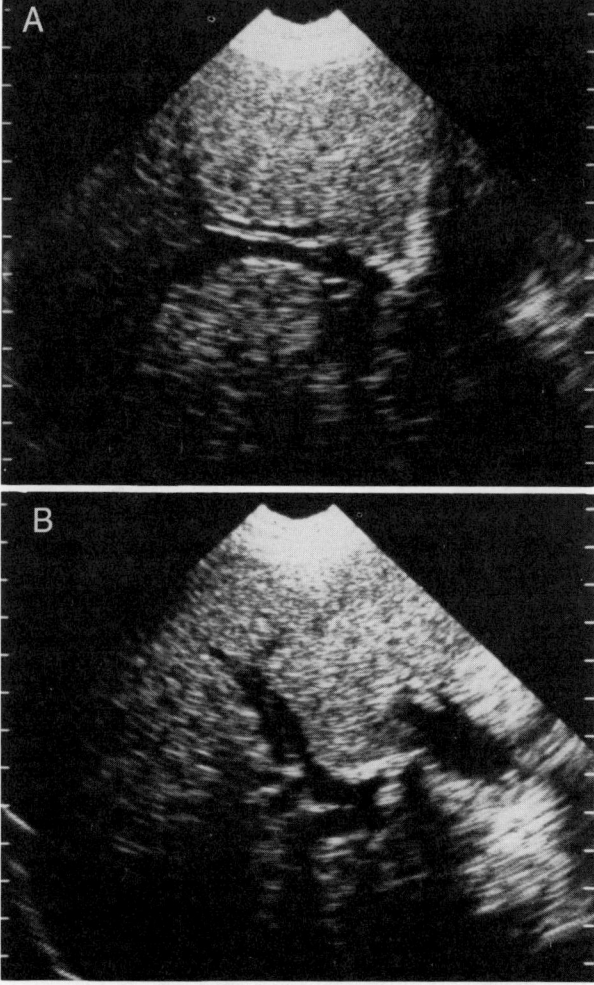

A, scan through the liver showing the usual parallel channel sign with preserved echoes from the walls of the bile duct and portal vein before parenteral nutrition. There is some degree of fatty change in the liver. **B,** the stilette sign is now seen after parenteral nutrition and more marked fatty change. (Courtesy of Ingram C, Joseph AEA: *Clin Radiol* 40:257–258, 1989.)

Subject Index

A

Abdomen
    cancer, organ cluster transplant in, 280
    organ cluster transplant in abdominal cancer, 280
    rectopexy for rectal prolapse, 189
    trauma
        jejunostomy feeding after, causing gastrointestinal symptoms, 154
        major, TEN vs. TPN after, 147
    tuberculosis, clinical features, 404
Achalasia
    esophageal resection in, indications and results, 7
    with esophageal sphincter relaxation, 3
    radiographic and manometric correlation in, 3
    treatment, current perspective, 6
Achlorhydria
    pentagastrin-fast, with duodenal ulcer, 401
Acquired immunodeficiency syndrome (see AIDS)
Adenocarcinoma
    in Barrett's esophagus (see Barrett's esophagus, adenocarcinoma in)
    colon, liver and lung metastases from, 200
    Crohn's disease and dysplasia, 141
    of gastric antrum, gastrectomy in, 75
Adenoma
    rectosigmoid villous, endoscopic laser for, 196
Adenomatous (see Polyposis, adenomatous)
Admissions
    for duodenal ulcer, changing pattern, 57
Adrenal
    -spleno-renal shunt after endoscopic sclerotherapy, 409
Aganglionosis
    colon, colectomy and ileorectal anastomosis in, 217
Aged
    chronic illness, nasogastric feeding tubes in, 152
    hospitalized, inadequate barium enema for, 403
    mesenteric infarction, acute, 130
    pancreatography of, retrograde, interpretation of, 361
AIDS
    (See also HIV)
    with cholangiopathy, 345
    with cholangitis, radiography of, 343
    esophagitis in, mycobacterial, 418
    Isospora belli infection in, 107

Air
    -fluid sign, gastric, in CT assessment of gastric wall thickening, 87
Albumin
    in cirrhosis with ascites and paracentesis, 255
    supplement for parenteral nutrition and hospital morbidity, 146
Alcohol
    effect on pancreatic secretion, meal-stimulated, 356
    gastric alcohol dehydration activity decrease and first-pass metabolism, 40
    high blood levels in women, 40
    pancreatitis due to, bile duct stenosis in, 414
Alcoholic
    cirrhosis with ascites, peritoneovenous shunt vs. medical treatment in, 256
    hepatitis, methylprednisolone in, 253
    pancreatitis, pancreatic resection in, 381
Alimentary tract
    duplications, surgery of, 116
Alkaline
    gastroesophageal reflux in Barrett's esophagus, 28
    reflux gastritis, atony after Roux-Y diversion, 66
    shift in gastric pH after cholecystectomy, 42
Alpha-interferon
    in hepatitis B, chronic, 237
Amino acid
    for protein sparing after surgery, 149
5-Aminosalicylic acid
    suppositories in ulcerative colitis, 404
Amiodarone
    hepatotoxicity, case review, 271
Ampicillin
    in cholangitis, 412
Ampulla
    tumors, 391
Anabolic
    steroid in early postoperative period, 148
Anal anastomosis (see Anastomosis, ileal pouch-anal)
Anastomosis
    ileal pouch-anal
        "ileal brake" in, 98
        quality of life after, 182
        results in polyposis and ulcerative colitis, 181

technique alterations, complications and outcome, 182
ileorectal in colonic aganglionosis, 217
Angelchik
prosthesis vs. Nissen fundoplication, 23
Antibiotic(s)
in appendicitis, acute nonperforated, for prophylaxis, 210
-associated diarrhea by *Saccharomyces boulardi*, prevention, 172
in peritonitis, bacterial, and polymorphonuclear cells, 407
Antibody(ies)
anti-carcinoembryonic antigen, in colon carcinoma (in mice), 200
to etiologic virus of hepatitis C, 241
HBs, after hepatitis B vaccination, 233
hepatitis B X gene, in liver disease, 239
hepatitis C (*see* Hepatitis C antibodies)
Anti-carcinoembryonic
antigen antibody $F(ab')_2$ fragments in colon carcinoma (in mice), 200
Antigen
anti-carcinoembryonic, in colon carcinoma (in mice), 200
hepatitis B e, mutation preventing formation of, 236
Antimitochondrial
autoantibodies in biliary cirrhosis, 285
Antinucleating factors
inhibiting $CaCO_3$ precipitation in biliary duct and gallbladder bile (in dog), 313
Antireflux surgery
Hill, results, 19
in reflux esophagitis, evaluations, 17
Aortic
reconstruction and colonic ischemia, 213
Appendicitis
acute
ileus of jejunum in, 207
nonperforated, antibiotic prophylaxis in, 210
ultrasound in, 208
surgery, consequences of constraints on, 210
"Apple peel" deformity
with jejunal atresia, 115
Ascites (*see under* Cirrhosis)
Atony
gastric, after Roux-Y diversion, 66
Atopic
dermatitis, histamine release from basophils and histamine-releasing factor in, 93
Atresia
biliary, surgery of, 347
jejunal, with "apple peel" deformity, 115
Atrophy

pancreatic, after pancreatitis, CT of, 364
Autoantibodies
in cirrhosis (*see under* Cirrhosis)
Autonomic
neuropathy and chronic liver disease, 406

B

Bacteremia
bilirubin and liver enzyme abnormalities in, 222
Bacteria
in gallbladder and gallstone formation, 315
Bacterial
peritonitis, antibiotics in, and polymorphonuclear cells, 407
Barium
enema, inadequate, in hospitalized aged, 403
Barrett's esophagus
adenocarcinoma in
development of, 27
study of, 29
cytometric abnormalities in, flow, 25
dysplasia in, 25, 27
gastroesophageal reflux and, alkaline, 28
Basophils
histamine release from, in atopic dermatitis and food hypersensitivity, 93
Benzodiazepine
receptor antagonist, flumazenil in hepatic encephalopathy, 266
Bile
acid(s)
alterations in intrahepatic cholestasis, 224
as feedback inhibitors of bile acid synthesis (in rat), 300
kinetics, cholecystectomy in, 299
duct
antinucleating factors inhibiting $CaCO_3$ precipitation and (in dog), 313
dilation in fatty liver, stilette sign, 430
stenosis in alcohol-induced pancreatitis, 414
duct stones
cholangiography and, endoscopic, before cholecystectomy, 339
endoscopic sphincterotomy for, catheter perfusion after, 335
ERCP in, 338
lithotomy with lithotripsy in, choledochoscopic electrohydraulic, 336
lithotripsy for, 337

Subject Index / 433

preoperative risk factors in, 336
sphincterotomy in, endoscopic, 338
duct tumors, distal, 391
gallbladder (*see* Gallbladder bile)
Biliary
atresia, surgery of, 347
cancer, liver transplant in, 278
cirrhosis (*see* Cirrhosis, biliary)
endoscopic therapy, endoscopic with percutaneous, 340
lipids during hormones for prostatic carcinoma, 311
Roux-en-Y biliary diversion, effect on *Campylobacter pylori*, 82
sludge, parenteral nutrition induced, cholecystokinin preventing, 413
strictures, benign postoperative, 346
tract dilatation in chronic pancreatitis, CT and ultrasound in, 380
Bilirubin
abnormalities in bacteremia, 222
Birth
weight, very low, cholestasis and enteral protein, 150
Bismuth
subcitrate, colloidal, in *Campylobacter* gastritis, 79
Bleeding (*see* Hemorrhage)
Bowel
inflammatory bowel disease
lymphoma of large intestine complicating, 405
refractory, methotrexate in, 134
6-mercaptopurine in, toxicity study, 136
irritable bowel syndrome
dietary fiber and rectosigmoid motility in, 203
food intolerance and, 205
ischemia, CT in, 214
rest and metabolic response to endotoxin, 151
short bowel syndrome
jejunostomy effluents in, and SMS 201–995, 110
outcome in newborn, 109
small
cancer, laparotomy in, 122
dilatation of, segmental, 94
obstruction, closed loop, enteroclysis in, 125
obstruction, postoperative, management, 126
Brooke
ileostomy, quality of life after, 182
Brush-border
assembly and differentiation, microvillus inclusion disease as inherited defect of, 101

Bypass
ileal, partial, in familial hypercholesterolemia, 119

C

$CaCO_3$ precipitation
antinucleating factors inhibiting, in biliary duct and gallbladder bile (in dog), 313
Calcifying
pancreatitis, protein messenger RNA in, 377
Campylobacter
gastritis with dyspepsia, 79
pylori
effect on Roux-en-Y biliary diversion, 82
gastritis, with gastric fold enlargement, 81
Cancer
abdomen, upper, organ cluster transplant in, 280
colon, hemoccult test evaluation, 194
duodenum, heterotopic gastric mucosa mimicking, 419
extrahepatic, after immunosuppression of hepatitis, 406
gastric, detected by mass screening, follow-up, 76
gastrointestinal, upper, with adenomatous polyposis, 121
hepatobiliary, liver transplant in, 278
liver
intraoperative ultrasound and preoperative imaging in, 275
primary, surgery and survival in, 273
recurrent, repeat hepatectomy in, 274
pancreas
CA19-9 in, 385, 386
CA19-9 radioimmunoassay in, 386
serologic marker in, 385
/polyp sequence in colon, radiography of, 194
rectum
clinical significance in young patients, 196
endosonography in, rectal, 191
hemoccult test evaluation, 194
radiotherapy for, preoperative, survival, 198
stomach, remnant, relationship to dysplasia, 65
CA19-9
in pancreatic cancer, 385, 386
Carcinoids
of duodenum, histology and immunohistochemistry, 77

Carcinoma
  cecal, CT for staging, 192
  colon, anti-carcinoembryonic antigen
    antibody F(ab')$_2$ fragments in (in
    mice), 200
  esophagus
    endosonography and CT in, 31
    multiplex with gastric metastases, 415
    preoperative classification vs. new TNM
      system, 31
    squamous cell superficial, case review,
      31
  gallbladder, experience with, 349
  hepatocellular, hepatitis C antibodies in,
    250
  pancreas, total pancreatectomy in, 392
  prostate, hormones for, biliary lipids
    during, 311
Catheter
  for methyl tert-butyl ether in cholesterol
    gallstones, 319
  perfusion after sphincterotomy of bile duct
    stones, 335
  vs. implanted reservoir for home nutrition
    support, 145
CCK (*see* Cholecystokinin)
Cecal
  carcinoma, CT for staging, 192
Cell(s)
  duodenal epithelial, ferritin lack in, in
    hemochromatosis, 96
  polymorphonuclear cells, and antibiotics in
    bacterial peritonitis, 407
Cephalic
  pancreatitis, duodenopancreatectomy in,
    382
Children
  gastroesophageal reflux, Nissen
    fundoplication in, 19
  reflux esophagitis, cimetidine for, 16
  of Southeast Asian refugees, hepatitis B in,
    234
Chloride
  sodium causing diarrhea after ileal and
    colonic resection, 159
Cholangiography
  endoscopic, and bile duct stones before
    cholecystectomy, 339
Cholangiopancreatography
  endoscopic retrograde, in bile duct stones,
    338
Cholangiopathy
  with AIDS, 345
Cholangitis
  with AIDS, radiography of, 343
  mezlocillin, ampicillin and gentamicin in,
    412
  sclerosing, study of, 341

Cholecystectomy
  in bile acid kinetics, 299
  cholangiography and bile duct stone
    removal before, 339
  gastric pH alkaline shift after, 42
  in sphincter of Oddi dysfunction,
    endoscopic sphincterotomy after, 328
Cholecystitis
  acute
    cholecystostomy in, percutaneous, 323,
      325
    cholescintigraphy of, 306
Cholecystokinin
  gastrointestinal motor functions and, 303
  infusion during cholescintigraphy and
    ultrasound of gallbladder emptying,
    305
  preventing parenteral nutrition induced
    biliary sludge, 413
  receptor antagonism by loxiglumide and
    gallbladder, 302
  receptor antagonists, effects on pancreatic
    secretions (in rat), 353
Cholecystostomy
  percutaneous, in acute cholecystitis, 323,
    325
Choledochoscopic
  electrohydraulic lithotripsy for stones in
    bile duct, intrahepatic duct and
    gallbladder, 336
Cholera
  seafood and, 402
Cholescintigraphy
  of cholecystitis, acute, 306
  of gallbladder emptying, 305
Cholestasis
  with enteral protein in very low birth
    weight, 150
  intrahepatic, bile acid alterations in, 224
Cholesterol
  absorption and serum level variations, 155
  gallstones, methyl tert-butyl ether for, 319
Cimetidine
  in reflux esophagitis in children, 16
Cirrhosis
  alcoholic, with ascites, peritoneovenous
    shunt vs. medical treatment in, 256
  with ascites, albumin in, and paracentesis,
    255
  biliary
    autoantibodies in, antimitochondrial,
      285
    autoantibodies to recombinant
      mitochondrial protein in, 283
    liver transplant in, 287
    liver transplant in, disease recurrence,
      410
    ursodeoxycholic acid in, 286

varices in, esophageal, 411
with variceal bleeding, 259
Cisapride
  in gastroparesis and intestinal
    pseudoobstruction, 85
Clostridium difficile
  diarrhea, bacteriotherapy of, 403
  infection with protein-losing enteropathy,
    405
  nosocomial infection, 171
Colectomy
  total, in colonic aganglionosis, 217
Colitis
  collagenous, vs. lymphocytic microscopic
    colitis, 175, 177
  diversion, fatty acid irrigation in, 179
  hemorrhagic, due to *Escherichia coli*, 165
  lymphocytic microscopic
    clinicopathology, 177
    histopathology, 175
    vs. collagenous colitis, 175, 177
  pseudomembranous, ulcer in, colonic
    aphthous, 427
  ulcerative (*see* Ulcerative colitis)
Collis
  -Nissen operation, continued assessment,
    20
Colon
  adenocarcinoma, liver and lung metastases
    from, 200
  aganglionosis, colectomy and ileorectal
    anastomosis in, 217
  cancer, hemoccult test evaluation, 194
  carcinoma, anti-carcinoembryonic antigen
    antibody F(ab')$_2$ fragments in (in
    mice), 200
  ischemia, clinical and endoscopic
    documentation, 213
  polyp/cancer sequence in, radiography of,
    194
  polyposis, lymphomatous, 425
  resection, sodium chloride causing
    diarrhea after, 159
  surgery without nasogastric
    decompression, 218
  trauma, penetrating, closure and
    colostomy in, 186
  ulcer, aphthous, in pseudomembranous
    colitis, 427
Colostomy
  in colon trauma, penetrating, 186
  after rectal injuries, with drainage, 185
Computed tomography
  in bowel ischemia, 214
  in cecal carcinoma staging, 192
  in esophageal carcinoma, 31
  in gastric wall thickening, gastric air-fluid
    sign in, 87

of liver hemangioma, giant cavernous, 292
of pancreatic atrophy after pancreatitis,
  364
in pancreatitis, chronic, with biliary tract
  dilatation, 380
of paraesophageal hernia, 34
in rectal villous tumors, 192
of sphincterotomy complications,
  endoscopic retrograde, 329
Corrosive acids
  ingestion, gastrointestinal tract after, 400
Corticosteroids
  in hepatitis in postmenopausal women,
    407
Cost
  of duodenal ulcer medical and surgical
    treatment, 56
Cricopharyngeal
  dysphagia, reflux-induced, myotomy in, 13
Crohn's disease
  with adenocarcinoma and dysplasia, 141
  chronic active, cyclosporine in, 138
  fistula and sinus tracts in, MRI of, 133
  hyperbaric oxygen in, 402
  obstructive, strictureplasty in, 140
  recurrence risk and reoperation in, 140
Cryptosporidiosis
  outbreak due to contamination of public
    water supply, 170
Cullen's sign
  in pancreatitis, acute, 360
Cyclosporine
  in Crohn's disease, chronic, 138
Cyst
  liver, hydatid, surgical results, 293
Cystic fibrosis
  gene, identification of, 367
Cytometry
  flow, abnormalities in Barrett's esophagus,
    25

D

Debridement
  in pancreatic necrosis, 372, 373
Delta (*see* Hepatitis, delta)
Dermatitis
  atopic, histamine release form basophils
    and histamine-releasing factor in, 93
Diarrhea
  chronic, after drinking untreated water,
    169
  Clostridium difficile, bacteriotherapy of,
    403
  osmotic, polyethylene glycol and lactulose
    causing, 161
  by *Saccharomyces boulardi*, antibiotic-

associated, prevention, 172
shigella, pathogenesis (in rabbit), 167
sodium chloride causing, after ileal and colon resection, 159
Diet
gallstone risk and, 309
regimens for gastric acidity reduction, 156
Dietary
fiber in irritable bowel syndrome, 203
Dihydrolipoamide acetyltransferase
of pyruvate dehydrogenase complex in biliary cirrhosis, 285
Diversion
colitis, fatty acid irrigation in, 179
Drainage
with colostomy after rectal injuries, 185
Drug(s)
IV users with chronic liver disease, hepatitis A in, 408
Duodenopancreatectomy
in chronic pancreatitis with pancreatic duct occlusion, 382
mortality and morbidity with, 389
Duodenum
cancer, heterotopic gastric mucosa mimicking, 419
carcinoids, histology and immunohistochemistry, 77
epithelial cells, ferritin lack in, in hemochromatosis, 96
injury with pancreatic injury, conservative management, 395
microgastrinoma, and Zollinger-Ellison syndrome failed surgery, 62
-preserving resection of pancreatic head in pancreatitis, 383
tumors, 391
ulcer (*see* Ulcer, duodenal)
Dyspepsia
in *Campylobacter* gastritis, 79
Dysphagia
cricopharyngeal, reflux-induced, myotomy in, 13
Dysplasia
in Barrett's esophagus, 25, 27
Crohn's disease and adenocarcinoma, 141

E

Elderly (*see* Aged)
Electrocoagulation
multipolar, in peptic ulcer, 73
Electrolyte
transport, intestinal, shiga toxin to villus cells of jejunum in (in rabbit), 167
Emergency
control of esophageal variceal bleeding, 261

Encephalopathy
hepatic, flumazenil in, 266
Endoscopic
biliary therapy, percutaneous with endoscopic, 340
cholangiography with stone removal before cholecystectomy, 339
gastrostomy, percutaneous, 154
laser of rectosigmoid villous adenoma, 196
retrograde cholangiopancreatography in bile duct stones, 338
sclerotherapy, spleno-adreno-renal shunt after, 409
sphincterotomy (*see* Sphincterotomy, endoscopic)
variceal sclerotherapy in variceal bleeding, 263
Endoscopy
in colon ischemia, 213
Endosonography
in esophageal carcinoma, 31
rectal, in rectal cancer, 191
Endotoxin
infusion and neutrophils for enteral and parenteral nutrition, 146
metabolic response to, TPN and bowel rest in, 151
Enema
barium, inadequate, in hospitalized aged, 403
Energy
requirements during hospitalization, and feeding tubes, 152
Enteral
nutrition, endotoxin infusion and neutrophils, 146
protein, and cholestasis in very low birth weight, 150
Enteritis
typhoid, perforated, surgery of, 173
Enteroclysis
in small bowel closed loop obstruction, 125
in small intestine hemorrhage, 402
Enteropathy
HIV-induced, 105
protein-losing, with *Clostridium difficile* infection, 405
Enzyme
liver, abnormalities in bacteremia, 222
Escherichia coli
colitis due to, hemorrhagic, 165
Esophagitis
mycobacterial, in AIDS, 418
reflux (*see* Reflux esophagitis)
Esophagus
Barrett's (*see* Barrett's esophagus)
carcinoma (*see* Carcinoma, esophagus)

gastroesophageal (see Reflux, gastroesophageal)
mucosal sensitivity to pH in gastroesophageal reflux, 15
paraesophageal hernia, CT of, 34
resection in achalasia, indications and results, 7
rupture, spontaneous, experience with, 33
spasm, radiographic and manometric correlation, 8
sphincter relaxation in achalasia, 3
variceal bleeding, sclerotherapy with staple transection in, 261
varices in biliary cirrhosis, 411
Estrogen
-induced gallstones in males, 311
Ethanol
first-pass metabolism, gastric origin of, 39

F

F(ab')$_2$ fragments
in colon carcinoma (in mice), 200
Famotidine
in duodenal ulcer, healing after, 45
in gastric ulcer, nocturnal acid secretion suppression in, 47
Fatty
acid irrigation in diversion colitis, 179
liver, stilette sign of bile ducts in, 430
Fecal
triglyceride excretion in pancreatic insufficiency, 357
Feedback
inhibitors, bile acids as, in bile acid synthesis (in rat), 300
Feeding
cholecystokinin receptor antagonism by loxiglumide and gallbladder contractions, 302
jejunostomy, gastrointestinal symptoms due to, 154
tubes
for energy requirements during hospitalization, 152
nasogastric, for chronic illness in aged, 152
Ferritin
lack in duodenal cells in hemochromatosis, 96
Fiber
dietary, in irritable bowel syndrome, 203
Fibrosis
cystic, gene, identification of, 367
Fistula
in Crohn's disease, MRI in, 133

FK 506
in liver, kidney and pancreas transplant, 277
Flumazenil
in encephalopathy, hepatic, 266
Food
hypersensitivity, histamine release from basophils and histamine-releasing factor in, 93
intolerance and irritable bowel syndrome, 205
iron absorption in hemochromatosis, 97
Fundoplication (see Nissen fundoplication)

G

Gallbladder
bacteria in, and gallstone formation, 315
bile
antinucleating factors inhibiting $CaCO_3$ precipitation in (in dog), 313
nucleation time and ursodeoxycholic acid, 312
carcinoma, experience with, 349
contractions, cholecystokinin receptor antagonism by loxiglumide and, 302
emptying, cholescintigraphy and ultrasound for, 305
motility and extracorporeal shock-wave lithotripsy, 320
Gallstone(s)
abdominal symptoms, epidemiology, 412
cholesterol, methyl tert-butyl ether for, 319
estrogen-induced formation in males, 311
formation and bacteria in gallbladder, 315
lithotomy with lithotripsy for, choledochoscopic electrohydraulic, 336
with pancreatitis during pregnancy, 369
partially calcified, lithotripsy with methyl tert-butyl ether in, 318
radiolucent, external shock-wave lithotripsy with ursodiol in, 315
recurrence after ursodeoxycholic acid, 322
risk of, weight and diet in, 309
Gastrectomy
in adenocarcinoma of gastric antrum, 75
gastric origin of ethanol first-pass metabolism and, 39
post-gastrectomy stomach, gastroscopic screening, 65
Gastric (see Stomach)
Gastrin
release by secretin increase in Zollinger-Ellison syndrome, 59

Gastrinoma
　microgastrinoma of duodenum and Zollinger-Ellison syndrome failed surgery, 62
Gastritis
　alkaline reflux, atony after Roux-Y diversion, 66
　Campylobacter
　　with dyspepsia, 79
　pylori, with gastric fold enlargement, 81
　histologic, and *Helicobacter pylori* infection, 80
Gastroesophageal reflux (*see* Reflux, gastroesophageal)
Gastrointestinal
　cancer, upper, with adenomatous polyposis, 121
　motor functions and cholecystokinin, 303
　sarcoidosis, radiography of, 422
　symptoms due to jejunostomy feeding, 154
　tract, upper, after corrosive acid ingestion, 400
　tumors, hormone-secreting, somatostatin in, 111
Gastroparesis
　cisapride in, 85
Gastroplasty
　vertical banded, assessment, 71
Gastroscopy
　screening of post-gastrectomy stomach, 65
Gastrostomy
　endoscopic, percutaneous, 154
Gene
　cystic fibrosis, identification of, 367
　X gene protein and antibody, hepatitis B, in liver disease, 239
Gentamicin
　in cholangitis, 412
Grey Turner's sign
　in pancreatitis, acute, 360
Gut
　diseases, somatostatin in, 111

H

Healing
　of duodenal ulcer after famotidine, 45
　of gastric ulcer after omeprazole and ranitidine, 48
Helicobacter pylori
　infection and gastritis, 80
Hemangioma
　of liver, giant cavernous, CT and MRI of, 292
Hemoccult test
　in colorectal cancer screening, 194
Hemochromatosis
　idiopathic
　　ferritin lack in duodenal epithelial cells in, 96
　　iron absorption in, food, 97
　MRI in, 428
Hemorrhage
　intestine, small, enteroclysis in, 402
　variceal (*see* Variceal bleeding)
Hemorrhagic
　colitis due to *Escherichia coli*, 165
Hepatectomy
　repeat, in recurrent liver cancer, 274
Hepatic (*see* Liver)
Hepatitis
　A, fulminant, in IV drug users with chronic liver disease, 408
　alcoholic, methylprednisolone in, 253
　B
　　in children of Southeast Asian refugees, 234
　　chronic, alpha-interferon in, 237
　　chronic, mutation preventing formation of hepatitis B e antigen in, 236
　　heterosexual activity and transmission of, 246
　　vaccination, HBs antibody after, 233
　　X gene protein and antibody in liver disease, 239
　C
　　antibodies in hepatocellular carcinoma, 250
　　antibodies among risk groups in Spain, 244
　　antibodies after transfusions, 242
　　assay for circulating antibodies to etiologic virus in, 241
　　chronic, interferon alfa in, 247
　　heterosexual activity in transmission of, 246
　　corticosteroids in, in postmenopausal women, 407
　D virus, IgM anti- and RNA, 411
　delta
　　in homosexual men, 409
　　interferon in, lymphoblastoid alpha, 410
　fulminant, prostaglandin E in, 228
　immunosuppression in, extrahepatic cancer after, 406
　non-A, non-B (*see* Hepatitis C)
Hepatocellular
　carcinoma, hepatitis C antibodies in, 250
Hepatotoxicity
　amiodarone, case review, 271
Hernia
　paraesophageal, CT of, 34
Heterotopic
　gastric mucosa mimicking duodenal cancer, 419
Hill antireflux surgery
　results, 19

Subject Index / 439

Histamine
  release from basophils in atopic dermatitis and food hypersensitivity, 93
  -releasing factor in atopic dermatitis and food hypersensitivity, 93
HIV
  (*See also* AIDS)
  -induced enteropathy, 105
  infection, small intestine in, 105
Home
  nutrition support with implanted reservoir, 145
Homosexual men
  hepatitis in, delta, 409
Hormone(s)
  for prostatic carcinoma, biliary lipids during, 311
  -secreting tumors, pituitary and gastrointestinal, somatostatin in, 111
Human immunodeficiency virus (*see* HIV)
Hydatid
  cysts of liver, surgical results, 293
Hyperbaric
  oxygen in Crohn's disease, 402
Hypercholesterolemia
  familial, partial ileal bypass in, 119
Hypersensitivity
  food, histamine release from basophils and histamine-releasing factor in, 93
Hypertensive
  portal venous system, effects of meal in, 258

I

IgM
  anti-hepatitis D virus, 411
Ileal
  bypass, partial, in familial hypercholesterolemia, 119
  pouch (*see* Anastomosis, ileal pouch)
  resection, sodium chloride causing diarrhea after, 159
Ileorectal
  anastomosis in colonic aganglionosis, 217
Ileostomy
  Brooke, quality of life after, 182
Ileus
  of jejunum in acute appendicitis, 207
Imaging
  magnetic resonance (*see* Magnetic resonance imaging)
  preoperative, in liver cancer detection, 275
Immunohistochemistry
  of duodenal carcinoids, 77
Immunosuppression
  of hepatitis, extrahepatic cancer after, 406

Implant
  of reservoir for home nutrition support, 145
Infarction
  mesenteric, in aged, 130
Inflammatory bowel (*see* Bowel, inflammatory bowel)
Interferon
  alfa in chronic hepatitis C, 247
  lymphoblastoid alpha, in delta hepatitis, 410
α-Interferon
  in hepatitis B, chronic, 237
Intestine
  (*See also* Gastrointestinal)
  electrolyte transport, shiga toxin to villus cells of jejunum in (in rabbit), 167
  large, malignant lymphoma complicating inflammatory bowel disease, 405
  pseudoobstruction, cisapride in, 85
  small
    hemorrhage, enteroclysis in, 402
    in HIV infection, 105
    viability, methods for assessment, 129
Intrahepatic
  cholestasis, bile acid alterations in, 224
  duct stones, lithotomy with lithotripsy in, choledochoscopic electrohydraulic, 336
Iodine 131
  monoclonal anti-carcinoembryonic antigen antibody $F(ab')_2$ fragments in colon carcinoma (in mice), 200
Iron
  absorption, food, in hemochromatosis, 97
  deposition, extrahepatic, and MRI in hemochromatosis, 428
Irradiation (*see* Radiography, Radiotherapy)
Irritable bowel syndrome (*see* Bowel, irritable bowel syndrome)
Ischemia
  bowel, CT in, 214
  colon, clinical endoscopic documentation, 213
  liver, and liver resection, 290
Isospora belli infection
  in AIDS, 107

J

Jaundice
  obstructive, diagnostic workup in, 221
Jejunal
  atresia with "apple peel" deformity, 115
Jejunostomy
  effluents in short bowel syndrome and SMS 201-995, 110

feeding, gastrointestinal symptoms due to, 154
Jejunum
  ileus of, in acute appendicitis, 207
  villus cells, shiga toxin to (in rabbit), 167

K

Kidney
  transplant, FK 506 in, 277

L

Lactulose
  diarrhea due to, osmotic, 161
Laparotomy
  small bowel cancer and, 122
Laser
  endoscopic, for rectosigmoid villous adenoma, 196
Leiomyosarcoma
  gastric, advanced, 76
Lipid(s)
  biliary, during hormones for prostatic carcinoma, 311
Lithotomy
  for stones in bile duct, intrahepatic duct and gallbladder, 336
Lithotripsy
  of bile duct stones, 337
  choledochoscopic electrohydraulic, for stones in bile duct, intrahepatic duct and gallbladder, 336
  extracorporeal shock-wave
    gallbladder motility and, 320
    with methyl tert-butyl ether for gallstones, 318
    with ursodiol for gallstones, 315
Liver
  cancer (see Cancer, liver)
  carcinoma, hepatocellular, hepatitis C antibodies in, 250
  cysts, hydatid, surgical results, 293
  disease
    chronic, in IV drug users, with hepatitis A, 408
    chronic, neuropathy and, autonomic, 406
    hepatitis B X gene protein and antibody in, 239
    nonalcoholic, sexual behavior in women with, 408
  dysfunction in Wilson's disease, 290
  encephalopathy, flumazenil in, 266
  enzyme abnormalities in bacteremia, 222
  failure, fulminant
    liver transplant in, 231
  prognosis, 227
  fatty, stilette sign in bile ducts in, 430
  function changes after transplant, 279
  hemangioma, giant cavernous, CT and MRI of, 292
  hemodynamics of, changes after transplant, 279
  intrahepatic (see Intrahepatic)
  ischemia and liver resection, 290
  metastases from colon adenocarcinoma, 200
  morphology, changes after transplant, 279
  resection
    under total vascular exclusion, 289
    vascular occlusions for, 290
  transplant (see Transplantation, liver)
  trauma, blunt, organ injury patterns in, 295
  uptake, pericholecystic, in cholescintigraphy of cholecystitis, 306
Loxiglumide
  cholecystokinin receptor antagonism by, and gallbladder contractions, 302
Lung
  metastases from colon adenocarcinoma, 200
Lymphocytic (see Colitis, lymphocytic)
Lymphoma
  malignant, of large intestine complicating inflammatory bowel disease, 405
  in polyposis of colon, 425

M

Magnetic resonance imaging
  in Crohn's disease of fistula and sinus tracts, 133
  in hemochromatosis, 428
  of liver hemangioma, giant cavernous, 292
Malignancy (see Cancer)
Manometry
  in achalasia, 3
  in esophageal spasm, 8
Meal
  effects in hypertensive portal venous system, 258
  -stimulated pancreatic secretion, effect of alcohol on, 356
6-Mercaptopurine
  in inflammatory bowel disease, toxicity study, 136
Mesenteric
  infarction in aged, 130
Metastases
  gastric, in esophageal carcinoma multiplex, 415
  liver and lung, from colon adenocarcinoma, 200

Methotrexate
  in inflammatory bowel disease, refractory, 134
Methylprednisolone
  in hepatitis, alcoholic, 253
Methyl tert-butyl ether
  for gallstones
    cholesterol, 319
    with lithotripsy, 318
Mezlocillin
  in cholangitis, 412
Microgastrinoma
  of duodenum and Zollinger-Ellison syndrome failed surgery, 62
Microvillus
  inclusion disease as inherited defect of brush-border assembly and differentiation, 101
Mitochondrial
  protein, recombinant, autoantibodies to, in biliary cirrhosis, 283
Monoclonal
  anti-carcinoembryonic antigen antibody F(ab')$_2$ fragments in colon carcinoma (in mice), 200
Morbidity
  in duodenopancreatectomy, 389
  hospital, and albumin supplement for parenteral nutrition, 146
  septic, after abdominal trauma, TEN vs. TPN in, 147
Mortality
  in duodenopancreatectomy, 389
  in pancreatitis, chronic, 379
Motor
  functions, gastrointestinal, and cholecystokinin, 303
MRI (see Magnetic resonance imaging)
Mutation
  preventing formation of hepatitis B e antigen, 236
Mycobacterial
  esophagitis in AIDS, 418
Myotomy
  in reflux-induced cricopharyngeal dysphagia, 13

N

Nasogastric
  feeding tubes for chronic illness in aged, 152
Necrosis
  pancreas (see Pancreas, necrosis)
  in pancreatitis, severe acute, 371
Neuropathy
  autonomic, and chronic liver disease, 406
Neutrophils
  and endotoxin infusion for enteral and parenteral nutrition, 146
Newborn
  short bowel syndrome, outcome, 109
Nissen
  -Collis operation, assessment, 20
  fundoplication
    gastric emptying after, delayed, 21
    in gastroesophageal reflux in children, 19
    vs. Angelchik prosthesis, 23
Normoamylasemia
  pancreatitis and, acute, 413
Nosocomial
  Clostridium difficile infection, 171
Nutrition
  home support, with implanted reservoir, 145
  IV, in early postoperative period, 148
  parenteral
    albumin supplement for, and hospital morbidity, 146
    biliary sludge due to, cholecystokinin preventing, 413
    total, and metabolic response to endotoxin, 151
  parenteral and enteral, endotoxin infusion and neutrophils, 146
  TEN vs. TPN after abdominal trauma, 147

O

Obesity
  morbid
    gastric banding in, 71
    gastric surgery for, complications and weight control, 69
    gastric surgery for, restrictive, 70
Omeprazole
  in gastric ulcer, benign, 48
  in Zollinger-Ellison syndrome, efficacy and safety, 60
Osmotic
  diarrhea, due to polyethylene glycol and lactulose, 161
Oxygen
  hyperbaric, in Crohn's disease, 402
Oysters
  raw, shigellosis due to, 166

P

Pain
  of pancreatic cancer, 386
Pancreas
  atrophy after pancreatitis, CT of, 364
  cancer (see Cancer, pancreas)

carcinoma, total pancreatectomy in, 392
duct occlusion with
  duodenopancreatectomy in
  pancreatitis, 382
head
  resection, duodenum-preserving, in
    pancreatitis, 383
  tumors, 391
insufficiency, fecal triglyceride excretion
  in, 357
necrosis
  debridement and closed cavity irrigation
    in, 373
  delayed debridement and external
    drainage of, 372
  pancreatography of, 359
pseudocyst, drainage, 374
resection in pancreatitis, chronic alcoholic,
  381
secretions
  effects of CCK receptor antagonists on
    (in rat), 353
  meal-stimulated, effect of alcohol on,
    356
stone protein messenger RNA in
  pancreatitis, 377
transplant (see Transplantation, pancreas)
Pancreatectomy
  distal, with splenectomy, 387
  total, in pancreatic carcinoma, 392
Pancreaticoduodenectomy (see
  Duodenopancreatectomy)
Pancreatitis
  acute
    Grey Turner's sign and Cullen's sign in,
      360
    high-risk patients, automated selection,
      370
    normoamylasemia and, 413
    pancreatic atrophy after, CT of, 364
    severe, necrosis in, 371
    severe, surgery of, 370
  alcohol-induced, bile duct stenosis in, 414
  chronic
    alcoholic, pancreatic resection in, 381
    biliary tract dilatation in, CT and
      ultrasound of, 380
    calcifying, pancreatic stone protein
      messenger RNA in, 377
    cephalic, duodenopancreatectomy with
      pancreatic duct occlusion in, 382
    mortality factors in, 379
    pancreatic head resection in,
      duodenum-preserving, 383
    pseudocysts in, surgical results, 380
  gallstone, during pregnancy, 369
Pancreatoduodenal
  injuries, conservation management, 395

Pancreatography
  dynamic, of pancreatic necrosis, 359
  retrograde, interpretation in aged, 361
Paracentesis
  total, in albumin for cirrhosis with ascites,
    255
Paraesophageal
  hernia, CT of, 34
Parenteral (see Nutrition, parenteral)
Pelvis
  revascularization in aortic reconstruction
    and colon ischemia, 213
Pentagastrin
  -fast achlorhydria with duodenal ulcer,
    401
Peptic (see Ulcer, peptic)
Perineal
  Crohn's disease, hyperbaric oxygen in, 402
Peritoneovenous
  shunt in alcoholic cirrhosis with ascites,
    256
Peritonitis
  bacterial, antibiotics in, and
    polymorphonuclear cells, 407
pH
  esophageal mucosal sensitivity to, in
    gastroesophageal reflux, 15
  gastric, alkaline shift after
    cholecystectomy, 42
Pituitary
  tumors, hormone-secreting, somatostatin
    in, 111
Polyethylene
  glycol causing osmotic diarrhea, 161
Polymorphonuclear
  cells, and antibiotics in bacterial
    peritonitis, 407
Polyp
  /cancer sequence in colon, radiography of,
    194
Polyposis
  adenomatous familial
    with gastrointestinal cancer, 121
    ileal pouch-anal anastomosis in, 181
  lymphomatous, of colon, 425
Portal
  venous system, hypertensive, effects of
    meal on, 258
Postoperative
  early postoperative period, anabolic steroid
    and IV nutrition in, 148
Postpartum period
  management of gallstone pancreatitis
    during, 369
Pregnancy
  gallstone pancreatitis during, 369
Prostaglandin
  E in fulminant viral hepatitis, 228

Subject Index / 443

Prostate
  carcinoma, biliary lipids during hormones for, 311
Prosthesis
  Angelchik, vs. Nissen fundoplication, 23
Protein
  enteral vs. IV, and cholestasis in very low birth weight, 150
  hepatitis B X gene, in liver disease, 239
  -losing enteropathy with *Clostridium difficile* infection, 405
  messenger RNA, pancreatic stone, in pancreatitis, 377
  mitochondrial, recombinant, autoantibodies to, in biliary cirrhosis, 283
  sparing after surgery, and amino acid, 149
  X of pyruvate dehydrogenase complex in biliary cirrhosis, 285
Pseudocyst
  pancreas, drainage, 374
  in pancreatitis, chronic, surgical results, 380
Pyruvate dehydrogenase complex in biliary cirrhosis, 285

Q

Quality of life
  after Brooke ileostomy and ileal pouch-anal anastomosis, 182

R

Radiography
  in achalasia, 3
  AIDS with cholangitis, 343
  in esophageal spasm, 8
  of polyp/cancer sequence in colon, 194
  in sarcoidosis, gastrointestinal, 422
Radioimmunoassay
  CA19-9, in pancreatic cancer, 386
Radiotherapy
  in rectal cancer, preoperative, survival, 198
Ranitidine
  for duodenal ulcer recurrence prevention, 50
  in gastric ulcer, benign, 48
Rebleeding: in variceal bleeding with cirrhosis, 259
Reconstruction
  aortic, and colon ischemia, 213
Rectopexy
  abdominal, for rectal prolapse, results, 189
Rectosigmoid
  motility in irritable bowel syndrome, 203
  villous adenoma, endoscopic laser for, 196

Rectum
  cancer (*see* Cancer, rectum)
  endosonography in rectal cancer, 191
  ileorectal anastomosis in colonic aganglionosis, 217
  injuries, colostomy with drainage after, 185
  prolapse, abdominal rectopexy results in, 189
  surgery without nasogastric decompression, 218
  tumors, villous, CT of, 192
Reflux
  esophagitis
    antireflux surgery in, evaluations, 17
    cimetidine for, in children, 16
    gastritis, alkaline, atony after Roux-Y diversion, 66
  gastroesophageal
    alkaline, in Barrett's esophagus, 28
    esophageal mucosal sensitivity to pH in, 15
    Nissen fundoplication in, in children, 19
  -induced cricopharyngeal dysphagia, myotomy in, 13
Renal
  -spleno-adrenal shunt after endoscopic sclerotherapy, 409
Revascularization
  colonic and pelvic, in aortic reconstruction with colon ischemia, 213
RNA
  hepatitis D virus and, 411
Roux-Y diversion
  for alkaline reflux gastritis, gastric atony after, 66
  effect on *Campylobacter pylori*, 82
Rupture
  esophagus, spontaneous, experience with, 33

S

Saccharomyces boulardi
  diarrhea, antibiotic-associated, prevention, 172
Sarcoidosis
  gastrointestinal, radiography of, 422
Schiatosomal
  variceal bleeding, shunt in, 260
Scintigraphy (*see* Cholescintigraphy)
Sclerosing
  cholangitis, study of, 341
Sclerotherapy
  endoscopic
    spleno-adreno-renal shunt after, 409
    variceal, in variceal bleeding, 263
    with esophageal staple transection in

variceal bleeding, 261
Seafood
  cholera and, 402
Secretin
  gastrin release by, increase in Zollinger-Ellison syndrome, 59
Septic
  morbidity after abdominal trauma, TEN vs. TPN in, 147
Septotomy
  transampullary, with sphincteroplasty in sphincter of Oddi dysfunction, 327
Sexual behavior
  in women with nonalcoholic liver disease, 408
Shigella
  diarrhea, pathogenesis (in rabbit), 167
Shigellosis
  oysters causing, raw, 166
Shunt
  peritoneovenous, in alcoholic cirrhosis with ascites, 256
  after sclerotherapy, endoscopic, spleno-adreno-renal, 409
  in variceal bleeding (*see* Variceal bleeding, shunt in)
Sigmoid
  volvulus, experience with, 190
Sinus
  tracts in Crohn's disease, MRI of, 133
SMS 201-995
  in gut diseases, 111
  jejunostomy effluents in short bowel syndrome and, 110
  in pituitary and gastrointestinal tumors, 111
Sodium
  chloride causing diarrhea after ileal and colonic resection, 159
Somatostatin
  analogue (*see* SMS 201-995)
  in gut diseases, 111
  in pituitary and gastrointestinal tumors, 111
Sonography (*see* Ultrasound)
Spasm
  esophageal, radiographic and manometric correlation, 8
Sphincter
  esophageal, relaxation in achalasia, 3
  of Oddi dysfunction
    cholecystectomy in, sphincterotomy after, 328
    sphincteroplasty with septotomy in, 327
Sphincteroplasty
  transduodenal, with septotomy in sphincter of Oddi dysfunction, 327
Sphincterotomy
  endoscopic
    in bile duct stones, 338
    of bile duct stones, catheter perfusion after, 335
    case review, 332
    after cholecystectomy in sphincter of Oddi dysfunction, 328
    retrograde, complications, CT of, 329
Splenectomy
  with pancreatectomy, distal, 387
Spleno
  -adreno-renal shunt after endoscopic sclerotherapy, 409
Splenorenal
  shunt (*see* Variceal hemorrhage, shunt in, splenorenal)
Staple
  transection of esophagus in variceal bleeding, 261
Stenosis
  bile duct, in alcohol-induced pancreatitis, 414
Steroid
  anabolic, in early postoperative period, 148
Stilette sign
  in fatty liver, 430
Stomach
  (*See also* Gastrointestinal)
  acidity reduction by dietary regimens, 156
  adenocarcinoma of antrum, gastrectomy in, 75
  air-fluid sign in CT of gastric wall thickening, 87
  alcohol dehydrogenase activity decrease and first-pass metabolism, 40
  atony after Roux-Y diversion, 66
  banding in morbid obesity, 71
  cancer detected by mass screening, follow-up, 76
  emptying after Nissen fundoplication, 21
  fold enlargement with *Campylobacter pylori* gastritis, 81
  leiomyosarcoma, advanced, 76
  metastases in esophageal carcinoma multiplex, 415
  mucosa, heterotopic, mimicking duodenal cancer, 419
  origin of ethanol first-pass metabolism, 39
  pH, alkaline shift after cholecystectomy, 42
  post-gastrectomy, gastroscopic screening, 65
  relationship of dysplasia to remnant cancer, 65
  surgery for morbid obesity
    complications and weight control, 69
    restrictive surgery, 70
  ulcer (*see* Ulcer, gastric)

wall thickening, gastric air-fluid sign in CT of, 87
Stones
  bile duct (*see* Bile duct stones)
  gallstones (*see* Gallstones)
  pancreatic stone protein messenger RNA in pancreatitis, 377
Strictureplasty
  in Crohn's disease, obstructive, 140

T

Tomography (*see* Computed tomography)
Toxicity
  hepatotoxicity of amiodarone, case review, 271
  of 6-mercaptopurine in inflammatory bowel disease, 136
Toxin
  shiga, to villus cells of jejunum (in rabbit), 167
Transfusion(s)
  antibody to hepatitis C after, 242
Transplantation
  abdominal organ cluster, in upper abdominal cancer, 280
  liver
    in cirrhosis, biliary, 287
    in cirrhosis, biliary, disease recurrence, 410
    in fulminant hepatic failure, 231
    in hepatobiliary cancer, 278
    liver function, hemodynamics and morphology changes after, 279
  liver, kidney and pancreas, FK 506 in, 277
  pancreas
    experience with, 397
    FK 506 in, 277
Trauma
  abdomen (*see* Abdomen, trauma)
  liver, blunt, organ injury patterns in, 295
Triglyceride
  excretion, fecal, in pancreatic insufficiency, 357
Tuberculosis
  abdominal, clinical features, 404
Tubes (*see* Feeding tubes)
Tumors
  ampulla, 391
  bile duct, 391
  duodenum, 391
  gastrointestinal, somatostatin in, 111
  pancreatic head, 391
  pituitary, somatostatin in, 111
  rectal villous, CT in, 192
Typhoid
  enteritis, perforated, surgery of, 173

U

Ulcer
  colonic aphthous, in pseudomembranous colitis, 427
  duodenal
    admissions and surgery for, changing pattern, 57
    cost of medical and surgical treatment, 56
    famotidine for, healing after, 45
    postbulbar, with pentagastrin-fast achlorhydria, 401
    ranitidine for recurrence prevention, 50
    refractory, after standard antacids, 401
  gastric
    benign, omeprazole and ranitidine in, 48
    famotidine in, nocturnal acid-secretion suppression with, 47
    perforated, need for definitive therapy, 55
  peptic
    electrocoagulation in, multipolar, 73
    perforated, nonoperative treatment, 52
Ulcerative colitis
  chronic, results of ileal pouch-anal anastomosis in, 181
  5-aminosalicylic acid suppositories in, 404
Ultrasonography (*see* Ultrasound)
Ultrasound
  in appendicitis, acute, 208
  endosonography
    in esophageal carcinoma, 31
    rectal, in rectal cancer, 191
  of gallbladder emptying, 305
  in liver cancer detection, intraoperative, 275
  in pancreatitis, chronic, with biliary tract dilatation, 380
Ursodeoxycholic acid
  in biliary cirrhosis, 286
  gallbladder bile nucleation time and, 312
  gallstone recurrence after, 322
Ursodiol
  with lithotripsy for gallstones, 315
US (*see* Ultrasound)

V

Vaccination
  hepatitis B, HBs antibody after, 233
Variceal bleeding
  with cirrhosis, study of, 259
  esophageal, sclerotherapy with staple transection in, 261
  schistosomal vs. nonschistosomal, shunt in, 260
  sclerotherapy in, endoscopic variceal, 263

shunt in
  splenorenal, selective distal, results, 266
  splenorenal vs. lienorenal, 265
Varices
  esophageal, in cirrhosis, biliary, 411
Vein
  portal venous system, hypertensive, effects of meal on, 258
Very low birth weight
  cholestasis and enteral protein in, 150
Vessels
  liver resection under total vascular exclusion, 289
  occlusion for liver resection, 290
Viruses
  in hepatitis (*see under* Hepatitis)
  HIV (*see* HIV)
Volvulus
  sigmoid, experience with, 190

W

Water
  drinking untreated, causing chronic diarrhea, 169
  filtered public supply, contamination causing cryptosporidiosis, 170
Weight
  birth, very low, cholestasis and enteral protein, 150
  control after gastric surgery for morbid obesity, 69
  gallstone risk and, 309
  loss in pancreatic cancer, 386
Wilson's disease
  with liver dysfunction, 290

X

X gene
  protein and antibody, hepatitis B, in liver disease, 239

Z

Zollinger-Ellison syndrome
  failed surgery and duodenal microgastrinoma, 62
  gastrin release by secretin increase in, 59
  omeprazole in efficacy and safety, 60

Author Index

A

Abecassis, M., 228
Abell, T.L., 85
Abernathy, G.B., 152
Abu-Elmagd, K.M., 260
Addiss, D.G., 169
Adham, N., 256
Adson, M.A., 273
Ainley, C., 332
Akrividis, E.A., 407, 408
Alai, F., 169
Alain Clavien, P., 413
Albrecht, J., 247
Alexander, G.J.M., 227
Alexander, W.J., 246
Alexander-Williams, J., 82
Allen, E., 385
Allen, J.I., 256
Allen, M.J., 256
Alter, H.J., 241, 242
Alter, M.J., 241, 246
Aly, M.A., 260
Amarri, S., 16
Amerson, J.R., 337
Anadol, E., 293
Anderson, R.P., 19
Angelin, B., 311
Ansari, A., 283, 285
Appleman, M.D., 80
Aran, P.P., 231
Arends, J.W., 79
Arosio, P., 96
Arrambide, K.A., 159
Arroyo, V., 255
Arunachalam, T., 130
Astolfi, R., 16
Attwood, S.E.A., 28
Aufses, A.H., Jr., 196

B

Bach, N., 408
Badalamenti, S., 255
Baddeley, R.M., 71
Bader, J.-P., 48
Baetz, A., 379
Bahgat, O.O., 260
Baillie, J., 332
Baker, A.L., 231
Baker, J.D., 256
Balart, L.A., 247
Ball, T.J., 134
Balli, F., 16
Bansky, G., 266
Baraona, E., 39, 40
Barbara, L., 322
Barber, A., 151
Bardhan, K.D., 57
Barlow, A.P., 28

Bauer, M., 80
Bauer, T., 210
Baum, R.A., 256
Bayless, T.M., 175, 177
Bazzoli, F., 322
Beahrs, O.H., 182
Beart, R.W., Jr., 181, 218
Beaver, S.J., 341, 406
Bechstein, W.O., 278
Beger, H.G., 383
Beglinger, C., 303
Behrns, K.E., 71
Bekaert, E., 141
Bekemeyer, W.B., 146
Bell, J., 94
Belluzzi, A., 404
Bender, C.E., 318, 319
Bendix, J., 211
Benotti, P.N., 70
Berci, S., 337
Berg, C.J., 234
Berger, H.J., 385
Berger, K., 241
Bergmeijer, J.-H., 217
Berman, R.S., 47
Bernades, P., 379
Bernard, J.-P., 377
Bernhisel-Broadbent, J., 93
Berr, F., 299
Beynon, J., 191
Bianchi, P., 138
Bias, W.B., 177
Bijleveld, C.M.A., 224
Binder, V., 138
Bishop, H.C., 116
Bismuth, H., 274, 289
Bistrian, B.R., 70
Bittner, R.R., 383
Blackburn, G.L., 70
Bland, K.L., 337
Blane, C.E., 19
Blaser, M.J., 80
Blendis, L.M., 228
Block, G.E., 391
Block, P., 369
Bodenheimer, H.C., Jr., 247
Boeckl, O., 338
Bogdal, J., 302
Bogomoletz, W.V., 31
Bond, J.H., 194
Bonino, F., 241
Bopp, C.A., 169
Bornman, P.C., 414
Bose, K., 57
Bothe, A., Jr., 70
Botoman, V.A., 134
Boverhof, R., 224
Bozatli, L., 293
Bradley, D.W., 241
Bradley, E.L., III, 359
Bradley, J.E., 146
Bradley, M., 194

Brady, C.E., 402
Braghetto, I., 17
Brannigan, T.C., 374
Bremner, C.G., 21, 28
Britt, L.G., 190
Broadbent, K.R., 93
Broelsch, C.E., 231
Brolin, R.E., 129
Brook, M.G., 237, 410
Brooks, D.C., 392
Brooks, J.R., 392
Brophy, C., 122
Brough, W., 370
Brown, M.L., 85, 98
Brown, M.R., 150
Brown, R.O., 146
Brown, T.H., 42
Browne, B.B., 234
Brunetaud, J.M., 196
Brunton, F.J., 194
Brynskov, J., 138
Buchanan, J.A., 367
Buchegger, F., 200
Büchler, M., 383
Buchwald, M., 367
Bunzendahl, H., 278
Burch, J.M., 185
Burke, A.P., 77
Burnett, D., 315
Burns, H.J.G., 148
Burroughs, A.K., 259, 261
Burton, A.H., 234
Bushman, E.D., 151
Buti, M., 244
Byrne, P.J., 23

C

Caballeria, J., 39
Cacioppo, J.C., 210
Cahow, C.E., 122
Cain, G.D., 256
Cairns, S., 332
Cairns, S.R., 340
Calvano, S., 146
Camara, D.S., 256
Cameron, J.L., 346
Cameron, R., 228
Camilleri, M., 85
Campanini, M.C., 138
Campbell, D., 203
Campieri, M., 404
Camus, Y., 290
Caniano, D.A., 109
Carey, W., 247
Carithers, R.L., Jr., 253
Carlson, R., 200
Carman, W.F., 236
Carrel, S., 200
Carr-Locke, D.L., 336
Carter, D.C., 148

Caruana, J.A., 256
Caruso, A., 271
Casola, G., 374
Castaing, D., 274, 289
Castell, D.O., 3, 8
Cello, J.P., 345
Chakravarti, A., 367
Chalmers, A.G., 373
Chapman, N.J., 98
Chawla, Y.K., 409
Cheadle, W.G., 42
Chen, Y.M., 3, 8
Chenoweth, J., 34
Cherian, G., 76
Chezmar, J.L., 428
Chiba, T., 59
Chinn, J., 172
Chisaka, O., 239
Choi, B.I., 292
Choo, Q.-L., 241, 242, 244, 250
Choudhri, A.H., 343
Christensen, K.C., 110
Christensen, M.R., 386
Christensen, R.R., 374
Chung, S.S.C., 52
Church, T.R., 194
Ciarleglio, C.A., 401
Clarke, M.P., 275
Classen, M., 48
Claunch, C., 145
Clouse, M.E., 275
Cochelard, D., 196
Coene, P.P., 31
Cohen, A.J., 207
Cohen, H., 80
Cohen, P., 31
Colditz, G.A., 309
Cole, F.H., Jr., 33
Coleman, J., 346
Coleman, P.J., 246
Collen, M.J., 401
Collins, S.M., 203
Colombo, M., 241, 250
Combes, B., 253
Comi, R.J., 111
Conti-Nibali, S., 16
Cook, I.J., 203
Cook, J.D., 97
Cooley, B.J., 402
Cooney, L., 403
Cooper, A., 283
Coppel, R., 283
Coppel, R.L., 285
Coran, A.G., 19
Corstens, F.H.M., 305
Cortés, C., 17
Cortot, A., 196
Cotton, P., 332
Cotton, P.B., 337, 340
Cox, C., 150
Cox, T.K., 367
Coyle, S.M., 151
Croce, M.A., 190
Crofton, M.E., 343
Crofts, T.J., 52
Croker, J., 332, 340

Crowson, M., 71
Csendes, A., 17
Cuan-Orozco, F., 266
Cucchiara, S., 16
Cummings, M.L., 170
Cust, G., 57
Cutz, E., 101
Cuvelier, C., 141
Czaja, A.J., 406, 407
Czinn, S.J., 81

D

Dagorn, J.-C., 377
Dahms, B.B., 81
D'Anna, L., 332
Danner, D., 283
Danner, D.J., 285
Davies, J.W.L., 148
Davis, G.L., 247
Davis, J.C., 402
Davis, J.M., 146
Davis, M., 415, 425
Dawes, L.G., 313
Dawson, K., 23
Dawson, P.J., 391
de Bernardinis, M., 370
Deboisblanc, R., 55
Dehn, T.C.B., 140
Deihl, A.M., 253
Del Ninno, E., 250
Delva, E., 290
DeMeester, T.R., 21, 28
Demetris, A., 280
Demetris, A.J., 277
Demirci, S., 293
Den Hartog Jager, F.C.A., 31
De Potter, C., 141
Derevjanik, N.L., 177
Deriaz, H., 290
Deugler, K.R., 402
Devine, R.M., 218
De Vos, M., 141
Dickson, E.R., 285, 287, 341, 411
Dickson, R., 283
Dienstag, J.L., 241, 247
Diettrich, N.A., 210
Dilawari, J.B., 409
Dineen, P., 146
Dioguardi, N., 250
di Padova, C., 39, 40
Ditschuneit, H., 300
Dodds, W.J., 328
Dodson, T.F., 279
Domizio, P., 121
Donato, M.F., 250
Donohue-Rolfe, A., 167
Donovan, I.A., 82
Donowitz, M., 167
Dooley, C.P., 80
Douglass, H.O., Jr., 349
Dowsett, J., 332
Dowsett, J.F., 340
Dozois, R.R., 181, 218

Driscoll, D.L., 349
Drumm, B., 101
Drumm, J., 82
Dudley, C.R.K., 205
Duhaney, R., 146
Dunham, C.M., 295
Dunn, D.L., 397
Durie, P.R., 101

E

Eckhauser, F.E., 62, 213
Ederer, F., 194
Einarsson, K., 311
Ekberg, O., 422
Elashoff, J.D., 50
El-Barbary, M.H., 260
El-Fiky, A.M., 260
Elmer, G.W., 172
Elsea, W.R., 234
Elwood, R.K., 404
Emde, C., 156
Emond, J.C., 231
Enarson, D.A., 404
Endoh, S., 76
Eraslan, S., 293
Eriksson, A., 311
Eriksson, S., 48
Erroi, F., 391
Ertan, A., 315
Esnaola, S., 263
Esteban, J.I., 244
Esteban, R., 244
Estes, N.C., 76
Ezzat, F.A., 260

F

Fabian, T.C., 190
Fagniez, P.L., 75
Fagniez, P.-L., 371
Fallon, H.J., 253
Farci, P., 410
Fargion, S., 96
Fathy, O.M., 260
Federspiel, B.H., 77
Feldberg, M.A.M., 360
Feliciano, D.V., 185
Fennerty, M.B., 25
Ferguson, C., 359
Fernandes, J., 224
Festi, D., 322
Fields, H.A., 409
Finkelstein, M., 165
Finucane, P.M., 130
Fiorelli, G., 96
Fischer, H., 286
Fischer, J.E., 327
Fisher, L.D., 341
Fishman, E.K., 329
Fitzgibbons, P.L., 80
Flamant, Y., 75
Fleming, T.R., 287, 341

Flendrig, J.A., 79
Fleshman, J.W., 198
Flores, M.C., 356
Fong, T.L., 407
Fong, Y., 146, 151
Fordtran, J.S., 159, 161
Forstner, G.G., 101
Fournier, K., 200
Frabboni, R., 322
Fracanzani, A.L., 96
Franks, A.L., 234
Frasca, P., 315
Freeark, R.J., 221
Freund, L., 138
Frezza, M., 39, 40
Frost, R., 340
Frucht, H., 60
Fry, R.D., 198
Fujita, T., 59
Fulenwider, J.T., 256
Fung, J., 277
Fusamoto, H., 239

G

Gadacz, T.R., 256
Galatius, H., 210
Gall, F.P., 382
Galloway, J.R., 279
Garden, O.J., 148, 289
Gardner, J.D., 60
Gardner, R.C., 165
Garewal, H.S., 25
Gatzen, M., 286
Gayet, B., 31
Gebhardt, C., 382
Geenen, J.E., 328
Gelfand, D.W., 3, 8
Gelfand, M.D., 134
Genescà, J., 244
Gerecht, W.B., 412
Gershwin, M.E., 283, 285
Gheissari, A., 116
Giardiello, F.M., 175, 177
Gibas, A., 247
Gilbertsen, V., 194
Giles, G.R., 265
Gillespie, G., 338
Ginès, P., 255
Ginn-Pease, M.E., 109
Ginsberg, H.N., 306
Gionchetti, P., 404
Giorgi, D., 377
Gitnick, G.L., 241
Glick, M.E., 256
Go, S.T., 233
Go, V.L.W., 98, 111
Gobio-Casali, L., 16
Goetz, F.C., 397
Goff, J.S., 339
Gogel, H., 415
Goldschmiedt, M., 401
Golub, L., 150
González, A., 244

Gonzalez, F., 55
Goodman, P., 418
Gorden, P., 111
Gordon, H., 181
Gordon, R., 280
Gorelkin, L., 169
Gores, G.J., 411
Gouzi, J.L., 75
Govindarajan, S., 411
Goyal, A.K., 258
Graham, D.Y., 15, 47
Graham, J.B., 337
Grambsch, P.M., 287, 341
Graversen, P., 211
Gray, G.R., 338
Greenberger, N., 315
Greene, F.L., 65
Greene, K.D., 166
Greenfield, L.J., 213
Greenholz, S.K., 347
Greenlee, H.B., 256
Greenough, W.B., 405
Greig, P.D., 228
Grendell, J.H., 353
Gruessner, R., 397
Guandalini, S., 16
Guardia, J., 244
Guetta, V., 222
Güldütuna, S., 286
Gunn, R.A., 169
Gupta, S., 411
Gyepes, M.T., 115
Gyves, J., 385

H

Hadler, S.C., 246, 409
Hadziyannis, S., 236
Hahn-Pedersen, J., 210
Hajnal, F., 356
Hak, L.J., 152
Hall, P.A., 405
Hall, R.J., 347
Haller, C.C., 76
Hameeteman, W., 27
Hamilton, E.S., 275
Hamilton, G., 261
Hammer, H.F., 161
Hammerman, A.M., 87
Han, M.C., 292
Han, M.H., 292
Handcock, M., 391
Hanna, W.M., 13
Hannoun, L., 290
Hansell, D.T., 148, 338
Hardin, C.A., 76
Hargrett-Bean, N., 169
Harig, J.M., 179
Hashiba, S., 312
Hatfield, A., 332
Hatfield, A.R.W., 340
Havinga, R., 224
Hay, J.M., 75
Hayashi, N., 239

Hayes, E.B., 170
Hayes, K.C., 309
Hayllar, K.M., 227
He, W., 151
Heck, C.F., 389
Hegnhøj, J., 110
Heimann, T.M., 196
Heinerman, P.M., 338
Heise, W., 105
Heizer, W.D., 152
Helbert, M., 343
Hellstern, A., 286
Helwig, E.B., 77
Hench, V., 85
Henderson, J.M., 279
Henderson, R.D., 13
Henderson, R.F., 13
Hendricks, P.J., 192
Hennessy, T.P.J., 23
Henriksson, P., 311
Henry, N.K., 412
Herlong, H.F., 253
Hermreck, A.S., 76
Hernández, J.M., 244
Hernandez-Muñoz, R., 39
Hertzler, G.L., 279
Hess, C.F., 133
Hesse, D.G., 146
Hewson, E.G., 8
Heyen, F., 189
Hildebrand, P., 303
Hill, L.D., 19
Hill, M.C., 380
Hinchliffe, R.F.C., 57
Hinder, R.A., 21, 28
Hobbs, K.E.F., 261
Hodnett, R.M., 55
Hoffenberg, E., 81
Höffken, G., 105
Hoffman, W.W., 412
Hofmann, A.F., 315
Hogan, W.J., 328
Holcomb, G.W., III, 116
Holcombe, B.J., 152
Holl, J., 321
Hollingshead, J., 70
Holm, B., 210
Hooks, M.A., 279
Hopert, R., 156
Hopman, W.P.M., 305
Hordijk, M.L., 140
Horiuchi, I., 412
Houghton, M., 241, 242, 244, 250
Housman, J.F., 428
Houthoff, H.J., 27
Howard, J.M., 372
Howard, L., 145
Huang, G., 357
Hübner, K., 286
Hughes, R.W., 71
Huguet, C., 290
Huguier, M., 75
Humberstone, D.A., 149
Humbert, P., 255
Humphries, T.J., 47
Huntington, D.K., 380

Hurwitz, E.S., 170
Hutcheon, D.F., 177
Hutner, E.B., 341

I

Ikeda, S., 336
Ilstrup, D.M., 181, 218, 273
Ilves, R., 19
Imediegwu, O.O., 173
Infante-Rivard, C., 263
Ingram, C., 430
Iovanna, J., 377
Irvine, E.J., 203
Ishak, K.G., 271
Ismail, T., 71
Isselbacher, K.J., 200
Iwatsuki, S., 280

J

Jackson, L.K., 271
Jacobson, I.M., 247
Jacyna, M.R., 236
Jafri, S.Z.H., 192
Jain, A., 277
Jakubowski, A., 404
James, K.E., 256
James, R., 205
Jansen, J.B.M.J., 303, 305
Jarnum, S., 110
Jennings, H., 279
Jensen, R.T., 60
Jenss, H., 133
Jessurun, J., 175
Jewell, D.P., 140, 205
Jewell, W.R., 76
Jiménez, W., 255
Joanes, F., 427
Joehl, R.J., 323
Johnson, W.D., Jr., 107
Johnson, W.H., 33
Jones, M.D., 207
Jones, R., 315
Jones, R.S., 337
Jones, S.N., 361
Jones, T.N., 147, 154
Jordan, P.H., 256
Jorgensen, T., 412
Joseph, A.E.A., 430
Juler, G.L., 256
Juranek, D.D., 170

K

Kadowaki, S., 59
Kajiyama, G., 312
Kalk, J.-F., 266
Kalvaria, I., 414
Kamada, T., 239
Kandel, G., 167

Kane, M.A., 234
Kane, R.A., 275
Kapelman, B., 408
Kaplan, G., 210
Karayiannis, P., 236, 237, 410
Karnel, F., 374
Karrer, F.M., 347
Kasahara, A., 239
Katayama, K., 239
Kaufman, H.S., 315
Kaufman, S.L., 346
Kawasaki, S., 279
Keane, P.F., 119
Keefe, B., 192
Keeling, P., 23
Keeney, G., 192
Keighley, M.R.B., 189
Keith, R.G., 381
Kelly, K.A., 71, 98, 181
Kelly, T.R., 369
Kelter, U., 311
Kennedy, W., 397
Kerem, B., 367
Kesäniemi, Y.A., 155
Kettlewell, M.G.W., 140
Keusch, G.T., 167
Keynan, A., 222
Khouri, M.R., 357
Kim, C.-W., 292
Kim, S.H., 292
Kirby, R.M., 71
Kivilaakso, E., 29, 380
Kiviluoto, T., 380
Kivisaari, L., 380
Klintmalm, G.B.G., 287
Knol, J.A., 213
Knuff, T.E., 47
Koch, R.A., 129
Kochhar, R., 400
Kodner, I.J., 198
Koea, J., 149
Koelbel, G., 133
Komorowski, R.A., 179
Konturek, J.W., 302
Konturek, S.J., 302
Koopman, B.J., 224
Korelitz, B.I., 136
Korn, O., 17
Korsten, M.A., 39
Koussouris, P., 266
Kozarek, R.A., 134
Kune, G.A., 370
Kracht, M., 371
Kramer, E., 246
Kristensen, E.S., 210
Krumholz, M.P., 136
Kueper, K., 133
Kuhlman, H.E., 329
Kuipers, F., 224
Kuo, C., 241
Kuo, G., 241, 242, 244, 250
Kurek, A., 302
Kuroda, Y., 336
Kurtz, W., 286
Kwork, R.Y.Y., 171

L

Lacaine, F., 75
Ladefoged, K., 110
Ladenson, P.W., 177
L'age, M., 105
Laine, L., 73
Lambert, M.E., 335
Lamers, C.B.H.W., 48, 305
Lange, J.F., 274
Lanza, F.L., 47
Lappas, J.C., 402
Larkai, E., 15
Larson, G.M., 42
LaRusso, N.F., 341
Larvin, M., 373
Laughon, B.E., 405
Launois, B., 75
Lauritsen, K., 138
Lazenby, A.J., 175, 177
Leditschke, J.F., 94
Lee, E.C.G., 140
Lee, K.K., 256
Lee, R.M., 126
Lee, W.C., 55
Lee, W.S., 241
Lees, W.R., 361
Leese, T., 274
Lefkowitch, J., 247
Lempinem, M., 380
LeRoy, A.J., 319
Leuschner, M., 286
Leuschner, U., 286
Levenson, H.L., 47
Levine, E.J., 177
Levine, J.D., 392
Levine, M.S., 422
Levy, G.A., 228
Levy, P., 379
Lewis, F., 187
Lewis, J.H., 271
Li, A.K.C., 52
Lieber, C.S., 39, 40
Liehr, R.-M., 156
Lienhart, A., 290
Liljeqvist, L., 182
Lillemoe, K.D., 315
Lilly, J.R., 347
Lindenauer, S.M., 213
Lindfors, K.K., 325
Lindquist, K., 182
Lindsay, K., 247
Lisle, D., 94
Little, K.H., 159
Livingstone, A.S., 256
Ljungdahl, I., 182
Llach, J., 255
Lllanger, J., 214
Lodge, J.P.A., 265
Loffeld, R.J.L.F., 79
Logsdon, G.S., 170
Long, E.G., 170
López-Talavera, J.C., 244
Low, D.E., 19
Lowry, P.W., 402
Lowry, S.F., 146, 151
Ludwig, J., 341
Luther, R.W., 146

Author Index / 451

Lynch, S.R., 97
Lyon, C., 57
Lyon, D.T., 47
Lysen, D., 210

M

McArthur, K.A., 60
McCarty, M., 343
MacCarty, R.L., 341
McCormick, P.A., 259
McCroskey, B.L., 147, 154
McCullough, A.J., 47
McCullough, J.E., 319
MacDonald, A.S., 138
McDowell, R., 145
McFarland, L.M., 402
McFarland, L.V., 171, 172
McGahan, J.P., 325
McGarvey, M.J., 236
McGregor, J.C., 335
Mach, J.-P., 200
McIntyre, N., 259, 261
Mackenzie, J.W., 129
Mackie, R., 315
McKinely, T.W., 170
MacLaren, D.M., 233
McLean, A., 385
Maclure, K.M., 309
McMahon, M.J., 373
McNeil, N.I., 361
Maddrey, W.C., 253
Magazzú, G., 16
Maglinte, D.D.T., 402
Magnuson, J.E., 364
Magnuson, T.H., 315
Maher, J.W., 337
Majer, M.C., 133
Makris, A., 236
Malagelada, J.R., 85
Malchow-Møller, A., 138
Malmfred, S., 211
Malpani, A.R., 34
Mamel, J.J., 154
Mandel, E., 246
Mandel, J.S., 194
Mangiante, E.C., 190
Maniscalco, W. M., 150
Manning, C., 115
Mansour, M.A., 395
Marano, M.A., 151
Margolis, H.S., 246
Markiewicz, D., 367
Marks, I.N., 414
Markus, B.H., 287
Marryatt, G., 13
Marsh, J.W., 279
Martin, D.F., 335
Martin, D.L., 166
Mascioli, E.A., 70
Masclee, A.A.M., 305
Mashhoor, N., 260
Mason, R.R., 340
Mast, B.A., 129

Maton, P.N., 60, 111
Matsubara, K., 239
Matsumoto, S., 336
Matte, T.D., 170
Mattox, K.L., 185
Mauer, S.M., 397
Maunoury, V., 196
Mavor, A.I.D., 265
Maxwell, G., 425
May, G.R., 319
Mayberry, J.F., 140
Mazzaferro, V., 287
Mazzella, G., 322
Meier, D.E., 173
Meier, P.J., 266
Meister, R., 382
Melpolder, J.C., 242
Meltzer, S.J., 136
Mercado, M.A., 266
Meschievitz, C., 247
Messina, L.M., 213
Meyer, B.M., 303
Meyer, J., 146
Meyer, P., 413
Meyers, M.A., 360
Mezwa, D.G., 192
Mezzanotte, G., 259, 261
Michelassi, F., 391
Mieles, L., 280
Miettinen, M., 29
Miettinen, T.A., 155
Milan, C., 379
Millar, M.A., 338
Miller, J.K., 246
Miller, L.S., 60
Milligan, F.D., 329
Millikan, W.J., Jr., 279
Millward, S., 427
Mirowitz, S.A., 87
Miyamura, T., 241
Mizuno, S., 312
Molas, G., 31
Moldaver, L.L., 151
Molenaar, J.C., 217
Molina, F., 138
Montanari, M., 370
Moody, F.G., 337
Moore, E.E., 147, 154, 395
Moore, E.W., 313
Moore, F.A., 147, 154, 395
Moore, J.B., 395
Moore, O.F., III, 190
Moore, P.B., 279
Morel, P., 397
Morishita, T., 59
Morrison, S., 81
Mortensen, N.J.M., 140
Motte, P., 200
Moudry-Munns, K.C., 397
Mowji, P.J., 207
Mullick, F., 271
Mulligan, M.E., 171
Munsell, W.P., 47
Munson, J.L., 337
Murakami, R., 76
Murphy, F., 359

Murray, W.R., 338
Myerson, R., 198

N

Nagi, B., 400
Nagorney, D.M., 273, 318
Nahrwold, D.L., 323
Najarian, J.S., 397
Najem, A.Z., 256
Nakamura, A., 59
Nance, F.C., 55
Nanda, R., 205
Nava, H.R., 349
Nelken, N., 187
Nelson, P.E., 319
Nelson, R.C., 428
Nemchausky, B.A., 256
Neoptolemos, J.P., 336
Neuberger, J., 410
Neumann, L., 222
Newbold, K.M., 82
Ng, S.-N., 357
Niederau, C., 353
Niederau, M., 353
Nivatvongs, S., 218
Noda, S., 391
Nolan, D.J., 125
Nommensen, F.E., 233
Nora, P.F., 210
Nordlinger, B., 290
Norton, L.W., 339
Nussbaum, M.S., 327

O

O'Brien, T.R., 170
Ochi, S., 256
O'Connor, H.J., 82
O'Dowd, J., 130
Oettinger, W., 383
O'Grady, J.G., 227
Oh, C., 196
Ohri, S.K., 119
Oldham, K.T., 19
O'Leary, J.P., 315
Olen, R., 221
Olesksy, J., 302
Oliphant, M., 360
O'Neill, J.A., Jr., 116
Onik, G., 275
Opekun, A.R., 15
Orringer, M.B., 7, 20
Ortego, T.J., 247
Oshima, A., 76
Østergaard Thomsen, O., 138
Ott, D.J., 3, 8
Ovaska, J., 29
Overby, L.R., 241
Owen, E.W., 33
Ozturk, M., 200

P

Palmer, J., 214
Panés, A., 255
Pape, J.W., 107
Pappas, J., 166
Paquet, J.C., 75
Paquet, K.-J., 266
Parc, R., 290
Paris, J.C., 196
Park, J.H., 292
Park, K.G.M., 52
Parsonnet, J., 169
Pate, J.W., 33
Pathy, M.S.J., 130
Patterson, D.E., 318
Patterson, D.J., 134
Paumgartner, G., 299, 321
Pauwels, C., 141
Pavia, A.T., 402
Payne, J., 247
Pearlman, N.W., 339
Peine, C.J., 318, 319
Pellegrini, C.A., 6, 389
Pemberton, J.H., 181, 182, 218
Pena, A.S., 140
Pennell, T.C., 337
Peracchia, A., 370
Pérez, C., 214
Perez-Perez, G.I., 80
Perlino, C.A., 279
Perozza, J., 47
Perrillo, R.P., 247
Petersen, B.T., 318, 319
Peterson, V.M., 147
Peterson, W.L., 401
Pfister, C., 200
Phillips, A., 259, 261
Phillips, M.J., 228
Phillips, R.K.S., 121
Phillips, S.F., 98, 182
Pichlmayr, R., 278
Pickleman, J., 126, 221
Pietrabissa, A., 391
Pignon, J.P., 379
Pimpl, W., 338
Pinero, S.S., 418
Pinsky, P.F., 170
Piper, D.W., 48
Piperno, A., 96
Pitt, H.A., 315, 346, 413
Planas, R., 255
Pleskow, D.K., 385
Podesta, L., 280
Podolsky, D.K., 385
Pokharna, D.S., 258
Polson, R.J., 410
Polydorou, A., 340
Portmann, B., 410
Potet, F., 31
Potters, H.V.J.P., 79
Pozzato, G., 40
Pratschke, E., 299
Present, D.H., 136
Prevel, F., 200
Price, J., 125
Prindiville, T., 285
Puig, J., 214
Purcell, R.H., 241, 242

Q

Quarto di Palo, F., 138
Quill, T.E., 152

R

Raasch, R.H., 152
Radley, S., 356
Raju, G.S., 409
Ramsay, R.C., 397
Ranard, R.C., 271
Ranzi, T., 138
Raper, S., 389
Rask-Madsen, J., 403
Rasmussen, S.N., 138
Ratcliffe, J., 94
Ravikumar, T.S., 275
Rawlinson, J., 194
Ready, R.R., 182
Reddell, M.T., 129
Reddy, S.N., 203
Redeker, A.G., 241, 408
Reedy, T.J., 50
Reeve, G., 166
Rege, R.V., 313, 323
Reynolds, J.C., 45
Rhoads, J.M., 101
Ricciardelli, E., 19
Richardson, D., 146
Richardson, D.Q., 387
Richter, J.E., 3, 8
Richter, J.M., 386
Riddell, R., 25
Riecken, E.O., 105, 156
Riederer, E., 266
Riis, P., 138
Rimola, A., 255
Ringe, B., 278
Rivkind, A.I., 295
Robert, J., 413
Roberts, E.A., 228
Robertson, R.P., 397
Robinson, J.E., Jr., 315
Robinson, P.J., 373
Roche, T.E., 285
Roda, E., 322
Rodés, J., 255
Roels, H., 141
Roget, M., 244
Romano, R., 96
Rommens, J.M., 367
Ronchi, G., 96
Roncoroni, L., 370
Root, J.K., 47
Roscher, R., 383
Rose, J.B., 170

Rosenbusch, G., 305
Rothmund, M., 208
Rotman, N., 371
Roufail, W.M., 47
Rouquier, S., 377
Rovati, L., 302
Rovati, L.C., 303
Royle, G.T., 194
Ruggeri, G., 96
Runyon, B.A., 407
Rüschoff, J., 208
Russell, C., 332
Russell, R.C.G., 340
Rustgi, A.K., 386
Rutgersson, K., 48
Rybolt, A.H., 405

S

Sackier, J.M., 119
Sackmann, M., 321
Saeed, Z.A., 60
Sagawa, H., 312
Saibil, F.G., 381
Salen, G., 315
Salmon, P., 332
Salonen, D., 427
Samanta, A.K., 256
Sampliner, R.E., 25
Sampson, H.A., 93
Santa Ana, C.A., 159, 161
Santangelo, W.C., 159
Sarles, H., 377
Sarr, M.G., 71
Sasaki, H., 312
Sasaki, Y., 239
Sato, N., 239
Sauer, L., 6
Sauerbruch, T., 321
Sax, H.C., 327
Schaffalitzky de Muckadell, O., 138
Schaffner, F., 408
Schechtman, K.B., 198
Scheibner, J., 300
Schiff, E.R., 247, 256
Schiller, L.R., 159, 161
Schlaeffer, F., 222
Schlegel, K.E., 152
Schmid, M., 266
Schmiedl, U., 133
Schneider, M.U., 382
Schneidman, D., 50
Schreyer, M., 200
Schroter, G.P.J., 347
Schuman, L.M., 194
Schwerk, W.B., 208
Scott-Conner, C.E.H., 387
Seeff, L.B., 271
Segura, J.W., 318
Sehonanda, A., 129
Selby, R., 280
Semmlow, J.L., 129
Shannon, S., 203
Shapiro, D.L., 150

Author Index / 453

Sharma, S.K., 258
Shaw, D.E., 336
Shaw, E.W., 253
Shaw, J.H.F., 149
Shekitka, K.M., 77
Shemesh, E.I., 198
Shenkin, A., 148
Shepherd, N.A., 405
Sheppard, R.H., 381
Sherman, P.M., 101
Shiau, Y.-F., 357
Shih, J.W., 242
Shires, G.T., 146, 151
Shivananda, S., 140
Shorter, N.A., 116
Shortsleeve, M.J., 165
Shouval, D., 200
Shuster, J.R., 241
Siegel, J.H., 295
Siegelman, S.S., 329
Siemens, F., 266
Sikes, R.K., 234
Sikuler, E., 222
Silk, Y.N., 349
Silverstein, M.D., 386
Sinar, D.R., 47
Sinclair, S.B., 228
Singer, J., 34
Skikne, B.S., 97
Skjoldborg, H., 211
Smith, H., 205
Smith, J.L., 15, 47
Smith, S.L., 279
Snover, D.C., 194
Sobin, L.H., 77
Soergel, K.H., 179
Sonnenberg, A., 56
Soper, N.J., 71, 98
Speelman, P., 172
Speizer, F.E., 309
Spengler, U., 321
Spigelman, A.D., 121
Stabile, B.E., 374
Stahlgren, L., 315
Staiano, A., 16
Stalder, G.A., 303
Stamm, W.E., 171
Stampfer, M.J., 309
Stanczak, V.J., 401
Stanley, J.C., 213
Stanley, M.M., 256
Starr, J., 109
Starzl, T.E., 277, 280, 287
Steele, G., Jr., 275
Steele, R.J.C., 52
Steffes, M.W., 397
Stein, H.J., 21
Steinberg, W., 380
Steinborn, P.A., 413
Steinbronn, K., 25
Stellaard, F., 299
Stellin, G.P., 347
Stephens, D.H., 364
Stevens, C.E., 241
Stevenson, W., 280
Stewart, M.T., 279

Stieber, A., 280
Stirling, M.C., 7, 20
Stizmann, J.V., 413
Stobberingh, E., 79
Stone, D.L., 403
Strange, E.F., 300
Strauss, A., 115
Strauss, W., 200
Strodel, W.E., 213
Strohmeyer, G., 353
Stuart, R.C., 23
Sultan, A.A., 260
Sun, J.H., 339
Sun, S., 200
Sundaram, M., 34
Surawicz, C.M., 172
Surh, C.D., 283, 285
Susman, N., 87
Sutherland, D.E.R., 397
Swayne, L.C., 306
Swift, I., 119

T

Tage-Jensen, U., 138
Tait, J., 94
Takahashi, H., 200
Talbot, I.C., 121
Tamburro, C., 247
Tanaka, M., 336
Tanton, R., 138
Taroni, F., 322
Tarpley, J.L., 173
Tartarian, A., 349
Tate, J.J.T., 194
Tauxe, R.V., 169
Tazuma, S., 312
Tegtmeier, G.E., 241
Teperman, L., 280
Terpin, M., 40
Thomas, H.C., 236, 237
Thomas, J.H., 76
Thistle, J.L., 318, 319
Thompson, G.R., 119
Thompson, H., 82
Thompson, N.W., 62
Thompson, R.E., 166
Thuluvath, P.J., 406
Thunberg, B.J., 150
Tibboel, D., 217
Timchalk, M., 145
Tinetti, M.E., 403
Tio, T.L., 31
Titó, L., 255
Todo, S., 277, 280
Tommasini, M.A., 250
Toouli, J., 328
Tracey, K.J., 146
Triger, D.R., 406
Trock, S.C., 169
Tsui, L.-C., 367
Turnage, R.H., 19
Tvede, M., 403
Tweedle, D.E.F., 335

Tytgat, G.N.J., 27, 31
Tzakis, A., 280

U

Ubukata, T., 76
Udding, J., 31
Ueda, K., 239
Ungar, B.L.P., 170
Ullrich, R., 105

V

Vaira, D., 332, 340
Valenzuela, J.E., 356
Valinluck, B., 411
van Belle, G., 172
van den Tweel, J.G., 27
Van Deventer, G.M., 50
Van de Water, J., 283
van Heerden, J.A., 218, 273
van Sonnenberg, E., 374
Van Spreeuwel, J.P., 79
Van Stiegmann, G., 339
Van Thiel, D.H., 247, 287, 315
Vargas, V., 244
Varney, R.R., 374
Vas, W., 34
Vasquez-Estevez, J.J., 347
Vassy L., 315
Venkataramman, R., 277
Vennits, B., 210
Venu, R.P., 328
Verdier, R.-I., 107
Viladomiu, L., 244
Villadsen, J., 211
Villanova, N., 322
Villeneuve, J.-P., 263
Vinayek, R., 60
Vinik, A.I., 62
Violi, V., 370
Viste, A., 397
Vogel, S.B., 66
Vogelzang, R.L., 323
Vonk, R.J., 224
Vuitch, F., 401

W

Wakefield, T.W., 213
Walan, A., 48
Walker, W.A., 33
Walsar, H., 266
Walsh, J.H., 50
Walshe, J.M., 290
Walton, G., 42
Walz, B.J., 198
Wands, J.R., 200
Wanek, E.A., 347
Wang, K.K., 406, 407
Warner, B.W., 327

Warner, M.A., 318
Warren, W.D., 279
Watt, G., 194
Way, D., 25
Way, L.W., 6, 337, 389
Weber, P., 133
Wechsler, R.J., 192
Weisfuse, I.B., 409
Welling, D.R., 181
Werbel, G.B., 323
Werth, B.A., 303
White, R.I., 346
Whitington, P.F., 231
Wichtrup, B., 208
Wiesner, R.H., 287, 341, 411
Wilhelmsen, F., 211
Willett, W.C., 309
Williams, C.B., 121
Williams, G.T., 405
Williams, H.J., 318, 319
Williams, N., 138
Williams, R., 227
Williams, S., 194, 332

Williamson, F.M., 57
Williamson, R.C.N., 119
Wilske, K.R., 134
Wilson, M.A., 170
Wilson, M.E., 165
Wittekind, C., 278
Wittich, G.R., 374
Wolf, D.C., 256
Wolff, B.G., 181, 218
Wolke, A., 136
Wolthers, B.G., 224
Wood, C.B., 119
Wood, C.J., 169
Wood, C.M., 179
Woodward, E.R., 66
Word, D.M., 170
Worley, W.E., 47
Wu, W.C., 3, 8

Y

Yale, C.E., 69

Yamaguchi, A., 59
Yamatani, T., 59
Yamazaki, H., 76
Yardley, J.H., 175, 177
Yoshida, M., 419
Yoshimitsu, K., 419
Yoshimoto, H., 336
Yoshioka, K., 189
Yurt, R.W., 146

Z

Zach, D., 303
Zargar, S.A., 400
Zeitz, M., 105
Zelenock, G.B., 213
Ziegler, W.H., 266
Zimmerman, H.J., 271
Zinsmeister, A.R., 85, 182
Zirngibl, H., 382